Temperance Lives

Temperance Lives

Life Assurance, Drink and Medicine in Britain, 1840–1918

James Kneale

BLOOMSBURY ACADEMIC
LONDON • NEW YORK • OXFORD • NEW DELHI • SYDNEY

BLOOMSBURY ACADEMIC
Bloomsbury Publishing Plc, 50 Bedford Square, London, WC1B 3DP, UK
Bloomsbury Publishing Inc, 1385 Broadway, New York, NY 10018, USA
Bloomsbury Publishing Ireland, 29 Earlsfort Terrace, Dublin 2, D02 AY28, Ireland

BLOOMSBURY, BLOOMSBURY ACADEMIC and the Diana logo are trademarks of Bloomsbury Publishing Plc

First published in Great Britain 2026

A catalogue record for this book is available from the British Library.

A catalog record for this book is available from the Library of Congress.

ISBN: HB: 978-1-3505-2971-7
ePDF: 978-1-3505-2972-4
eBook: 978-1-3505-2973-1

Typeset by Newgen KnowledgeWorks Pvt. Ltd., Chennai, India

For product safety related questions contact productsafety@bloomsbury.com.

To find out more about our authors and books visit www.bloomsbury.com and sign up for our newsletters.

Dedicated to Marjorie Kneale, and to the memory of John Kneale,
who chose the 'Dogs Home' over the Rechabites.

Contents

Figures

Maps

Tables

Acknowledgements

There are many people I need to thank for critical comments, support and the opportunity to develop my ideas. Some of this material has been presented at conferences organized by the Alcohol and Drugs History Society, the International Conference of Historical Geographers, the International Conference of the European Society for the History of Science, the German Society for the Study of British Culture, the Royal Geographical Society and Institute of British Geographers (RGS-IBG) and the American Association of Geographers. Thanks also to Matthew Ingleby and Matthew Kerr for including me in the Coastal Cultures of the Long Nineteenth Century conference, and to Iain Smith for the invitation to address the Royal College of Psychiatrists' Faculty of Addiction Psychiatry's annual conference. A presentation at the Portsmouth Liver Symposium at Queen Alexandra Hospital Portsmouth also allowed me to engage with new audiences.

The networks established by Phil Withington and Angela McShane (Intoxicants and Intoxication in Historical and Cultural Perspective), and Mark Hailwood and Deborah Toner (the Drinking Studies Network – DSN), provided many opportunities to present some of this material to the most sympathetic and knowledgeable audiences I could ever hope for. The DSN's Time and Temporalities cluster meetings have, under Steven Earnshaw's generous leadership, been particularly stimulating and enjoyable. We'll always have Vlonders! Annemarie McAllister's Radical Temperance conference at the University of Central Lancashire also offered an important opportunity to develop some of this book's arguments.

Smaller workshops allowed me to focus on particular elements of this project at the Universities of Oxford (courtesy of the Cambridge Socio-Legal Group), Cambridge, Leicester, Exeter and King's College London, and the Victoria and Albert Museum (thanks to Spike Sweeting), as did seminars at Birkbeck (Food History), the Institute of Historical Research (Metropolitan History), London School of Hygiene & Tropical Medicine (Centre for History in Public Health), UCL (Health Humanities, Geography) and Exeter, Glasgow, Cambridge (all Geography). Thanks also to the Historical Geography Research Group of the RGS-IBG for asking me to present at the Practising Historical Geography conference.

I have also been lucky enough to have the opportunity to present some of this work at public events, including a Lunchtime Lecture at UCL; a talk at the National Temperance Hospital (with Martin Austwick, Duncan Hay and Carina Schneider), before it was demolished to make way for a temporary lorry park; a contribution to the Torbay Heritage Day at Torquay Museum (thanks to Barry Chandler); and a Bright Club comedy event at the Royal Botanic Gardens, Kew, where I tried to involve a group of international visitors who had never heard of Bruce Forsyth in a mid-afternoon game of 'Play Your Temperance Life Assurance Cards Right'.

Among the many brilliant PhD students I have been lucky enough to work with, I learned a lot about drink, public health, Victorian Methodism and Turkish Baths from Hang Kei Ho, Linda Ng, Sadie Boniface, Ruth Slatter and Charlotte Jones. Thanks also to former undergraduate and postgraduate students who have taken up these ideas, especially Matt Lawrence for drawing my attention to some of the Temperance Hospital material discussed in this book, and Shuks Esmene for Teetotal Street.

Vital archive assistance was provided by Anna Stone at Aviva, John Porter at the Prudential, David Raymont at the Institute and Faculty of Actuaries, and Barry Chandler at Torquay Museum – huge thanks to all of them and countless staff at the London Archives; the Records Offices for Bristol, Essex, Hertfordshire and Manchester; the Wellcome Library and its Special Collections; the Library of the Society of Friends at Friends House, London; the National Art Library; the Salvation Army International Heritage Centre; and University College Hospital Archives. I am very grateful to David Boardman of manchesterhistory.net for the source for Figure 2.1.

Ideas, comments and support have come from many researchers working on drinking studies and related fields: Virginia Berridge, Andrew M. Butler, Kris Butler, Magnus Copps, Dorota Dias-Lewandowska, Laura Fenton, Sam Goodman, Paul Jennings, Mark Hailwood, Nigel Jeffries, Claire Markham, Phil Mellows, Alex Mold, Stella Moss, Emily Nicholls, James Nicholls, Noelle Plack, Richard Robinson, Amit Singh, Iain Smith, Stephen Spencer, Tom Thurnell-Read, Debbie Toner, Sivamohan Valluvan, Jennifer Wallis and Henry Yeomans. The brilliant Liz McFall's Wellcome Trust Seed Award–funded project 'Insuring Healthcare in a Digital World' proved to be enormously stimulating, and I'd like to thank Liz, Shaun French, Zsuzsanna Vargha and David Moats for teaching me almost everything I know about life assurance (Timothy Alborn's wonderful *Regulated Lives* provided me with the rest). I have also learned a great deal from Trev Broughton, Nancy Henry, Jane Hamlett and Elly McCausland, my talented and patient co-editors on the *Journal of Victorian Culture*. Thanks also to James Gregory for permission to use his paper on William Horsell.

Among the geographers who have listened to me discuss this topic are Gail Davies, Catherine Brace, David C. Harvey, Philip Howell, Stephen Legg, Divya Tolia-Kelly, Felix Driver and Miles Ogborn. In my own department the writing days organized by Jacob Fairless Nicholson and others in the Culture and Migration research cluster gave me the chance to draft and discuss several of these chapters. Miles Irving patiently drew and redrew the brilliant maps, and Nick Mann provided invaluable support. Jenny Robinson has been a fantastic mentor; thanks also to Jason Dittmer and Alan Ingram for comments on a paper related to this material, William Stewart and Caterina Liberace for many stimulating conversations, and Tatiana Thieme for book chats and general positivity. Tariq Jazeel proved to be exactly the company I needed on a productive writing retreat, and Caroline Bressey was always ready to discuss writing and method and was an early audience for some of the arguments explored in this book. Richard Dennis provided me with the model of historical-geographical scholarship I have been working with for over thirty years now, and I am immensely grateful to him. Ann Varley and Hugh Clout have also been supportive colleagues over many years – thank you! I wish I had begun this project earlier, so I could have discussed it with Hugh Prince and John Adams, and I would give anything for the chance to ask Russell Hitchings what he made of this book. Claire Dwyer's characteristically perceptive advice helped me fix a problem I was having with the material in Chapter 6; I miss her good sense and unrivalled ability to provide perspective, among many other things.

Many thanks also to the Bedford Way Picket for providing a glimpse of a better university. No thanks to the people who claim to lead UKHE – without you this book would have been finished several years earlier, and some of the people I've thanked here would still be making important contributions to scholarship and teaching.

Special thanks are due to a few particularly helpful people. Among the drinking studies crowd I owe a huge debt to David Beckingham, Steven Earnshaw, Mark Hailwood, Pam Lock, Dan Malleck, Annemarie McAllister, Angela McShane, Debbie Toner and Ryosuke Yokoe, for organizing sessions and conferences, sending me things to read, producing great work, convincing me that I was on the right track (but also telling me when I wasn't) and generally being lovely people and brilliant scholars. Working with the equally wonderful Sam Randalls resulted in a parallel project on weather and climate insurance, but if this book owes its existence to a single person, that would be Shaun French, who first brought temperance life assurance to my attention – in a pub, of course – and who co-authored several papers with me at what turned out to be the start of this bigger project. Thanks, Shaun.

Finally, I would like to thank Siobhan for her encouragement and love, and my family, which has contained both ordinary drinkers and teetotalers—as I suspect many twentieth-century families did—plus several insurance workers. My paternal grandmother, Lydia Kneale, was a Rechabite, and my maternal grandfather, John Dutton, was a grocer who later worked for the Prudential. The lives described in this book are not really all that different to theirs. Thank you to those ordinary, special people.

Abbreviations

B&FSSI	British and Foreign Society for the Suppression of Intemperance
BWTA	British Women's Temperance Association
CCB	Central Control Board (Liquor Traffic)
CETS	The Church of England Temperance Society
NB&FTS	New British & Foreign Temperance Society
NTS	National Temperance Society
UKT	The life assurance office known as the United Kingdom Life Assurance Association until 1847, and then as the United Kingdom Temperance and General Provident Life Institution
UMFC	United Methodist Free Churches
WTAU	Women's Total Abstinence Union

Part 1

Ordinary Temperance

Introduction: A man walks into a life assurance office

This book concerns the relationships between drink, temperance and health in Britain and the Anglophone world between 1840 and 1918, a period in which attitudes to drinking changed enormously as alcohol consumption rose and fell. These relationships have attracted attention from historians and others over the past fifty years, but the story presented here is different because it draws on historical material relating to life assurance firms. The book focuses on three British life assurance companies: the United Kingdom Temperance and General Provident Institution (UKT[1]), the Sceptre Life Association and the Whittington Life Assurance Company, but also considers other firms in North America, Australia and New Zealand. In doing so it aims to contribute to recent work on the importance of finance to Victorian society and culture, which has traced the role finance played in the expansion of imperial capitalism while transforming understandings of the relations between Christianity and commerce, economic activity and political agency, and questions of value, including – in the case of life assurance – the meaning and value of life itself.

As Mary Poovey put it, 'much of the writing that seems most characteristically Victorian grappled with the way that the invisible movement of capital was already beginning to transform the distribution of political and economic power, both within Great Britain and across the globe, by challenging the way value was conceptualized and circulated'.[2] Historians, literary critics, historical geographers and others have sought to trace these movements and transformations through the nineteenth century; in doing so, as Francis O'Gorman pointed out, they have shifted critical attention from the 'factory-dominated world' to 'the institutions and instruments of high finance'.[3]

One of the central arguments of this book is that finance also transformed the values associated with drinking, providing unexpected support for arguments in favour of temperance. The sale of temperance life assurance policies provided the opportunity to reflect upon ideas of health and risk in scientific and everyday discussions of drinking and abstinence. Life assurance companies changed their practices to reflect the ways ordinary men and women engaged with alcohol, and they proved to be remarkably productive in *shaping* those changes. As commercial enterprises, they were driven by different motivations than other temperance organizations, because their records showed that the teetotalers they assured enjoyed longer lives; as a result, those abstainers received a greater financial return on their policies. The firms assuring them also prospered, because their longer-lived policyholders paid their premium payments for longer, while the company had to make fewer payments to policyholders who died earlier than expected. Temperance advocates noted that abstainers seemed to make better 'lives', as assurance firms referred to their policyholders, making use of this evidence in their arguments with politicians and physicians. Historians have suggested that life assurance helped shape understandings of the risks of opium consumption and the aetiology of tuberculosis, as well as the modern medical examination itself; this book will argue that it also offered a new way of thinking about drinking.[4]

Tracing the influence of insurance ideas and practice on understandings of the risks associated with alcohol also requires a reconsideration of the way we write about drink and temperance. The scattered field that covers the history of alcohol and drugs is undergoing something of a revival, but – with honourable exceptions – in much of this work, temperance is treated simply as a movement that sought to regulate drinking, rather than a thing of interest in its own right. While the principles of moderation and abstinence are probably as old as the use of alcoholic drinks in human societies, the development of societies dedicated to the collective pursuit of temperance date from the United States in 1813, followed by the establishment of societies in Ireland and Scotland in the 1820s, and then England and Wales. These were originally 'moderationist' societies abstaining from distilled spirits alone, but in 1832 total abstinence or 'teetotalism' was adopted by a group of men in Preston, and societies on this model sprung up across the UK.

By 1853 the movement included a parliamentary pressure group, the UK Alliance for the Suppression of the Traffic in All Intoxicating Liquors, which became focused on the passing of a Permissive Bill for 'Local Veto' or 'Local Option' which would allow voters to decide on whether the sale of drink should be allowed in their district. In the 1870s the Alliance made great efforts to pass the Permissive Bill through Parliament, with the support of some sections of the Liberal party, while the movement began to gain support within the established church. By the 1890s the Liberals had adopted the Permissive Bill as an official policy, though many other alternatives were discussed by reformers.

Historians concerned with British temperance have tended to concentrate on the political aspects of the 'drink question', however, following Brian Harrison's lead; others have examined its social and cultural lives.[5] The annual general meetings of major temperance firms have received much less attention, and little has been said about the sense of belonging that might have been associated with life assurance – the UKT was a 'mutual' firm, for example, so policyholders had voting rights, were addressed as 'members' and shared profits between them in the form of regular bonuses. Something of the scale and significance of temperance life assurance can also be seen in the people these firms employed – the physician Dr John Snow, shoemaker James Clark and travel agent Thomas Cook all worked for the UKT. These firms also assured Liberal prime minister David Lloyd George (Scottish Temperance), the fraudulent MP and businessman Jabez Balfour (UKT) and Sir Alfred Joseph Doughty-Tichborne (Sceptre), whose death in 1867 set in train the saga of the 'Tichborne claimant'.

We will return to the under-researched world of temperance business, and the wider context of 'ordinary temperance', after we have considered the origins of temperance life assurance in London in 1840. This makes it clear just how far attitudes to drinking changed over the period covered by this study.

Temperance life assurance: 'One man's bright idea'?

Sometime in 1840 a young London Quaker named Robert Warner applied for a life assurance policy, perhaps intending to provide security for his new wife and future family.[6] Robert was both prudent and prosperous – just the sort of 'life' assurance companies wanted.[7] Later accounts differed, but at least one firm would only assure him if he paid a sizeable addition or extra annual premium, which usually reflected company concern about the health or habits of the applicant. As a Canadian tract explained forty years later, Warner was told, 'You are a teetotaller; and the directors consider teetotal lives are worse than ordinary lives.'[8] Or in the livelier prose of American temperance writer Vance Thompson:

> The total abstainer was looked upon as a maniac who was playing a dangerous, suicidal game with his health … The directors held a meeting; the learned doctors were called in; and this was the decision: the policy would be granted only if the Quaker paid ten per cent more than the ordinary premium, because 'he was thin and watery and mentally cranked in that he repudiated the good things of God as found in alcoholic drinks'.[9]

Warner's abstinence challenged medical, business and temperance orthodoxies. Influenced by the work of the German chemist Justus von Liebig, which suggested that alcohol was a food, physicians like Robert J. Graves and Robert Bentley Todd developed systems for prescribing alcohol to treat fevers and tuberculosis in the early 1830s.[10] While Timothy Alborn found that 65 per cent of a sample of 110 medical forms from 1850 asked if the applicant for life assurance was 'sober, moderate, and/or temperate', it remained unclear how intemperance would be defined.[11] Alcohol was also a taken-for-granted part of the working life of assurance businesses. The directors of the Prudential ordered cognac for the office to help them ward off the dangers of cholera in 1849, for example, and the County office provided its shareholders with a pint of wine each at its inaugural general meeting in 1848.[12] The Royal Farmers office (originally the Farmers and General Fire and Life Insurance Company) forbade its clerks from drinking porter, ale, wine or spirits in the office from 1844; intemperance and debt were the two issues that most concerned clerks' employers.[13]

Robert Warner was also out of step with others involved in temperance. The first organized British groups dedicated to the moderate consumption of alcohol – specifically abstinence from spirits – appeared in the 1820s, with the rival principle of 'teetotalism', or total abstinence from all alcoholic drink, growing in the early 1830s. The opposition between these viewpoints came to dominate national discussions of temperance in the 1840s, exacerbated by differences in class, denomination and regional identity. Broadly speaking, these moderationists tended to be middle-class or genteel Anglicans, and their societies were strongest in London and the south, while teetotalers tended to be nonconformists and were particularly strong in Lancashire and Yorkshire.[14] As a teetotal Quaker, Warner was out of place within the moderationist currents of metropolitan temperance. He sought support from members of the British and Foreign Society for the Suppression of Intemperance (B&FSSI) but was told that it would be financially risky to assure teetotalers, 'a large proportion of them having been for many years habitual drunkards [whose] constitutions must have sustained some severe shock from their former habits'. Worse, it would be impossible for the B&FSSI to work 'at all pleasantly or efficiently' with the UKT, because the latter's board had fallen out with the B&FSSI over the 'short pledge' controversy, which allowed teetotalers to offer alcoholic drinks to guests – something the genteel committee of the B&FSSI wished to retain.[15] Medical, insurantial and temperance differences made the UKT look like a risky proposition.

The temperance historian P. T. Winskill explained that Warner decided 'that if there was any truth in temperance principles, the action of these directors should have been the very reverse of what it was ... he determined that temperance people ought to and should have an office for themselves'.[16] That would mean a 'class office' for teetotalers, on the model of other firms who assured only members of a particular profession, like lawyers, clergymen, doctors or military officers, or specific religious denominations, like Friends Provident, established for members of the Society of Friends in 1832.[17] Friends Provident might well have been one of the firms Warner applied to in 1840, as Quakers were still divided over temperance at this time – several large breweries, like London's Barclay Perkins, were in part Quaker businesses – and temperance 'was strongest among Friends from the North and West, and weakest in London'.[18] Friends Provident might well have agreed that Warner was too much of a risk.

Warner's response may have been encouraged by his personal networks, which included his friend Theodore Compton, who had been working in life assurance at the National Provident Institution since 1837.[19] Compton then consulted the treasurer, secretary and collector of the New British and Foreign Temperance Society (NB&FTS), respectively the Quaker William Janson (a banker and Lloyds underwriter), the Reverend William R. Baker (a Congregationalist minister) and James Ellis (a draper and lacemaker).[20] Warner, Baker, Ellis and Janson became four of the eleven original directors of the UKT, with Compton as secretary. From this point on the UKT and NB&FTS were closely intertwined, with Compton acting as secretary to both institutions and their offices sharing the same building. When the NB&FTS became part of the National Temperance Society (NTS) in 1842, Warner and Janson joined its executive committee.[21] The temperance societies that emerged across Britain from the 1830s provided the UKT with agents to sell its policies, medical referees to examine applicants and a national market of abstainers.

The United Kingdom Total Abstinence Life Association was established at the end of 1840, with offices in the City of London at 39 Moorgate Street, and issued its first policy – to Robert Warner – in January 1841. As a mutual company, it had no shareholders; the firm's profits would be returned to members in the form of quinquennial bonuses (paid every five years).[22] Members had to prove that they had signed the pledge, and backsliding was punished, as a prospectus from 1840 made clear:

> Every person assuring in this Association must be a member of a Total-Abstinence Society ... Every member of this Association, who breaks his pledge to abstain from intoxicating beverages, will be required to pay a fine of ten shillings for every £100 assured to him.
>
> Every member persisting in the use of intoxicating beverages, or refusing to renew his pledge, will forfeit all the privileges of membership, and be required to pay an additional premium of ten per cent, or two shillings for every pound of the ordinary rate.[23]

This additional premium for pledge-breaking 'was the very reverse of the proposal put to Mr. Warner by the directors of the company he proposed to join', as Winskill noted – a penalty for drinking, not abstinence.[24]

Later histories of the firm emphasized the UKT's challenge to established insurance practice and medical belief: 'The medical profession almost to a man was against them', as Winskill put it, 'and who were they to set themselves up against such learned authorities?'[25] By 1847 the new firm was indeed struggling, and the decision was taken to open membership to applicants who were not abstainers.[26] From this moment on the firm operated a General section and an Abstainers' or Temperance section, and the name was changed to the United Kingdom Temperance and General Provident Institution to reflect this. The new business model proved more successful, and the UKT prospered, particularly between 1856 and 1865 when the number of new policies approved exceeded 2,500 every year.[27] By 1864 it was already being described as one of Britain's 'principal temperance commercial institutions', alongside the Temperance Permanent Building Society, which encouraged teetotalers to save to buy property.[28] In 1890 the UKT was the eighth largest life office in Britain, in terms of premium income; by 1898 it was the sixth largest, in terms of its accumulated funds.[29] In 1918, at the end of the period covered by this book, it assured over 5,000 new policies, the largest amount of new business in the company's history. That year there were around 72,000 policies of all kinds in force, and the firm's total funds amounted to over £11 million.[30]

The growth of the General section made abstainers the minority from 1847 until the 1890s. Only forty-seven of the 273 policies issued in 1847 were for General members, but by 1850 the number of new General policies issued exceeded the number of new Abstainers' policies.[31] Teetotalers made up between 30 and 40 per cent of the total number of lives assured from 1855 through to the early 1880s, and an average of 52.7 per cent of new lives assured by the company in 1891, 1896 and 1901.[32] General policies were more likely to lapse, though, and between 1882 and 1902 the number of active policies in the Abstainers' section grew by 29 per cent, while the number of General lives fell by 23 per cent.[33] The Temperance section was still in operation in 1952, so it is quite possible that some abstainers' policies were in force in 1986, when the firm merged with Friends Provident, itself taken over by Aviva in 2015.[34] The UKT, like Robert Warner, lived a long and prosperous life, and the story of its founding would later be described by one paper as 'the story of the growth of one man's bright idea'.[35]

The UKT as experiment

The new structure introduced in 1847 brought additional challenges, however. The General section needed to be policed very carefully: applications from drink sellers and makers were automatically rejected, while other applicants were screened for excessive drinking. The board remained confident that their experiment would pay off, as the company was more careful than other assurers:

> Though the public generally may not at present admit the superior longevity of Teetotalers, the Directors think it must be plain to everyone capable of taking a candid view of the subject, that an office which is entirely exempt from all losses by intemperance, and by what is called free living, must stand upon a much more favourable basis, than offices subject to such risks.[36]

There was another, unintentional consequence of this model, which made it an experiment of sorts, well known within and beyond temperance circles. Actuarial tables predicted the life expectancy of people at different ages, telling the firm how many of their policyholders would die in a particular period; because the two sections kept separate records it was possible to compare the firm's populations of abstainers and moderate drinkers. It soon became apparent that the former lived longer on average than the latter. The temperance historian and statistician James Dawson Burns explained it this way:

> Expectancy of life is made the basis of the rates of premium in the tables used in insurance offices; and a mortality below that expectancy is, therefore, an evidence of special longevity and vigour. Out of so many persons a given number are expected to die; and if fewer die, then the body of members as a whole is proved to be possessed of special vitality; and by applying the same standard to two bodies we get at a certain index of their relative vital force.[37]

Burns presented the UKT's tables showing the comparative mortality of its two sections for every year between 1866 and 1882 as part of his analysis of 'the vital statistics of total abstinence'.[38] Over that period the number of actual deaths in the General section was 98.4 per cent of the predicted number, while the number of deaths in the Abstainers' section was only 70.4 per cent of the expected total. Burns pointed out that the number of deaths in the General section exceeded expectations in six different years, while the Abstainers' section was *always* lower than expected. These figures suggested the universal adoption of total abstinence in England, Scotland and Ireland would save nearly 190,000 deaths every year.[39]

This had financial implications for the firm's assurers, too. Warner's 'bright idea' assumed that a company that only insured abstainers would pay fewer claims every year because abstainers were less likely to die unexpectedly. Fewer deaths meant there was always more money available for bonuses for abstainers; more frequent claims in the General section meant a reduction in the profits returned to surviving members.

Put simply, abstainers lived longer, and the value of their policies grew faster. Here, it seemed, was proof of the medical and financial benefits of abstinence, of longer life and greater wealth – proof that temperance activists would make good use of.

Burns set out the many successes of the UKT in his unpublished history of the office:

> Drawing its chief sustenance from the Middle and Humbler classes, it has been intrusted with the hopes, the fortunes, and the happiness of many thousands of persons, and in not a single case have those hopes been disappointed, or that happiness been destroyed. Conducted on principles of commercial integrity and prudence, it has received its natural reward. And the benefit received has been diffused. It has set a light in darkness, and been to the desolate and bereaved a comfort and a stay. *It has furnished to the advocate of Temperance an argument that no sophistry can turn aside*; and by its encouragement of habits of thrift, it has cultivated one of the virtues that make nations vigorous and self-reliant.[40]

In this passage Burns touched on many of the aspects of life assurance promoted by the wider industry: its promise of security against disaster and of hope and happiness in the form of a significant return on the investment of premiums paid.[41] Life assurance also encouraged 'habits of thrift' through the regular payment of premiums. This form of life assurance had a novel twist, though; it also offered an argument in favour of temperance.

The story of the UKT's founding was retold in print and at public meetings in Britain, Ireland, the United States, Canada, Australia and New Zealand from the late 1850s into the twentieth century.[42] It seems likely that its continuing appeal reflected the fact that it captured a sea-change in attitudes towards abstinence and drinking over this period. Until the 1870s, mainstream medical opinion saw alcohol as a harmless or useful element of diet and medicine. As life assurance companies asked doctors to vet applicants for problem drinking, charging publicans and others in the drink trade extra premiums, many – but not all – doctors began to wonder if abstinence might be healthier than moderate drinking.

It seems likely that firms like the UKT may well have played a part in this, persuading doctors with the evidence supplied by their life expectancy statistics. Supporters certainly retrospectively represented the firm as an experiment designed to demonstrate the healthiness of abstinence. For Vance Thompson, for example, the firm's success, Warner's own longevity and changing attitudes in medicine and insurance were all vindications of Warner's apparently 'suicidal' behaviour in 1840. Similarly, Samuel Kerr, the firm's representative in Belfast, claimed that 'it was started by its present and only chairman Mr Robert Warner, in 1840, *to test this very question*'.[43]

In approaching this as the story of an experiment, this book seeks to apply insights from science and technology studies to this historical development, as a study of the making of markets.[44] Gerald Wayne Olsen noted that teetotal doctors who challenged orthodox thinking before 1855 attracted like-minded patients, so that 'every teetotal society became a kind of *unofficial outdoor laboratory*, supplementing the more directly scientific studies of the medical community with hundreds of case histories of their teetotal "guinea pigs" '.[45] By 1847 the UKT had already issued 2,627 life assurance policies to teetotalers, and the firm's statistical understanding of their mortality made it another 'unofficial outdoor laboratory'. These case histories and tables of comparative mortality could then be put to use by temperance activists keen to demonstrate that alcohol was not essential for health, travelling beyond medicine into speeches, tracts and personal conversations. Life assurance offices became testing grounds for controversies about health and risk decades before epidemiological studies of public health. In 1840 teetotalers saw doctors as hostile adversaries; by 1918 medical opinion had largely accepted abstinence and was arguing for a form of moderation defined by relatively modest levels of consumption.

The success of an experiment can never be guaranteed, however. In his account of the development of the Kodak camera, Bruno Latour pointed out that its popularity could not have been predicted from the outset: 'At many other steps in the story the innovation was highly flexible, negotiable, at the mercy of a contingent event.'[46] Robert Warner's idea for a temperance life assurance company might well have failed – indeed it did fail, as an institution for assuring *only* abstainers. It was also threatened, as we will see, by directors with troubled financial pasts, by fraudulent agents, by 'reformed drunkards' whose health had been ruined by drinking before they took the pledge, and by criticism from rival insurance offices, hostile ministers and sceptical doctors.

At the same time, we should resist the temptation to see this as 'one man's bright idea'. Warner's idea succeeded because the firm and its networks worked to counter these and other challenges, constantly 'tinkering', in John Law and Evelyn Ruppert's sense of iterative problem-solving and bricolage, of trying new combinations of elements within a wider assemblage of people, objects and ideas.[47] The numerical evidence produced by the UKT helped to establish trust; as Theodore Porter suggests, 'quantification is a technology of distance', and the firm's tables of comparative mortality travelled easily, as what Latour called 'circulating references', through the firm's networks and out into a wider public sphere of print and discussion.[48] At the same time, just as Kodak's success relied not just on the invention of a mass-market camera but also the creation of a mass market for it, we have to see the UKT's success as contingent on other changes in medicine, temperance and alcohol consumption, which allowed for a larger market for this strange new product.

This also has implications for the way we think about the development of temperance in this period. In a much-quoted passage Latour argued that we should avoid the temptation to *totalize* in our descriptions of any given scenario:

> Take some small business-owner hesitatingly going after a few market shares, some conqueror trembling with fever, some poor scientist tinkering in his lab, a lowly engineer piecing together a few more or less favourable relationships of force, some stuttering and fearful politician; turn the critics loose on them, and what do you get? Capitalism, imperialism, science, technology, domination – all equally absolute, systematic, totalitarian.[49]

Latour's point is not that we should sympathize with these capitalists and imperialists, but that a totalizing analysis of this kind 'renders its practitioners powerless in the face of the enemy, whom it endows with fantastic properties'.[50] Warner came from a successful family of capitalists, was well connected in the business world and could afford to invest in this risky enterprise; but those assets did not grant him fantastic powers. For Latour, power *emerges* from a successful network, it does not *drive* it. Similarly, even if British temperance had been a purely bourgeois enterprise – and Chapter 1 will question that idea – its power over working-class drinkers was not guaranteed. Focusing attention on the contingent ways in which temperance life assurance became an unlikely success reminds us that this history might have turned out very differently and was not simply the outcome of structural forces.

Temperance and the actuarial imaginary

Warner's 'bright idea' also offers an excellent example of what François Ewald called the 'actuarial imaginary', 'the ways in which, in a given social context, profitable, useful and necessary uses can be found for insurance technology'.[51] Ewald's work was part of the study of governmentality – those techniques developed to understand and direct the behaviour of populations and individuals – inspired by the work of Michel Foucault. Governmentality is broadly concerned with 'the conduct of conduct', conceived, as Margo Huxley explains, as 'a generalized power that seeks to fashion and guide the bodily comportments and inward states of others and of the self; a form of action on the actions and capacities of the self and of others'.[52] As this suggests, governmentality covers everything from police power to discipline, the fashioning of the self and the biopolitical regulation of populations, but one of the crucial insights of this work is that governing is also done by market institutions like life assurance companies.

Modern life assurance is often dated to the end of the eighteenth century, when the actuaries of the Equitable office began to analyse records of mortality using the mathematical insights offered by the 'probabilistic revolution'.[53] Their aim was to ensure that the premiums they received would cover the amount claimed at death – without this calculation, firms risked making a loss if the premium income did not cover outgoing claims; after it, actuaries began to wonder if 'laws of mortality' might be uncovered that governed how many policyholders would die each year. As firms accumulated records of the life expectancy of their own policyholders and shared data with other firms and the General Register Office, actuaries became more confident about predicting normal life expectancy.

Additional risks like tuberculosis or childbirth which might shorten life and threaten the firm's profitability required additional charges. As Daniel Defert put it: 'You aren't inoculated for smallpox? A supplement. You travel? A classification of countries is drawn up according to their dangerousness, to fix your additional premium.'[54] These additions were not always based on careful actuarial calculations, however; other ideas of risk were used to determine the necessary supplement. Fire insurance, for example, was characterized by what O'Malley and Roberts called 'cumulative dangerousness', 'a practical epistemology that sought to identify as many hazards as possible in pursuit of identifying bad risks'.[55] A more subjective evaluation would have to be made in these cases, as statistical experience was often lacking, making actuarial practice a combination of expert judgement and mathematical proficiency.

The principle of insurers rewarding those who were a lower risk for the company, and banning others altogether, was already well established. The Sceptre refused policies for miners, railway guards and those in the 'liquor traffic', for example.[56] The Prudential, which specialized in 'industrial policies' for working-class customers, reassessed the risks associated with drinking from the 1870s. The firm's agents for industrial assurance were warned not to recommend potential policyholders 'as are, or have been, noted for *intemperance*'. Noting that 'the Company had sustained considerable loss from the early deaths of publicans & those immediately connected with public house trade', the firm added this occupation to the list of risks that demanded an extra charge, alongside prior illness, military service and foreign travel. In 1874 this addition was 15 shillings per £100 assured; by 1896 this had been increased to £2 for whole-life policies and was extended to wine and spirit merchants, including some grocers. Publicans with industrial policies worth £50 or more would be charged an extra sixpence per cent per week.[57] These rates were still in place, unchanged, in 1922 and might well have continued beyond that point.[58]

The actuarial imagination was put to work in dealing with drink, though not simply to punish drinkers. Ewald suggested the actuarial imaginary created 'profitable, useful and necessary uses' for insurance; temperance life assurance created income from the lives of teetotalers, and the Prudential's extra charge was a necessary response to a loss-making phenomenon. However, both responses could also be described as 'useful', in the sense that they made other things happen. Insurance is considered to be a form of governmentality because it encourages thrift; Jeremy Bentham suggested that liberalism needed to 'accustom men to submit to the yoke of foresight', to consider future risks and to guard against them.[59] As O'Malley points out, insurance was 'a governing technology for instilling and institutionalizing thrift'.[60] Insurance 'responsibilizes' policyholders in other ways; the UKT insisted that members remain teetotal, giving them another reason to keep their pledge, and many firms discouraged potential applicants from working in the licensed trade.

The UKT's abstainers really did live longer than its moderate drinkers, on average, and the firm prospered because abstinence was a sound investment. Walter Priestman, the vice-president of one of the UKT's rivals, the Abstainers and General life assurance company, told a temperance meeting in Swansea in 1895 that 'total abstainers held that the teetotaller was like a slated house, whilst the moderate drinker was like a thatched article, and they claimed the same distinction with respect to life as was made by the fire offices with respect to the insurance of houses'.[61] Fire insurers instructed their agents to charge an additional premium or refuse thatched properties, because of the additional risk.[62] Drinkers, like thatched roofs, were simply more of a risk.

The implications of the difference between the UKT's sections were captured in a pithy phrase that was to serve as an excellent advertisement for abstinence and temperance life insurance. *Wings*, the journal of the British Women's Temperance Association, retold the familiar story of the establishment of the UKT by 'a few obstinate teetotalers' and the difference in life expectancy between the two sections.[63] The difference between the bonuses paid to abstainers and moderate drinkers had apparently been discussed at one of the UKT's annual general meetings. One member had asked 'on what principle … are the profits divided?' The firm's actuary had replied by saying that 'they are not divided on any "principle", they divide themselves; the fact is, *those who don't drink don't die so fast*; and that is the explanation of the difference our friend refers to'.[64] The questioner may have suspected that the firm favoured abstainers, choosing to pay them larger bonuses, but the reply made it clear that this was simply a consequence of a chain of facts: abstainers lived longer, so the company paid out fewer claims than expected, and so a larger surplus would to be returned to the abstainers. In firms without a separate section for abstainers, their sacrifice would go unrewarded as the money saved would be shared with moderate or heavy drinkers. The striking phrase 'those who don't drink don't die so fast' would be used again in 1922, by long-time temperance assurance worker William Bingham.[65]

The UKT's model would turn out to be so successful that several other British firms were established on this principle. While these companies were all 'interested in total abstinence as a commercial advantage', as Walter Priestman put it, they went about it in different ways.[66] Some, like the Whittington, followed the UKT in offering abstainers better bonuses; others, like Scottish Temperance or Sceptre, also offered cheaper premiums. By 1901 there were temperance life firms or sections in the United States, Canada, Australia and New Zealand.[67] Older firms that might well have been suspicious of the UKT in 1840 also began to acknowledge the risks of insuring drinkers, many charging extra for those in the drink trade. As one supporter noted, this was simply good business sense:

> The hard-headed business sagacity that directs these institutions is not very likely to be influenced by any merely sentimental considerations, and yet the companies, that some time ago looked with suspicion upon teetotallers, now seek after them as insurers with the utmost eagerness, and even offer them special inducements. Why do they do this? Simply because IT PAYS.[68]

In these discussions questions of morality and piety are often entirely absent; these are straightforward appeals to commonsense. In fact, it seems likely that it did not matter whether actuaries, agents, applicants for life assurance, or doctors knew about, or believed, arguments about the relationships between drink and mortality. To remain within this assemblage – to be given or claim a policy, or to receive payment as a director, medical referee, agent, or actuary – individuals had to fit the places prescribed for them. Networks of life assurance rewarded *practice*, not belief, zeal, or faith. Given the widespread appeal of commonsense understandings of temperance as a moral or religious movement, this might prompt us to consider whether these Victorians were really as 'civilized' as temperance tracts or autobiographies might lead us to believe.[69] Comparative tables of mortality and the greater return on abstainers' premiums presented different forms of evidence about drinking and abstinence that were immensely appealing to temperance advocates – and they appeared to be matters of fact, rather than opinion. And while questions were asked about other factors that might explain these facts, they seem to have been largely accepted by 1900.

Lives, temperance and otherwise

To these companies the phrase 'temperance lives' would have meant the people assured in their Abstainers' section; to the policyholder the word 'life' carried a reminder of their own mortality.[70] Both of these meanings are important, but there is another way of thinking about temperance lives, and that is as biographical accounts of people associated with temperance life assurance. This book presents a series of these accounts in order to provide a sense of 'ordinary', rather than spectacular, forms of temperance.

Life writing is a well-established tradition in temperance history. The prosopographical approach Brian Harrison adopted for *Drink and the Victorians*, the *Dictionary of Temperance Biography*, and his study of the UK Alliance's subscribers involved researching the biographies of nearly four hundred prominent teetotalers active between 1833 and 1872.[71] Some of those men and women are famous enough to be listed in the *Dictionary of National Biography*, or wrote autobiographies, like Thomas Whittaker, father of Thomas Palmer Whittaker, MP and chair of the UKT from 1898. Many more appear only in late nineteenth- or early twentieth-century temperance biographies and histories, like those produced by Peter Turner Winskill, himself briefly an agent for the UKT in Belper, or are almost impossible to trace.[72] Biographical studies have also appeared in more recent histories of drink and temperance, from David Beckingham's study of Father Mathew to Annemarie McAllister's analysis of the careers of seven temperance writers, and Dorota Dias-Lewandowska and Pam Lock's 'microherstories' of Polish and British women's drinking.[73]

This book considers some of these individuals, with a special emphasis on the temperance lives assured by these firms, including many men and women who were not prominent temperance activists. There are twenty longer 'lives' here – fourteen teetotalers and three drinkers, plus a set of towns, a bundle of forms and some buildings – and many more are briefly considered. Life assurance firms keep very good records because the security of their funds depends on it, but archival records relating to individual policies are rarely retained. The ledgers of the Sceptre office present an important exception, providing us with very detailed records – names, ages, addresses, policy types and other information – for thousands of teetotal policyholders assured between 1865 and 1881. Chapter 7 includes an analysis of a sample of nearly a thousand of these lives, and brief biographies of others appear throughout the book.[74] Board meeting minutes provide further details, as applications were discussed and policies claimed, or as policyholders, agents, directors and others created problems. With the help of digitized resources, particularly newspapers, it is often possible to provide some account of lives visible in the archives in these ways.

These lives – some teetotal, others decidedly not – are presented here for five reasons. First, they illustrate the issues considered in each chapter; in Chapter 3 a controversial preacher and a drunken baronet show the difficulties temperance and drinking created for assurance, for example. In keeping with the wider argument of this book, which takes this business to be a material as well as a social network, some of these biographies concern objects – policy forms, buildings – as well as people. Second, they present us with stories of ordinary temperance of a kind rarely seen in histories of this topic – with a few decidedly unusual lives, admittedly. Third, some of these lives demonstrate that Victorian attitudes to temperance and drink could be complicated and sometimes contradictory. Fourth, they go some small way towards offsetting the masculine character of much of this material. The absence of women from board rooms and medical schools left them few roles to play in the world of temperance life assurance, in contrast to their important role in the wider movement.[75] A small number of women assured their own lives or the lives of their husbands, just as British women bought shares, saved and speculated through the nineteenth century.[76] While their stories are often tangled up in their relationships with their spouses and other men, they provide some sense of women's engagement with temperance and drink. Finally, these lives can often be spatialized in useful ways, so that biography and place shed light on one another, as they have done in recent historical-geographical work.[77] As David Beckingham and Charles Watkins note, 'place was foundational to the temperance movement'; the biographies of key figures like Lady Elizabeth Biddulph and Lady Henry Somerset are intertwined with local histories in ways that created 'distinctive arenas for temperance action that united landowners and labourers'.[78]

The first of the lives examined in this book is that of Robert Warner, holder of the UKT's first policy.

Temperance lives: Robert Warner (1815–1896)

Robert Warner was born into a large Quaker family whose main concern was the Crescent Foundry on Jewin Crescent, Cripplegate, London, established by Robert's grandfather Jacob Warner in 1739. The firm cast the first Big Ben bell for Parliament in 1856, won a medal at the 1862 International Exhibition and later expanded into hydraulic and sanitary engineering.[79] Robert married Mary Ann Greenwood in 1837, and they had two sons and two daughters. He took sole charge of the Crescent Foundry in 1869, selling it within the family in 1891. In the 1870s Robert built a new foundry at Walton-on-the-Naze, developing his father's land and property in the Essex resort town. He was made an Associate of the Institute of Civil Engineers in 1870, for the sea defences he built at Walton, earning him the ironic title 'Conqueror of the German Ocean'.[80] Besides the UKT and his properties in Essex and London, Robert's other business interests included Brooks Wharf, off Upper Thames Street.[81] He was reported to own 176 acres in 1873, with an estimated rental value of £1,174.[82]

Warner appears to have been a shrewd capitalist, taking charge of investing the UKT's funds. His decision to found the UKT was described as showing his 'characteristic pluck and energy', and one obituarist noted his 'extraordinary business capacities and keenness'.[83] He was also quick to make use of the capital generated by the lives of those assured in the office for his own business ventures, beginning in 1844 by borrowing £1000 from the UKT at 5 per cent interest, secured against railway shares and other securities.[84] Stepping down as chairman and director at the firm's fifty-fifth annual general meeting in 1896, Warner was awarded an annual pension of £500 by the office; as the *Financial Times* noted, 'Pleasant although such a recognition may be, we imagine that Mr. Warner values still more the triumphant success of the institution

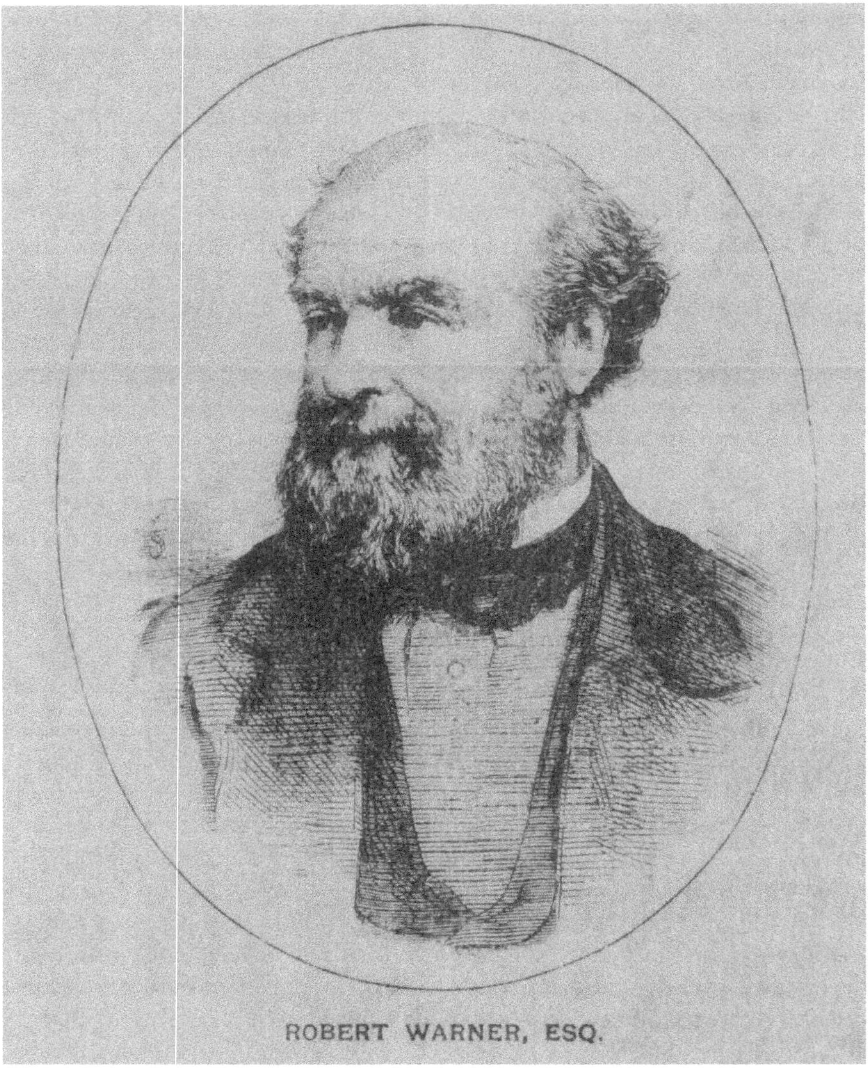

Figure 0.1 Robert Warner, *Hand and Heart Illustrated. A Family, Social and Temperance Journal*, May 1883, n.p.

Source: Aviva Archives.

which it has been his privilege to guide.' At his death Robert left a sizeable estate valued at over £100,000.[85]

Robert does not seem to have been very active in temperance before the UKT was founded, however, and even as an executive director of the NTS he seems to have been most effective behind the scenes. Characteristically, his most important contribution to the NTS may well have been organizational and financial, as he oversaw the payment of the existing debts of its constituent societies after they merged.[86] The fact that Robert became the owner of two fully licensed hotels in Walton-on-the-Naze, as we will see in Chapter 6, would seem to further undermine his commitment to temperance.[87] Similarly, Robert does not seem to have been a lifelong Liberal like many temperance workers, voting for the Whig candidate in the North Essex election of 1847 but chairing a meeting in support of the local Conservative MP in 1885.[88] Though he remained a member of the Society of Friends, his faith seems to have been a private matter. While the meetings of some temperance societies began with prayers, the UKT's board meetings were strictly business.

Robert Warner was clearly a successful businessman and organizer. However, we know little about his commitment to temperance, the strength and character of his religious beliefs, or his devotion to Liberal or radical causes – the key aspects of many temperance biographies. Robert's life is a reminder that temperance life assurance might not simply be driven by morality or piety. For him this experiment may well have been an attempt to fill a gap in the market that only existed because no one else thought this 'product' would work. If he was testing the question of the risks of temperance and drinking, that may have been as much to do with the chance to make money as it was to disseminate new information about the health benefits of abstinence.

We will return to these questions throughout the book, meeting other lives with different relations to these ideas of prosperity and piety, but now we turn to the shape of the narrative and the argument of each chapter.

Examining temperance life assurance

The book's Part 1 considers life assurance businesses as a key form of *ordinary temperance*, a term explored further in Chapter 1. It provides an overview of the book's key arguments, introductions to the main firms, and examples of some very different temperance lives and temperance towns across England. Arguing that work that approaches temperance as a primarily political movement misses a good deal of what made it important, Chapter 1 looks first at temperance's radical roots, which influenced the movement into the twentieth century. It then considers temperance life assurance as an example of the important but neglected temperance businesses that made the movement an ordinary part of the everyday lives of tens of thousands of people. The chapter outlines the histories of the three offices that form the main focus of the book (the UKT, 1840–1986; Whittington, 1855–94; Sceptre, 1864–1917), and their rivals in the UK and elsewhere, suggesting that by putting the actuarial imaginary to work to deal with alcohol and abstinence these firms had a much wider influence. Lives covered in this chapter include the abolitionist and businessman Samuel Bowly and two of the UKT's first policyholders.

Chapter 2 considers the idea of *mapping* this ordinary temperance in towns and cities across Britain. Temperance support and activity was unevenly spread, and tensions existed between the metropolitan centre of political life and the strongly teetotal northern heartlands of the early movement; while the Alliance arguably fared better in its attempts to organize nationwide political pressure, its headquarters were in

Manchester while the subject of its efforts were in Westminster. Similarly, while most of the firms selling temperance life assurance were based in London, their business was widely scattered. The chapter offers a quick tour of temperance Manchester to demonstrate the value of mapping ordinary temperance, before turning to more scattered, messier geographies. The records of temperance life assurance firms allow us to locate some of the applicants, policyholders, agents and medical referees they dealt with in particular towns and cities. Two local clusters are presented in more detail: first, the 'life' of a set of mill towns in northeast Lancashire which were home to both ordinary teetotalers and key figures in the labour movement, and second a more surprising cluster of teetotalers in Exeter, a city far less supportive of temperance. The life of Edward Vivian of Torquay further illustrates the difficulties facing temperance in Devon. The chapter concludes by turning to East London to consider a tiny temperance enclave, demonstrating that ordinary temperance might rapidly fade from public visibility.

Part 2 of the book explores the development of the UKT's experiment over the firm's first ten years (1840–50), as temperance networks became insurantial ones during a decade when temperance – already socially marginal – was riven by internal conflict, and the life assurance industry was beset by fraud and failure. Chapter 3 asks how the UKT survived the 1840s, a decade in which dozens of assurance firms collapsed – some in scandalous circumstances. The firm faced many challenges and struggled to recruit 'good' teetotal lives. However, the establishment of a General section for moderate drinkers in 1847 both widened its market and generated greater trust in its business and in total abstinence. This chapter includes the lives of James Ellis, one of the UKT's founding directors, who was forced to leave the company, and the controversial minister Joseph Barker.

Chapter 4 explores the ways in which the claims made by temperance life assurance companies circulated within public discussions of the risks associated with drinking, and were translated into forms of knowledge that differed from the religious or moral arguments that characterized other temperance discourse. In doing so it develops insights from science and technology studies by shifting its attention from facts to forms of knowledge, from claims about the world to the social relationships and material things that made those claims effective. These firms contributed to the 'avalanche of printed numbers' so characteristic of Victorian public life, though these numbers did not *borrow* authority from the powerful but actively *produced* it as they travelled through firms' networks.[89] Drawing on work on the turn to numbers as a way of working at a distance, the chapter describes firms' efforts to manage the internal tensions within life assurance identified by Timothy Alborn.[90] Lives described here include Robert Charleton, factory owner and statistician, and a bundle of forms assuring one Whittington life.

Chapter 5 describes the formation of these social-material networks, considering two key types of actor – agents and medical referees – who ensured that the temperance principles and medical knowledge of the directors and medical officers were put into practice. Medical directors and boards urged local agents and doctors to follow particular practices; those agents and referees had to navigate conflicting loyalties, and a good deal of ongoing tinkering was needed to keep these networks running. The

UKT's review of its first fifteen years found that the firm had relaxed its usual prudence in order to 'do as much moral good … as possible' by offering policies to a few reclaimed drunkards.[91] This reminds us that the UKT was not simply driven by the quest for actuarial and medical truths but was concerned with a much broader sense of the values of temperance: socialized risks, the promotion of individual responsibility and careful investment. The lives presented in this chapter include the Manx temperance missionary turned UKT agent, James Teare, two generations of a family of Leicester agents and two early medical referees.

Part 3 of the book explores the success of these firms between 1850 and 1918, beginning in Chapter 6 with an examination of the aims of temperance life assurance. Was it a form of governmentality aimed at improving behaviour, a flexible 'affective technology' producing feelings of security, a progressive source of what might now be called 'ethical finance', or a straightforward business decision that took advantage of the natural prudence of temperance lives, while purifying the symbolic and actual filth generated by all this filthy lucre?[92] It seems likely it was thought to be all of these things. At the same time, though, the worldly complications of business could become entangled with temperance principles, and there can be no better example of this than the fact that the UKT and its directors somehow became the owners of several pubs. The lives included in this chapter include the UKT's first physician, Robert Dundas Thomson; the soldier-tailor Edward Cahill; and the UKT's office buildings.

Chapter 7 looks at ordinary temperance lives, based largely on a sample of nearly a thousand teetotalers assured by Sceptre between 1865 and 1881. The sample includes a few gentlemen, professionals and merchants, but is dominated by men and women in lower middle-class occupations, alongside a significant number of more straightforwardly working-class lives, not all of them artisans of the sort usually associated with temperance. Alongside aspiring nonconformists with strong temperance convictions there are many more modest men and women whose engagement with the movement is harder to discern. There is only one full temperance life in this chapter, that of Caroline John, though many others are considered in brief.

Temperance assurance also influenced medical arguments about alcohol and abstinence, as Chapter 8 illustrates. The evidence collected and disseminated by these firms provided new ways of knowing and representing the dangers of drinking, rivalling both newer work in physiology and medical practitioners' existing experience. Some teetotalers argued that medicine simply confirmed what life assurance had already proven, and some doctors supported teetotalism through 'medical temperance'.[93] Insurers learned from medicine, too, as attempts to establish a safe daily limit for alcohol consumption became part of insurance practice in the United States and elsewhere. This suggests not only broad agreement about the risks of drinking between actuaries and doctors, but also the dissemination of this understanding through insurance networks. By the beginning of the twentieth century, the life assurance view of excessive drinking was widely shared by doctors, though scepticism remained in more conservative quarters. This chapter's lives include royal physician Sir Thomas Barlow and the health writer Joseph Mortimer Granville.

An emphasis on temperance as a political, prohibitionist movement has prompted historians to see the end of the First World War as the end of the temperance movement. The final chapter of this book (Chapter 9) suggests instead that this period represents the beginning of a new way of thinking about alcohol and temperance. In 1918 a government report concluded that the experience of life assurance firms did not prove that abstinence was necessarily the cause of increased longevity; the publication of Raymond Pearl's *Alcohol and Longevity* (1926) further shifted the consensus of medical and insurantial opinion towards the acceptability of moderation. The scientific debate continued, now framed by a new emphasis on moderation, which would dominate twentieth-century research. Temperance life assurance could be said to have anticipated and influenced that conclusion, as well as the statistical approach some used to investigate this question. An acceptance of moderation meant a partial victory for temperance. It was no longer possible to argue that drink was necessary for health, as had been common until the 1870s. At the same time, the principle of carefully selecting 'good' lives even amongst moderate drinkers had become accepted; firms were unanimous in their rejection of heavy drinkers. In essence the UKT had reached this conclusion in 1847, though its acceptance of moderate drinking was forced upon them for business reasons. Life assurance had made 'a very business-like argument for the value of temperance', as the *Manchester Guardian* put it in 1906, and in the process had made temperance an ordinary, taken-for-granted aspect of everyday life.[94]

Notes

1. The firm was originally called the United Kingdom Total Abstinence Life Association, changing its name to the United Kingdom Temperance and General Provident Institution in 1847. 'UKT' will be used to refer to both, though where it is worth distinguishing between them 'UKTALA' refers to the firm between 1840 and 1847, and 'UKT&GPI' after that date.
2. Mary Poovey, 'Economics and Finance', in *The Cambridge History of Victorian Literature*, edited by Kate Flint (Cambridge: Cambridge University Press, 2012), 388–404.
3. Francis O'Gorman, 'Introduction', in *Victorian Literature and Finance*, edited by Francis O'Gorman (Oxford: Oxford University Press, 2007), 1–16. For some of the key work in this field see Margot C. Finn, *The Character of Credit: Personal Debt in English Culture, 1740–1914* (Cambridge: Cambridge University Press, 2003); Mary Poovey, ed., *The Financial System in Nineteenth-Century Britain* (New York: Oxford University Press, 2003); Nancy Henry and Cannon Schmitt, eds, *Victorian Investments: New Perspectives on Finance and Culture* (Bloomington: Indiana University Press, 2009); and O'Gorman's collection. For a classic work of economic sociology which considers nineteenth-century developments in a similar light, see Viviana A. Zelizer, *Economic Lives: How Culture Shapes the Economy* (Princeton, NJ: Princeton University Press, 2011).
4. Virginia Berridge, 'Opium Eating and Life Insurance', *British Journal of Addiction* 72 (1977), 371–7; Ray Jureidini and Kevin White, 'Life Insurance, the Medical Examination and Cultural Values', *Journal of Historical Sociology* 13 (2000), 190–214; Timothy Alborn, 'Insurance against Germ Theory: Commerce and Conservatism in Late-Victorian Medicine', *Bulletin of the History of Medicine* 75 (2001), 406–45; James Kneale and Shaun French, '"The Relations of Inebriety to Insurance": Geographies of

Medicine, Insurance and Alcohol in Britain, 1840–1911', in *Intoxication: Problematic Pleasures*, edited by Jonathan Herring, Ciaran Regan, Darin Weinberg and Phil Withington (Basingstoke: Palgrave Macmillan, 2013), 233–49; Shaun French and James Kneale, 'Excessive Financialisation: Insuring Lifestyles and Everyday Geographies of Social Excess', *Environment and Planning D: Society and Space* 27, 6 (2009), 1030–53.

5. Brian Harrison, *Drink and the Victorians* (London: Faber, 1971); John Greenaway, *Drink and British Politics since 1830: A Study in Policy-Making* (Basingstoke: Palgrave Macmillan, 2003); James Nicholls, *The Politics of Alcohol: A History of the Drink Question in England* (Manchester: Manchester University Press, 2009); Lilian Lewis Shiman, *The Crusade against Drink in Victorian England* (Basingstoke: Macmillan, 1988); Annemarie Mcallister, *Demon Drink: Temperance and the Working Class* (London: Faber, 2014); David M. Fahey, *Temperance Societies in Late Victorian and Edwardian England* (Newcastle upon Tyne: Cambridge Scholars, 2020).
6. M. J. Senter and A. M. Senter, *Walton-on-the-Naze: The Warner Story* (Colchester: M. J. & A. M. Senter, 1997), MS 127/3, Library of the Society of Friends; 'One of the Pioneers at Walton-on-the-Naze', *Essex Standard, West Suffolk Gazette, and Eastern Counties' Advertiser*, 26 May 1883, 6.
7. For histories of nineteenth- and twentieth-century life assurance in Britain and the United States, see Timothy Alborn, *Regulated Lives: Life Assurance and British Society, 1800–1914* (Toronto: University of Toronto Press, 2009); Sharon AnnMurphy, *Investing in Life: Insurance in Antebellum America* (Baltimore, MD: Johns Hopkins University Press, 2010); Liz McFall, *Devising Consumption: Cultural Economies of Insurance, Credit and Spending* (London: Routledge, 2019); and Dan Bouk, *How Our Days Became Numbered: Risk and the Rise of the Statistical Individual* (Chicago: University of Chicago Press, 2015).
8. *Temperance, Longevity, Insurance. A Tract for the Times* (Toronto: Canada Citizen Publishing, 1884).
9. Vance Thompson, *Drink and be Sober* (New York: Moffat: Yard, 1915), 42.
10. Peter T. Winskill, *The Temperance Movement and Its Workers: A Record of Social, Moral, Religious, and Political Progress*, vol. 1 (London: Blackie, 1891), 7–9; John Harley Warner, 'Physiological Theory and Therapeutic Explanation in the 1860s: The British Debate on the Medical Use of Alcohol', *Bulletin for the History of Medicine* 54 (1980), 235–57; Jonathan Reinarz and Rebecca Wynter, 'The Spirit of Medicine: The Use of Alcohol in Nineteenth-Century Medical Practice', in *Drink in the Eighteenth and Nineteenth Centuries*, edited by Susanne Schmid and Barbara Schmidt-Haberkamp (London: Pickering and Chatto, 2014), 127–40.
11. Alborn, *Regulated Lives*, 225.
12. 'Brandy for Directors during the Cholera of 1849', 6 September 1849, Minute Book 1, Prudential Archives; Letter to shareholders, County Hailstorm Insurance Company, 1 May 1848, Hertfordshire Record Office 7257/1.
13. Board meeting, 12 November 1844, Royal Farmers, Minute Book 5, CLC/B/192/MS14989/001, London Archives; Gregory Anderson, *Victorian Clerks* (Manchester: Manchester University Press 1976), 33–5.
14. Norman Longmate, *The Waterdrinkers: A History of Temperance* (London: Hamish Hamilton, 1968); Gerald Wayne Olsen, 'From Parish to Palace: Working-Class Influences on Anglican Temperance Movements, 1835–1914', *Journal of Ecclesiastical History* 40, 2 (1989), 239–52.
15. Copy of letter from H. Rickman to Robert Warner, December 1840, FL357, Aviva Archives.

16. Peter T. Winskill, *The Comprehensive History of the Rise and Progress of the Temperance Reformation from the Earliest Period to September 1881* (Warrington: P.T. Winskill, 1881), 248.
17. Alborn, *Regulated Lives*, 34–7.
18. David Tregoning and Hugh Cockerell, *Friends for Life: Friends' Provident Life Office 1832–1982* (London: Melland, 1982); Elizabeth Ischei, *Victorian Quakers* (Oxford: Oxford University Press, 1970), 238.
19. 'One of the Pioneers', *Essex Standard*; 'Theodore Compton', *The Annual Monitor for 1910, Being an Obituary of Members of the Society of Friends of Great Britain and Ireland, From October 1, 1908, To September 30, 1909* (London: Headley Brothers, 1910), 36–53.
20. Brian Harrison, *Dictionary of Temperance Biography* (Coventry: Society for the Study of Labour History, 1973), 70; Winskill, *Temperance Movement*, vol. I, 217–19.
21. Peter T. Winskill, *The Temperance Movement and Its Workers: A Record of Social, Moral, Religious, and Political Progress*, vol. 2 (London: Blackie, 1891), 147.
22. Cornelius Walford, 'History of Life Assurance in the United Kingdom, 5. Life Assurance 1825 to 1843', *Journal of the Institute of Actuaries* 26 (1886–7), 302–15.
23. Prospectus, 'The United Kingdom Total Abstinence Life Association', volume of prospectuses of Assurance Societies sent by the Clerical, Medical and General Life Assurance Society, R826-G, 2, Institute and Faculty of Actuaries Library.
24. Winskill, *The Temperance Movement*, vol. 2, 120.
25. Winskill, *Comprehensive History*, 249.
26. Board meeting, 8 January 1847, UKT Minute Book 1, MS FL108, Aviva Archives.
27. See the appendix.
28. 'Review of *Tweedie's Temperance Yearbook of Facts and History for 1864*', *Daily News*, 26 December 1864, 2.
29. Alborn, *Regulated Lives*, table 1.1, 27; 'Twenty-Seven Years' Progress. Accumulated Life Assurance Funds (Ordinary and Industrial) of British Life Offices in 1871 and 1898', supplement to *The Review*, 25 January 1899, Prudential Archives.
30. *The Times*, 14 January 1920, 19; 22 April 1920, 24.
31. Burns, company history, 1896, 25, MS FL368, Aviva Archives. Burns's document remained unpublished, though it provided the basis for Hartley Withers's official history of the UKT, *Pioneers of British Life Assurance*.
32. *Bristol Mercury*, 24 March 1855, 6; *Leicester Chronicle*, 25 October 1862, 3; *Quiver* 8, 370 (1873), 716; *Morning Post*, May 23, 1877, 3; 'The Effect of Alcohol on Human Life', *Isle of Man Times and General Advertiser*, 29 September 1883, 2; Arthur Newsholme, 'The Possible Association of the Consumption of Alcohol with Excessive Mortality from Cancer', *Journal of the Institute of Actuaries* 38, 4 (1904), 347–53.
33. Central Control Board (Liquor) Advisory Committee, *Alcohol: Its Action on the Human Organism* (London: H. M. Stationery Office, 1918), 118.
34. Hartley Withers, *Pioneers of British Life Assurance* (London: Staples Press, published for the UK Provident Institution, 1951); Advantages of the temperance policy, United Kingdom Temperance and General Provident Institution, Prospectus, 1952, MS C Uni Livesey Collection.
35. *Essex Standard*, 26 May 1883, 6.
36. Report of Sixth Annual Meeting, 1 January 1847, 2, United Kingdom Temperance & General Provident Institution Annual Reports and Balance Sheets 1840–1910, MS 1232, Aviva Archives.

37. James Dawson Burns, *The Vital Statistics of Total Abstinence* (London: National Temperance Publication Depot, 1883).
38. Burns, *Vital Statistics*, 4–5.
39. Ibid., 5–6.
40. Burns, company history, 9–10, emphasis added.
41. See Alborn, *Regulated Lives*, especially 8–9.
42. See, for example, *Leicester Chronicle*, 23 September 1857; 1; 'Lecture at the Exchange Hall', *Nottinghamshire Guardian*, 24 October 1862, 3; *Aberdeen Weekly Journal*, 10 December 1891, 4; 'Swansea Gospel Temperance Union. Total Abstinence and Life Assurance', *Cambrian*, 8 March 1895, 7; *Belfast News-Letter*, 5 November 1889, 6; 'Religion and Temperance', *Bendigo Independent*, 6 January 1900, 2; 'Statist', 'Who Slew All These?' *Evening Star*, 15 August 1903, 7.
43. S. P. Kerr, *Belfast News-Letter*, 5 November 1889, 6, emphasis added.
44. Koray Çalişkan and Michel Callon, 'Economization, Part 2: A Research Programme for the Study of Markets', *Economy and Society* 39, 1 (2010), 1–32; Michel Callon, *Markets in the Making: Rethinking Competition, Goods, and Innovation*, trans. Olivia Custer (Brooklyn, NY: Zone Books, 2021).
45. Gerald Wayne Olsen, '"Physician Heal Thyself": Drink, Temperance and the Medical Question in the Victorian and Edwardian Church of England, 1830–1914', *Addiction* 89 (1994), 1167–76, emphasis added.
46. Bruno Latour, 'Technology Is Society Made Durable', in *A Sociology of Monsters: Essays on Power, Technology, and Domination*, edited by John Law (London: Routledge, 1991), 103–31.
47. John Law and Evelyn Ruppert, 'The Social Life of Methods: Devices', *Journal of Cultural Economy* 6 (2013), 229–40.
48. Theodore Porter, *Trust in Numbers: The Pursuit of Objectivity in Science and Public Life* (Princeton, NJ: Princeton University Press, 1995), ix; Bruno Latour, *Pandora's Hope* (Cambridge, MA: Harvard University Press, 1999).
49. Bruno Latour, *We Have Never Been Modern* (New York: Harvester Wheatsheaf, 1993), 125–6.
50. Ibid., 126.
51. Francois Ewald, 'Insurance and Risk', in *The Foucault Effect: Studies in Governmentality*, edited by Graham Burchell, Colin Gordon and Peter Miller (Hertfordshire: Harvester Wheatsheaf, 1991), 197–210.
52. Margo Huxley, 'Geographies of Governmentality', in *Space, Knowledge and Power: Foucault and Geography*, edited by Stuart Elden and Jeremy Crampton (Oxford: Routledge, 2007), 185–204.
53. Geoffrey W. Clark, *Betting on Lives: The Culture of Life Insurance in England, 1695–1775* (Manchester: Manchester University Press, 1999).
54. Daniel Defert, '"Popular Life" and Insurance Technology', in *The Foucault Effect*, 211–33.
55. Pat O'Malley and Alex Roberts, 'Governmental Conditions for the Economization of Uncertainty', *Journal of Cultural Economy* 7 (2014), 253–72; Samuel Randalls and James Kneale, 'A Fragile Network: Effecting Hail Insurance in Britain, 1840–1900', *Enterprise & Society* 22, 3 (2020), 833–48; James Kneale and Samuel Randalls, 'Making Climate Risks Work: Governmentality and "Foreign Residence" in British Life Assurance, 1840–1940', *Transactions of the Institute of British Geographers* 45, 4 (2020), 739–69.

56. Board meeting, 27 February 1896, Board of Directors, Minute Book 4, CLC/B/005/SC01/05/01/004, London Archives.
57. *Special Instructions and Tables*, February 1884, 116, Agents' instructions: 1B Special for superintendents, 1870–1922, 1314; Board meeting, 20 February 1896, Minute Book 24, 20 February 1896–29 July 1897, Prudential Archives.
58. *Special Instructions*, December 1922, Agents' instructions: 1B Special for superintendents, 1870–1922, 1314; Board meeting, 22 October 1874, Minute Book 4; Board meeting, 20 February 1896, Minute Book 24, Prudential Archive.
59. Jeremy Bentham, *The Works of Jeremy Bentham*, vol. 1 (New York: Russell and Russell, 1962), 31.
60. Pat O'Malley, 'Imagining Insurance: Risk, Thrift and Industrial Life Insurance in Britain', *Connecticut Insurance Law Journal* 5 (1999), 676–705.
61. 'Swansea Gospel Temperance Union'.
62. See, for example, Board meeting, 5 September 1854, Royal Farmers Minute Book 14, MS14989/14, London Archives.
63. George Lynas, 'Why will ye die?', *Wings*, 1 July 1893, 219.
64. Ibid., emphasis added.
65. William J. P. Bingham, *Alcohol and Life Assurance* (London: United Kingdom Alliance, 1922).
66. 'Swansea Gospel Temperance Union'.
67. *New York Times*, 9 June 1901, 14.
68. 'Temperance, Longevity, Insurance', 1, original emphasis.
69. Peter K. Andersson, 'How Civilized Were the Victorians?', *Journal of Victorian Culture* 20, 4 (2015), 439–52.
70. Alborn, *Regulated Lives*, 7–12.
71. Harrison, *Drink*; *Dictionary of Temperance Biography*; 'The British Prohibitionists 1853–1872: A Biographical Analysis', *International Review of Social History* 15, 3 (1970), 375–467.
72. Winskill, *Comprehensive History*; *The Temperance Movement*; and Peter T. Winskill, *Temperance Standard Bearers of the Nineteenth Century. A Biographical and Statistical Temperance Dictionary*, 2 vols. (Liverpool: Winskill, 1897 and 1898).
73. David Beckingham, 'The Press and the Pledge: Father Theobald Mathew's 1843 Temperance Tour of Britain', *Historical Geography* 42 (2014), 93–110; Annemarie McAllister, *Writing for Social Change in Temperance Periodicals: Conviction and Career* (New York: Routledge, 2023); Dorota Dias-Lewandowska and Pam Lock, 'Women, Home, and Alcohol: Constructed Façades and Social Norms in Nineteenth-Century Polish and British Representations of Female Drinking Practices', *Journal of Victorian Culture* 28, 2 (2023), 227–42.
74. The Sceptre sample is described in more detail in the appendix, but is based upon the following documents: Sceptre Life Association Limited Policy Ledger 1, MS SC04/01/01; Sceptre Life Association Limited Policy Ledger 2, MS SC04/01/02; Sceptre Life Association Limited Policy Ledger 3, MS SC04/01/03; Sceptre Life Association Limited Policy Ledger 4, MS SC04/01/04; Sceptre Life Association Limited Policy Ledger 5, MS SC04/01/05, London Archives.
75. See Ros Black, *Scandal, Salvation and Suffrage: The Amazing Women of the Temperance Movement* (Kibworth Beauchamp: Matador, 2015) and McAllister, *Writing for Social Change*.
76. For example, Nancy Henry, '"Ladies Do It?" Victorian Women Investors in Fact and Fiction', in *Victorian Literature and Finance*, edited by Francis O'Gorman

(Oxford: Oxford University Press, 2007), 111–31; George Robb, 'Ladies of the Ticker: Women, Investment, and Fraud in England and America, 1850–1930', in *Victorian Investments: New Perspectives on Finance and Culture*, edited by Nancy Henry and Cannon Schmitt (Bloomington: Indiana University Press, 2009), 120–40.

77. See Jake Hodder, 'On Absence and Abundance: Biography as Method in Archival Research', *Area* 49, 4 (2017), 452–9; David Lambert, 'Reflections on the Concept of Imperial Biographies', *Geschichte und Gesellschaft* 40 (2014), 22–41; Miles Ogborn, *Global Lives: Britain and the World 1550–1800* (Cambridge: Cambridge University Press, 2008); Caroline Bressey, *Empire, Race and the Politics of Anti-Caste* (London: Bloomsbury, 2015).
78. David Beckingham and Charles Watkins, 'Temperance Lives and Landscape: Lady Elizabeth Biddulph, Lady Henry Somerset, and Late Nineteenth-Century Ledbury', *Rural History* (2024), 1–22.
79. Senter and Senter, *The Warner Story*; 'Obituary, Robert Warner 1815–1896', *Minutes of the Proceedings of the Institution of Civil Engineers* 128 (1897), 363–4; *Cassell's Illustrated Family Paper Exhibitor: Containing about Three Hundred Illustrations, with Letter-Press Descriptions of All the Principal Objects in the International Exhibition of 1862* (London: Cassell, Petter and Galpin, 1862), A.17.11, National Art Library; 'Notes of the Quarter', *Essex Review* (1897), 15.
80. 'Notes of the Quarter', 16.
81. Ibid., 15; *London Gazette*, 8 April 1879, 2713.
82. Essex Local Government Board and John Lambert, *Return of Owners of Land, 1873* (London: Her Majesty's Stationery Office, 1875), 45.
83. 'Temperance Notes and News', *Quiver* 687 (1899), 663; 'Notes of the Quarter', 16.
84. Board Meeting, 2 February 1844, UKT Minute Book 1, Aviva Archives.
85. 'Wills and Bequests', *Morning Post*, 18 February 1897, 10.
86. Winskill, *Temperance Movement*, vol. 2, 146, 147.
87. Anthony Warner, *John Warner. Some Notes on His Family* (Lowewood Museum, 1990).
88. 'North Essex Election', *Essex Standard*, 20 August 1847, 4; *Essex County Chronicle*, 19 June 1885, 7.
89. Ian Hacking, *The Taming of Chance* (Cambridge: Cambridge University Press, 1990).
90. Porter, *Trust in Numbers*; Dan Bouk, *How Our Days Became Numbered: Risk and the Risk of the Statistical Individual* (London: University of Chicago Press, 2015); Latour, *Pandora's Hope*; Alborn, *Regulated Lives*.
91. Joseph T. Mitchell, *Report of the Medical Director to the Directors of the Temperance and General Provident Institution*, 16 September 1856, 13, FL293, Aviva.
92. Nigel Thrift, *Non-representational Theory: Space, Politics, Affect* (London: Routledge, 2008).
93. John Granville Woolley and William E. Johnson, *Temperance Progress in the Century* (London: Linscott Publishing, 1903), 379.
94. 'Disappointing the Undertakers', *Manchester Guardian*, 17 February 1906, 10.

1

Ordinary temperance

Introduction: Varieties of temperance

When E. Dawson King of the Manchester and Salford Temperance Society gave a lecture in the Trinity Wesleyan Schoolroom at Whanganui, New Zealand, in 1892, he listed three 'epoch-making movements' in the history of English temperance: the United Kingdom Alliance, the most significant political temperance organization of the nineteenth century; the Band of Hope, a children's temperance group that claimed to have 3.5 million members by 1901; and the UK Temperance and General Provident Institution.[1] The Alliance and Band of Hope have attracted some attention from historians over the past fifty years, but the UKT remains obscure in comparison.[2] On the whole, historians have focused on temperance as a social, cultural or political phenomenon and have neglected the history of temperance businesses. This lack of interest in temperance companies is puzzling because teetotalers established many important firms in Victorian Britain: Thomas Cook's travel agency, publishers like Cassells, manufacturers of chocolate (the Cadburys), biscuits (Huntley and Palmer, Peek Freans), and shoes and boots (Clarks). However, there has been little research on firms established by temperance supporters beyond their company histories.

This chapter seeks to broaden our understandings of temperance by emphasizing the *ordinariness* of some aspects of the movement. At the same time, it seeks to illustrate the *variety and complexity* of that movement. The UKT, which played an important part in the growing ubiquity of temperance, drew on surprisingly radical roots in its first decades and continued to work alongside progressive elements of Victorian and Edwardian society. The life of Samuel Bowly, a director of the UKT for over forty years, exemplifies this mixture of radicalism and commercial enterprise, and the chapter then expands upon the histories of the most important temperance life assurance offices. Brief accounts of the lives of some of the UKT's early agents and policyholders explore the place of total abstinence in everyday life. The chapter concludes by asking what is to be learned from focusing on ordinary temperance away from parliament and the metropolis.

Ordinary temperance

Despite its breadth and variety, we have become used to thinking of British temperance as a *political* movement. To some extent this reflects the influence of a particular understanding of temperance borrowed from the United States. As Harry G. Levine put it, 'The passage of constitutional Prohibition and the experiences of the 1920s have so affected American consciousness that they have determined the shape and content of virtually all subsequent historical inquiries.'[3] Levine suggested that Prohibition is seen as a rare and short-lived episode of political intervention into alcohol control, as if what went before it and what came after it were not also political schemes for managing drinking. Similarly, accounts of nineteenth-century temperance that see it as simply the road to Prohibition – what Mark Lawrence Schrad calls 'a rudimentary "if temperance, then prohibition" logic' – elide a much longer, more complicated and more interesting history.[4] American temperance and the campaign for Prohibition are thought to be characterized by middle-class evangelism, moral piety and nativist politics, which does not explain the simultaneous appearance of prohibitionist laws in very different places like Canada, Russia or Scandinavia, as Schrad points out. The path taken by temperance in the United States certainly does not parallel the development of the movement in Britain.

Brian Harrison's classic study *Drink and the Victorians* might also be said to encourage this reading. The period studied by Harrison's book ends with the Licensing Act 1872, the first real sign, in hindsight, that the UK Alliance, established in 1853 to bring temperance arguments to parliament, would fail in its efforts to pass legislation allowing local districts to ban the sale of alcohol. The title of the final chapter – 'the End' – suggests that temperance was only this political campaign for 'Local Option' or 'Local Veto'. Harrison, chiefly but not exclusively interested in these institutional efforts, listed temperance among other 'unsuccessful reforming movements' in the introduction to *Drink and the Victorians*, stating that 'the temperance movement also failed'.[5] Concluding the book, he suggested that 'temperance ceased to be a live political issue after the first world war', noting that its societies began to decline from that date, and explored the criticisms of temperance developed by socialists around the turn of the century.[6] As moral arguments gave way to 'environmental' ones, temperance was reduced to just one element of wider structural reform.

Temperance was never simply a campaign for prohibition, however. Alternative forms of alcohol control were discussed and adopted in many countries at the turn of the century, especially the state control of drinking places in Scandinavia, Britain, Southern and East Africa and Australia under some form of the 'Gothenberg' system of 'disinterested management'; Canadian provinces adopted similar principles after prohibition ended.[7] Harrison briefly mentions this policy of 'municipalization' in his account of 'the end' of UK temperance, contrasting the broad support it received from Liberal and Conservative MPs as well as from socialists with 'the temperance movement's exaggerated claims for its panacea' of prohibition.[8] But Gothenberg was also a form of temperance, one which influenced British breweries, who encouraged the building of 'improved' pubs, promoting eating and socializing over drinking. The British state also took control of many aspects of drinking during the First World War;

the 'afternoon gap' during which pubs in England and Wales were closed from 3 to 5 p.m. lasted until 1988, and the pubs covered by the 'Carlisle system' were still in state control when Harrison published his monograph.[9] Temperance reform meant much more than prohibition, and many of the ideas supported by members of the broader social movement came to fruition.

Crucially, there was no single 'Temperance Movement' in Britain, as David Fahey explained in 1971, but rather 'a myriad of organizations and policies and prickly personalities'. British temperance was shot through with different, shifting and sometimes competing interests and loyalties, linked to class, gender, religious beliefs, personal antagonisms, friendship and support networks and party membership. This was further complicated by local political cultures, as we will see in Chapter 2. Even if we restrict our interest to temperance as a political movement, its members differed about how best to answer the 'drink question', including 'advocates of persuasion and example and advocates of coercive legislation, proponents and opponents of compensation, friends of Sunday Closing, partisans of disinterested management by municipalities or philanthropic trusts, zealots for the "improved" public house, popularizing the membership of licensing authorities, shorter hours, high license, national prohibition, and Local Veto'.[10]

The prevailing wisdom has been that it was these differences within temperance that caused it to fail. While she recognizes that British temperance sought cultural as well as legislative change, for Virginia Berridge 'temperance as a social movement was in decline before the First World War' because 'there was no longer unamity about what its main aim should be'.[11] Other historians have supported Harrison's argument that the Alliance might have been more successful had it not been wedded to the single political principle of Local Option. Historians who have taken the Alliance to be the political expression of a social movement have tended to equate British temperance with the campaign for Local Option. Henry Yeomans's discussion of the movement's influence on British society takes a longer and wider perspective; legislation falling short of prohibition was still significant, and Yeomans describes the reforms enacted by the Licensing Act 1872 as 'the birth of the modern licensing system'.[12] He concludes that a focus on prohibitionist tendencies in British temperance has become 'something of a distraction that encourages academics to focus on the achievement (or non-achievement) of absolute campaigning goals. This search for a defining temperance victory, a British 18th Amendment, is erroneous. In Britain, the temperance movement placed greater emphasis on individual behavioural solutions, rather than collective legal coercion, and achieved more incremental legal measures'.[13]

Temperance was a failure only if we see it as 'a social movement with a political programme', as Berridge defines it, where this movement was a homogenous and coherent body with a single objective, and where 'politics' means the passing of national legislation.[14] The diversity of aims and groups visible in late Victorian temperance reflects in part some of its marginal and occasionally radical roots. There is still, in some quarters, an assumption that temperance was essentially conservative, a reaction to drastic social change that sought to impose bourgeois values of respectability and sobriety on ordinary people, aided by those sections of the working class who subscribed to these values out of a desire for self-improvement. For one group of social historians in the 1970s, this was part of the 'social control of leisure', where nineteenth-century entertainment was both subject to discipline (through the new police) and an agent of that discipline (as leisure became a civilizing force through the provision of 'rational recreation').[15] Gramcsi's argument that US Prohibition was a drive for industrial efficiency – 'the struggle against alcohol, the most dangerous agent of destruction of laboring power, becomes a function of the state' – follows a similar logic.[16]

However, as Berridge explains, British temperance was not 'a diversion from the real aims of working-class politics', nor 'a way of imposing middle-class culture and manners on the working class, as something which "civilized" them and drew them away from radical thoughts'.[17] Aristocratic and middle-class supporters tried to shape temperance but lost many battles to total abstainers. Genteel Anglican distrust of the working-class and nonconformist roots of teetotalism delayed the formation of the Church of England Temperance Society (CETS) until 1873. Clergymen who adopted total abstinence in the decades before the CETS, therefore, 'reversed somewhat the proposition enshrined in the evangelical tradition that true moral reform depended upon the leadership of the privileged classes and the compliance of their social inferiors', because they followed calls from below rather than from the church hierarchy.[18] In short, the tensions within British society that more conservative temperance campaigners sought to tame also shaped the movement they claimed to speak for, and those tensions are visible within temperance history. Nineteenth- and early twentieth-century temperance also maintained and developed connections to many progressive movements, including campaigns for the abolition of slavery and the slave trade, for women's suffrage and for the labour movement. Two brief sketches of temperance in its first decades and again in the 1870s help demonstrate that while its spirit was domesticated as the movement widened, its later claims to radicalism were not always simply rhetorical.

From its earliest days the broader movement included those who looked beyond the main currents of British political life. In 1841, for example, Queen Victoria reported that Lord Melbourne had told her that 'it was a very singular thing, but that almost all these Temperance people, were Radicals'.[19] Some temperance activists were active in the campaigns for the abolition of the trade in enslaved people and for emancipation, for example; as Brian Harrison put it, 'the antislavery movement was long regarded as a model by temperance reformers, who met in the same premises, used the same arguments, [and] attracted the same individuals'.[20] In the Victorian labour movement 'from Chartism and the Rochdale Pioneers, continuing through to the formation of the T.U.C. *(Trades Union Congress)* and the modern Labour party, temperance ideas played an important part in policy formulation'.[21] Typographical societies pursued total abstinence as part of a programme of self-improvement, while the Owenite socialist and cooperative pioneer John Finch declared that 'every Co-Operative Society was … a Temperance Society also'.[22] Teetotalers like Paisley's Reverend Patrick Brewster or the Birmingham Quaker Joseph Sturge were influential in both abolition and Chartism.[23] And in Ireland, temperance united Daniel O'Connell's Irish Repeal Association and the campaign of Father Mathew, 'the Father of Irish Temperance'.[24]

The first decades of British temperance also saw it mingle with more marginal causes. The son of a publican, William Horsell signed the moderation pledge in 1833 but must have been teetotal by 1840 as he became an agent for the UKT that year in Great Horwood, Buckinghamshire. He lectured on temperance at Aylesbury but was better known as the first secretary of the Vegetarian Society from 1837 and as founder of the first vegetarian newspaper in Britain.[25] Horsell was also a supporter of hydropathy, and the 'water cure' had other adherents within temperance; the Irish Quaker and temperance reformer James Haughton described hydropathy and teetotalism as 'almost twins by birth' in 1847.[26]

By the 1870s temperance had become more acceptable to the Church of England, and the Alliance was becoming increasingly influential within the Liberal Party – though this influence would also be blamed for Gladstone's defeat at the 1874 General Election. Following Harrison's arguments, described earlier, this moment could be seen as the beginning of the end for the movement, a narrowing of objectives to a single cause: the passing of a Permissive Bill allowing Local Option. The list of guests invited to the laying of the first memorial stone for the London Temperance Hospital's new building on Hampstead Road five years later in 1879 presents a different story, though.[27] Of the forty guests who hoped to be there, nineteen were MPs. These were a varied lot, including Jacob Bright, MP for Manchester and brother of John Bright, from a Quaker cotton-manufacturing family of radicals, feminists and teetotalers; George Palmer, MP for Reading and co-owner of the Huntley & Palmer biscuit firm; Thomas Burt, the Radical MP for Morpeth, a miner's son and trade unionist and one of the first working-class MPs; Henry Richard, Liberal MP for Merthyr, and minister, journalist and secretary to the Peace Society; Alexander Martin Sullivan, Irish nationalist MP; Benjamin Whitworth, MP for Kilkenny, an Irish linen manufacturer who was chair of the United Kingdom Alliance Executive Committee, and another UKT director; and William Shaw, Liberal MP for Cork and co-founder and early leader of the Home Rule movement.

Another ten guests were ministers of different denominations, including Canon Henry John Ellison, chaplain-in-ordinary to Queen Victoria from 1879 and founder of the CETS. Several of the others were campaigners for non-sectarian education, like the Baptist Reverend John Clifford, a former lace worker who took four degrees at University College London and led opposition to the Second Boer War, and the Reverend J. Hirst Hollowell. Other guests included James Barlow, a Bolton mayor, mill owner and philanthropist who will be mentioned again in Chapter 2; Vice-Admiral Sir William King Hall KCB, president of the Royal Temperance Naval Society, veteran of the Crimean and Second Opium Wars and a director of the UKT; and T. B. Smithies, founder of the *Band of Hope Review* and the *British Workman* temperance newspaper. Other temperance business representatives included John Broomhall, another UKT director, and G. H. Frean of Peek Freans Biscuits.

These guests illustrate something of the breadth and diversity of temperance in 1879, bringing together nonconformists and Anglicans, Liberals and Conservatives, pacifists and military veterans to celebrate the hospital's opening. Addressing them, however, Sir Wilfrid Lawson, the Alliance's spokesman in parliament, spoke to temperance's radical roots by noting that the Exchequer made £33 million a year from drink, 'and with it kept up the army and the navy, which were now engaged in killing the Zulus with the ostensible purpose of Christianising them afterwards'.[28]

Something of this strange mix of commercial enterprise and radicalism can be seen in the life of Samuel Bowly, one of the UKT's longest-serving supporters.

Temperance lives: Samuel Bowly (1802–1884)

Samuel Bowly was born in Cirencester in 1802. One obituarist wrote that he 'early developed that shrewdness and aptness for business which is, we suppose, characteristic of a Quaker education', establishing his first business in his twenties.[29] Bowly began to invest in banks and railways, becoming one of the founders of the Bristol and Birmingham Railway and director of the Gloucestershire Banking Company. A member of Gloucester's corporation, Bowly founded the town's first Land and Building Society with another Friend, Joseph Sturge of Birmingham. His political activism began in the anti-slavery movement, supporting Sturge's Central Negro Emancipation Committee and speaking and publishing on abolition. Drawing-room meetings and boycotts of 'slave sugar' also provided equally important but less visible support.[30] One of Bowly's biographers noted that the Friends of that generation who became active in abolition 'had become, most of them, total abstainers from the products of slave-grown cotton, and from slave-grown cane-sugar'.[31] Bowly is one of the subjects of Benjamin Robert Haydon's painting of *The Anti-Slavery Society Convention*, recording the meeting of the British and Foreign Anti-Slavery Society in 1840.

Bowly also supported British and Ragged Schools, associations for the relief of the poor, penny banks and mechanics' institutes.[32] However, an obituarist noted that 'the cause with which his name will be permanently identified is that of Temperance … *[after Abolition]* this fresh field of public service opened before him as a religious duty'.[33] Bowly pledged for moderation in 1830 and total abstinence in 1835. A founder of the National Temperance League in 1856, he became its president in 1862 and was an early supporter of the London (later National) Temperance Hospital.[34] He was one of the first directors of the UKT, chairing his last AGM in 1882 at the age of eighty.[35] Dawson Burns said Bowly 'brought to the cause a reputation for business ability and benevolent energy'.[36] Up until his death, on his eighty-second birthday, 'his personal appearance and indefatigable labours as an octogenarian were indisputable evidence of the physical soundness of the principles he upheld'.[37] Bowly was said to have addressed over a hundred meetings.[38] He was a keen advocate for teetotalism within the Society of Friends after 1850, though his youngest brother Edward, who left the Society for the Church of England, was a brewer.[39] After his wife, Jane Dearman Shipley, died in 1868, he married Louisa Cotterell, the widow of Jacob Henry Cotterell of Bath, an important supporter of the Rechabites – teetotal friendly societies – and an early agent for and then director of the UKT.[40]

Bowly's funeral brought Gloucester to a standstill; even pubs were closed. The procession was headed by the mayor and members of the corporation, and representatives of many different temperance organizations and businesses paid their respects, including Thomas Cash, the UKT's secretary, director and then managing director.[41] The UKT's annual report for 1884 acknowledged, 'The prominent and unique position Mr Bowly held in the Temperance world, and the influence of his commercial and Christian character, render his death no ordinary loss.'[42]

Samuel Bowly's temperance life was both radical and ordinary. In reminding us that teetotalers referred to 'the liquor traffic' – as they did in the full name of the United Kingdom Alliance for Suppression of the Liquor Traffic – because they identified it with the trade in enslaved Africans, he makes clear that some in his generation of teetotalers simply extended their campaigning from one focus to another. Boycotts of slave-grown sugar represented the first campaigns of consumer activism, and temperance drew on their methods. Temperance could be a radical cause.

Bowly also presents an interesting contrast to Robert Warner, his friend and co-worker in the UKT and the National Temperance Society. A preacher from the 1850s, Bowly's faith seems to have been vitally important to him, unlike Warner's. Like Warner, he was a successful capitalist, though one of his biographers was careful to separate this 'legitimate and Christian commerce which uplifts the masses as it ennobles those engaged in it' from other lower forms of commerce.[43] His daughter Maria thought that Bowly sometimes struggled to hold these things apart, as he had 'felt the temptation of worldly ambition' in the 1830s. Perhaps his work for the UKT allowed Bowly to combine promoting total abstinence with a form of 'legitimate and Christian commerce', seeing the many AGMs he chaired as temperance work.

It is time to say a little more about the business of temperance life assurance and the firms that are the focus of this book.

The business of temperance life

The *idea* of temperance savings predated the UKT. In 1839 an anonymous article in the *Manchester Guardian* instructed the drinker to 'see how much he might save by giving up his little drops', pointing out that saving a shilling and sixpence a week would add up to more than £120 after twenty years.[44] Savings banks opened for working-class families from the early nineteenth century, including 'penny banks' aimed at the poorest, and their success was only curtailed by the opening of the Post Office Savings Bank in 1861.[45] Many had connections to philanthropic and often religious institutions, and it is easy to see them as part of a wider set of middle-class responses to working-class need and the problem of 'pauperism' (Chapter 6).

Anthony Dingle's classic explanation of fluctuations in British alcohol consumption suggested that until late in the century, working men were likely to spend any extra income on drink, because there were few financial or social incentives for saving it, and few alternative commodities to spend it on.[46] However, savings banks, building societies and friendly societies all offered savings opportunities for working- and lower-middle-class households. Duncan Ross's examination of Glasgow's penny banks indicates that 'considerable saving was taking place, and that "penny banks" operated both as short-term liquidity stores and as vehicles for longer-term and larger-amount savings'.[47] Linda Perriton and Josephine Maltby's analyses of savings banks for better-off working-class savers also indicates that more was saved than might be assumed to be the case, with particular consequences for the household economy and women's agency.[48]

Members of building societies like the Temperance Permanent Building Society (TPBS) pooled their savings to build or buy housing. The TPBS shared many of the aims of the temperance life assurance firms discussed in this chapter. Its originator, the London solicitor William Shaen, thought 'a great business might be raised' through such a firm, one that would also advance 'the great cause of temperance'.[49] Shaen was a middle-class Unitarian, educated at University College London, who campaigned for abolition, women's education and female suffrage; he acted for the Jamaica Committee and for Josephine Butler's Association for the Repeal of the Contagious Diseases Acts.[50] The temperance publisher William Tweedie was a founding director of the firm, as was Thomas Hudson, an erstwhile UKT agent.[51] Later directors included William Bingham, who also worked for the Alliance and for the Sceptre office, and Frederick William Dimbleby, newspaper editor and owner, and grandfather of the journalist and broadcaster Richard Dimbleby. For a few years at the start of the twentieth century, the TPBS was the largest building society in Britain.[52] It merged with Barclays Bank in the 1970s.

British friendly societies were established as sick or burial clubs for working-class families, emphasizing collective risk-sharing and reciprocity rather than individual saving.[53] The Independent Order of Rechabites (Salford Unity) was founded in Salford in 1835, originally as a burial society. It offered its members the benefits offered by friendly societies like the Oddfellows or Ancient Order of Foresters, without expecting them to meet in pubs.[54] Friendly societies were treated with suspicion by assurance offices because payments were not based on actuarial calculations, making them more vulnerable to periods of sickness; they were largely unregulated until the 1840s, but their 'fraternal commitments provided a safety net in a world that was not always reducible to calculable risks'.[55] The Rechabites claimed to have 250,000 members worldwide by 1900 and 450,000 by 1910.[56] Their American equivalent, the Sons (and later Sisters) of Temperance, was founded shortly after the Rechabites, reaching Britain by 1849.[57] These organizations offered something a little like the 'industrial' life assurance offered by the Prudential and others from the middle of the century.

Temperance life assurance firms differed from friendly societies, however, because they considered actuarial calculations of risk, meaning that firms could be reasonably sure that the premiums they charged their members would more than cover the payments that had to be made when policies matured or the policyholder died – something that could not be said for friendly societies. Drink was seen as a risk, and these firms dealt with it in two ways. Temperance life assurance offered an incentive to abstainers – and therefore an incentive to abstain – by paying them larger bonuses, charging teetotalers lower premiums or a combination of the two. The other strategy, adopted by firms who did not go out of their way to court abstainers, was to charge higher premiums for applicants who were suspected of having damaged their health through drinking.

The nine most significant UK temperance life firms are listed in Table 1.1.

The UKT was the oldest and most successful temperance life office and grew strongly after its first decade, particularly in the late 1850s and early 1860s, and again at the turn of the century (Table 1.2).

Table 1.1 British companies offering temperance life assurance

Name	Start	Office	End, Acquired by
UK Total Abstinence Life/UK Temperance & General Provident Institution (UKT)	1840	London	1986, Friends Provident
British Empire Mutual Life Assurance Company	1847	London	1902, Pelican
Emperor Life Assurance Society	1852	London	1885, Whittington
The Briton Life Association	1853	London	1892, Sun Life
Whittington	1855	London	1891, National Life Assurance
Victoria Mutual Assurance Society	1860	London	1909, Norwich Union Life
Sceptre	1864	London	1917, Eagle and British Dominions
Scottish Temperance	1883	Glasgow	*Renamed* Scottish Mutual 1952
Blue Ribbon	1883	Birmingham	*Renamed* Abstainers and General Association 1890, Beacon, 1933

Source: Firms' archives, newspapers and appendix 1 of Alborn, *Regulated Lives*.

Table 1.2 UKT business, 1841–1905 (Figures Are Five-Year Averages)

Five-year period	New policies issued per annum	Sum assured per annum (£)	New policy value (£)	Accumulated capital (£)
1841–5	373	34,117	92	3,679
1846–50	601	94,522	150	26,090
1851–5	1,308	203,336	159	94,631
1856–60	2,794	423,130	151	250,161
1861–5	2,915	543,597	187	563,491
1866–70	2,235	433,327	194	1,036,189
1871–5	2,105	489,590	232	1,640,045
1876–80	2,143	548,714	256	2,475,917
1881–5	2,229	597,845	268	3,407,800
1886–90	2,421	661,266	273	4,434,335
1891–5	2,678	805,210	300	5,592,047
1896–1900	2,481	808,587	327	6,849,497
1901–5	2,970	975,138	326	7,751,822

New policies assured by the UKT, 1841–1914.
Source: Burns' company history; annual reports and balance sheets 1840–1910; newspapers 1910–18.

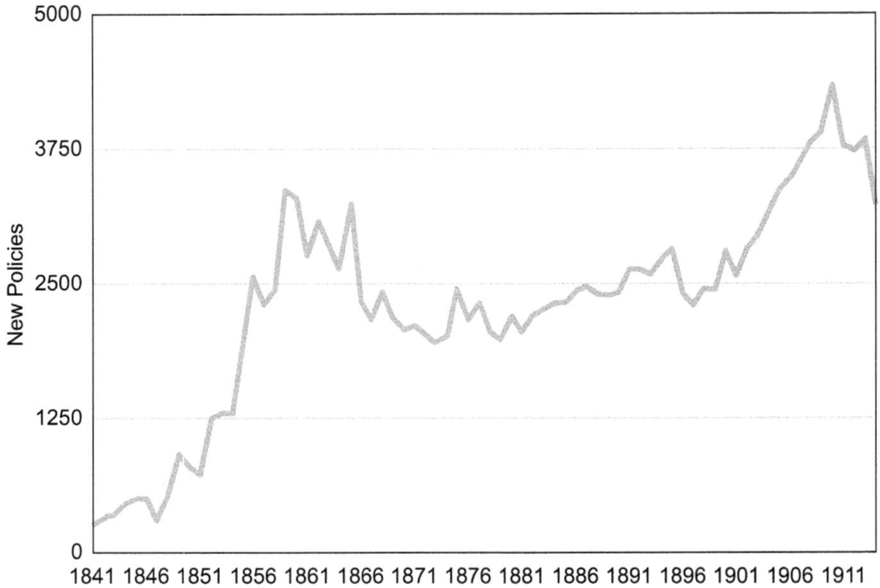

Figure 1.1 New policies assured by the UKT, 1841–1914.

Source: As Table 1.2.

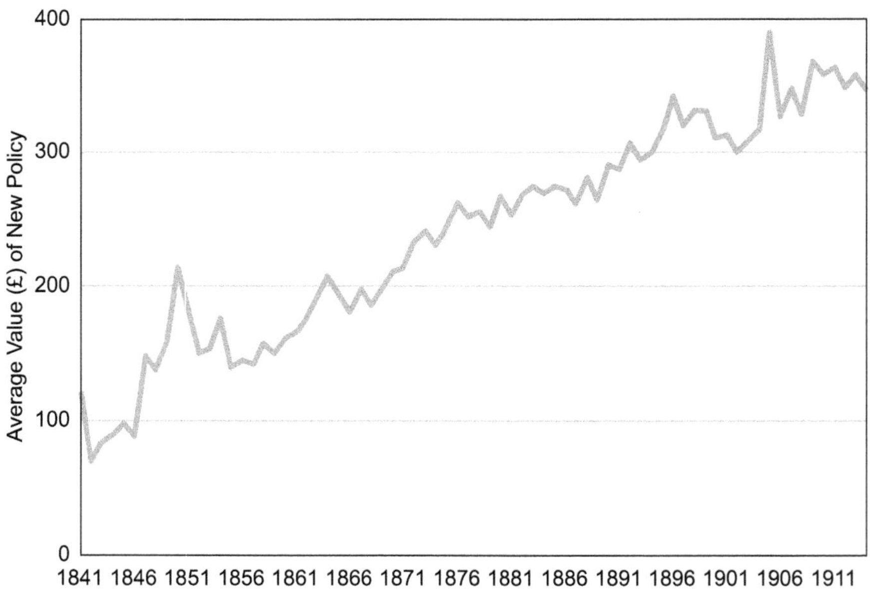

Figure 1.2 Average value (£) of new policies assured by the UKT, 1841–1914.

Source: As Table 1.2.

From 1855 onwards these five-year periods match the firm's quinquennial divisions of profits. This was the moment when it became possible to compare the Abstainers' and General sections (Chapter 4), and the second half of the 1850s continued the rapid growth in new policies that had begun in 1852 (Figure 1.1). Sales then declined from 1865, before picking up again from 1882. The average value of new policies established did not rise as quickly in these years, though, suggesting that this new business was made up of a larger number of smaller policies (Figure 1.2). In 1875 the actuary M. A. Black of the Australian Mutual Assurance Society told the New York *Spectator* that the UKT's business was 'peculiar – something between industrial and ordinary life assurance business', because the average size of its policies was so much smaller than other UK firms. Black continued, 'I entertain no doubt whatever that the bulk of their policies are for sums below £100, and that their temperance section is chiefly composed of mechanics, small trades people and such like … the holders of small policies.'[58] Compared to other life assurance firms, the UKT's policyholders, and especially its teetotalers, came from modest backgrounds.

By 1919 the UKT was assuring 72,000 policies altogether, suggesting perhaps 50,000–60,000 members.[59] When it was acquired by Friends Provident in 1986, the firm covered 300,000 policyholders. Its life business was still healthy, and the problems which led the firm to seek amalgamation stemmed from unwise speculations in British commercial property and North American oil and gas.[60]

We return now to the firm's first year of business and the first death of one of its policyholders.

Temperance lives: John Laverock (1796–1841)

One of the UKT's first agents and the first member to die, John Laverock was born in Warrington, Lancashire, in 1796.[61] Marrying Ellen Reade in 1813, John was described as a tailor in their daughter Emma's baptism records in 1822.[62] John was a Wesleyan Methodist, listed among the travelling preachers and society stewards of the Liverpool District's Missionary Auxiliary Society in 1820, and a subscriber to the Warrington Branch Society.[63] By 1828–9 he was a draper and tailor, with a shop on Bridge Street, and a shareholder in the Manchester and Liverpool District Banking Company.[64] In April 1841 the UKT's Standing Committee approved John's application for the Warrington agency, issuing him with a £200 policy.[65] The first census, conducted in June while the board was considering John's application, found the Laverocks at home on Bridge Street with their children.[66] At the end of August the Standing Committee received a letter announcing John's death, and the board agreed to pay the claim, deducting £10 – possibly due to the short period between the policy's establishment and payment – and a further deduction for the probate office, once the policy was surrendered (transferred) to the UKT. The claim was paid six months later.[67]

In the 1851 census, Ellen was listed as a widow and annuitant, living with two of her daughters.[68] Her son James, a draper and member of the town council, was charged with interfering with Warrington's municipal elections in 1869, but the outcome of this is not clear.[69] James had clearly prospered, inheriting his father's banking shares and his business, though his death in 1871 led to the sale of the shop on Bridge Street.[70] Ellen lived until 1874, dying in Warrington aged eighty-five, presumably supported by John's estate and her children's assistance.[71]

These brief details sketch the outline of a temperance life, or part of one at least. John Laverock was employed by the UKT for only six weeks, and he may not have sold any policies in that time. The office's first death offered an object lesson in the value of life assurance, though, with the report of the UKT's first annual meeting noting that Laverock 'was in the prime of life, and a few days before his death, had been, apparently, in perfect health'. For the board 'this instance affords a striking illustration of the advantages of Life Assurance in providing against casualties, which no human prudence can avert'.[72] We do not know what other assets John possessed beyond his banking shares, or how successful his business was, or whether Ellen inherited anything from her parents, but Ellen lived another thirty-three years and her children – especially James – seem to have done well enough. John's Wesleyan connections are also interesting, suggesting an aspirational nonconformist outlook. So far, so typical, perhaps, of the UKT life.

There is no mention of John's temperance activity in these fragmentary details or in the standard temperance histories, however; John's short-lived UKT agency is his only recorded link with the movement. That is all the more interesting because Warrington was an active temperance town at this time; its temperance society, founded at the Independent Methodists' Providence Chapel at Stockton Heath in 1830, was the second established in England after Bradford's. From its manifesto it seems to have been the first total abstinence society, though it returned to moderation after 'men of a higher social grade became its official leaders'. A breakaway teetotal society formed in 1834, centred around the Friar's Green Independent Methodist chapel, which was happy to host it when other places of worship, including Wesleyan chapels, rejected teetotalers. Temperance and nonconformity were both strongly associated with Independent Methodism in the area as a result.[73] Friar's Green Chapel is a short walk from Bridge Street, and John had just returned from a walk to Stockton Heath on the Sunday that he died, so he was close to both of the chapels associated with local temperance.

Far more ordinary than Warner or Bowly, as the UKT's first claim, John Laverock stands in for a particular type of temperance life: a reasonably well-off salesman whose business remained in the family for another thirty years, and a nonconformist of either respectable (Wesleyan) or more radical (Independent) tendencies. But John Laverock was also so ordinary that it is hard to say much more beyond that. It is time to return to the other temperance businesses that made up this aspect of ordinary temperance.

The UKT's rivals

The Whittington Life Assurance Company was a 'mixed' office, paying shareholders from surplus funds before using the remainder to pay a triennial bonus to its policyholders. The office was established in 1855 but did not open a separate Abstainers' section until 1862, returning a larger bonus to its teetotalers from 1872.[74] It had temperance connections: Samuel Pope, secretary of the United Kingdom Alliance for nearly fifty years, was engaged as standing counsel, and Dawson Burns spoke at a general meeting.[75] It is difficult to establish the relative size of the Abstainers' section, though. Again, its data – showing lower mortality in the Abstainers' section – was used by temperance activists to support their claims for the safety of teetotalism, though this evidence was rarely mentioned in the society's annual reports.

The Whittington was smaller than the UKT, averaging perhaps 700 new policies a year between 1866 and 1890. It grew by absorbing four other companies between 1858 and 1885, including Emperor Life, the second firm to offer temperance policies. The Whittington was absorbed into the National Life Assurance office, which then merged with the Mutual Life Assurance Society in 1896 to form the National Mutual Life Assurance Society, surviving until 2001. The company's records include materials not available for other firms of this kind, including detailed medical notes on applicants and a completed set of policy and reference forms (Chapter 4).

The third significant firm, the Sceptre Life Association, was established in September 1864. It was closely linked to Methodism, particularly those denominations that had parted ways with the Wesleyans – the United Methodist Free Church (UMFC), Methodist New Connexion, Bible Christians, and Primitive Methodists – and it actively courted their ministers and congregations while lending money to build dozens of chapels across England.[76] Not surprisingly, the temperance writers John Granville Woolley and William E. Johnson later described the company as being organized 'to insure for the most part members of religious bodies'.[77] Two years after their first board meeting, Sceptre's directors 'resolved that in future a special section and separate account be kept for Total Abstainers'.[78] Sceptre was another 'mixed' office, paying different bonuses to the two sections after reserving a portion of each year's income to pay its shareholders. In 1883 abstainers made up 40 per cent of new policies, rising to 58 per cent by 1889 and 65 per cent by 1892.[79] In the years before the First World War this proportion reached 81 per cent.[80]

Sceptre was a much smaller company than the UKT, though. While it established over a thousand new policies a year in its early years and briefly managed this again at the start of the 1880s, in the years before the First World War this fell to between 500 and 600 policies per annum. It became a small but very specialized business, selling life assurance to perhaps 400 total abstainers every year. In 1917 it was bought by a larger office, Eagle & British Dominions, which turned Sceptre into a special board for abstainers only, offering lower premiums.[81] More than twice as many policies were issued in 1919 compared to 1913, which probably reflected pent-up demand but also suggested that there was still life in this specialist section.[82] Renamed Eagle Star in 1937, the office is now part of Zurich Life. The Sceptre office was always a small concern, becoming increasingly reliant on teetotalers, but its separate sections, like the UKT's, supported claims made about the relative risks of abstinence and moderate drinking.

In the 1880s these three firms were joined by others offering temperance assurance at discounted premiums.[83] British Empire Mutual Life was still advertising its Temperance section in 1889, but it does not seem to have been a significant part of this market.[84] The Emperor Life Association remained small, with average policies of only £55 in its first dozen years; its business was transferred to the Whittington when it was wound up in 1886.[85] The Briton Life Association offered abstainers cheaper policies from the early 1880s but was plagued by the problems of its insolvent predecessor, the

Briton Medical and General, and its business was transferred to Sun Life in 1892.[86] A fourth competitor, the Victoria Mutual office, began as a friendly society. It ran a small Abstainers' section; in 1876 the office had issued 1,405 policies in the last eleven months, 252 of them to teetotalers.[87] Its secretary later admitted to Dawson Burns that its Temperance section was too small to allow a meaningful comparison of longevity to be made.[88]

Two more focused and successful temperance life offices were established forty years after the UKT. The Scottish Temperance office, founded by Adam Keir Rodger, the son of a brewer, borrowed Warner's strategy of converting a temperance network into a business one.[89] Writing to ask support from Sir William Collins, Provost of Glasgow and a key figure in the city's temperance organizations, Rodger suggested that lower premiums and higher bonuses would increase the attractiveness of temperance life assurance.[90] Collins was a director of the UKT, and Rodger promised that Scottish Temperance would not compete with the older office, but 'would rouse them to a better use of their undoubted resources while the outside public would be led to realise in a way that they have not yet that Abstainers were a superior class of lives'.[91] The annual report for 1887 stated that 917 policies had been issued; that for 1898, 1,428; and for 1918, 1,243.[92] Scottish Temperance did not become a significant rival to the UKT, but it was more successful than the Sceptre or Whittington. It changed its name to Scottish Mutual in 1951.

The Blue Ribbon office also opened in 1883, growing out of the eponymous mass movement. Advertising as 'the Total Abstainer's own Assurance Agency', it offered a discount of up to 15 per cent on premiums, but changed its name to the Abstainers and General in 1890 when it was forced to offer policies to those who were not total abstainers, like the UKT before it.[93] The Abstainers and General claimed to have 'a larger classified number of abstainers than any other office'.[94]

The British market for temperance life assurance was dominated by five firms: the UKT, Sceptre, Whittington, Scottish Temperance and the Abstainers and General. Of these, the latter two were established after the wider industry had recognized the potential risks of heavy drinking, a conviction which may have been strengthened by the experience of the first three firms. Other offices advertised Abstainers' sections from the 1880s onwards – for example, the London, Edinburgh and Glasgow; Imperial Life; Scottish Imperial; and British Equitable – but it is difficult to know how successful they were.[95] At least one major temperance organization sold its own life assurance, after the Salvation Army took over the Methodist and General Office in 1891, but it is not clear whether they offered specifically *temperance* forms of assurance.[96] By this point, major assurance firms had been persuaded that heavy drinkers represented a significant risk, and some were refusing to assure workers in the licensed trade. Thomas Whittaker explained the significance of this:

> What a lesson the positive refusal to insure a publican's life contains! These offices will insure sailors, pilots, fishermen; they will insure coal- miners, engine drivers, stokers, and railway guards, and indeed almost anybody and everybody, especially if they pay a little extra premium to cover any little special risk they may run, but they will not have a publican at any price. Why? There are more storms in the

public house than at sea; and there is more destruction in the bottle than in the winds of heaven.[97]

The industry's growing support for arguments about the relative risks of drinking and abstinence is explored further in Chapter 8.

Temperance life assurance had also begun to spread through the Anglophone world. Charles A. Jenney's report on insurance for the 1890 census lists temperance insurers and benefit associations in Chicago, Kansas, Maryland, Missouri and Pennsylvania, most established in the 1880s; Lisa M. F. Andersen suggests that in the United States 'there were at least 5 to 10 providers offering dry life insurance at any point between 1890 and 1905, from among the 100 or so industrial life insurance companies and several hundred fraternal and assessment providers', listing twenty offices operating over this period.[98] The American Temperance Life Insurance Company only assured teetotalers, and the Equitable Life opened a section for total abstainers in 1901.[99] Only one of these offices was closely linked to temperance, though, and that firm – Chicago's Total Abstinence Life Association – failed spectacularly in 1893 after investing in land bonds. Andersen suggests that the failure of these firms to 'engage in fiery pro-prohibition rhetoric' was down to their sense of themselves as insurance firms first and foremost, and to the fact that the industry had been screening heavy drinkers for some time; 'there were no pathbreaking pitches because the product itself was not radically new, at least from insurance companies' points of view'.[100] Temperance life assurance was ordinary in the United States too.

The UKT's model was replicated across and beyond the British Empire. Toronto's Temperance and General Life Assurance Company of North America opened in 1884. The Australasian Temperance and General Mutual Life Assurance Society, established in 1876, was described as 'the largest ordinary-industrial life society confining its operation to Australia and New Zealand' in 1931.[101] New Zealand Life, established and guaranteed by the Government Insurance Department in 1869, opened a Temperance section in 1883, disciplining members much as the UKT did, as well as charging more for lives employed in the drink trade.[102] At the end of 1893 there were 4,553 temperance policies in force, though the ratio of general to temperance policies issued that year was five to one.[103] In 1920 the department was described as 'probably the most successful (one might almost say the only successful) attempt the world has known in applying national enterprise to life insurance'.[104] Temperance health insurance also appeared in Sweden from the 1880s; temperance assurance firms were not restricted to Anglophone countries and could develop in countries with strong temperance activity.[105]

By the 1890s, then, temperance life assurance was a relatively minor but still successful life assurance 'product', with companies in Britain, Ireland, North America, Australia and New Zealand; British firms like the Whittington operated branches in Amsterdam, Brussels, Grenada, Hamburg, Jamaica, Mauritius, Réunion, Sydney and Trinidad.[106] Not all of these firms or branches conducted a significant amount of business, but smaller firms like Sceptre, Whittington or Abstainers and General filled profitable niches. None of these firms had been able to concentrate solely on assuring total abstainers, and some of their Temperance sections were small, but they contributed – to a greater or lesser extent – to debates about the relative value of drinking and abstinence through comparisons of the mortality of those assured in Abstainers' and General sections.

What Dawson Burns called 'the vital statistics of total abstinence' abstracted individual temperance lives into the firms' 'experience', of course, distancing us from the people assured. For Burns and others this was exactly the point, allowing them to make significant generalizations about the risks of moderate drinking, but for our purposes it is worth returning to the life of one woman. Though women were much less likely than men to assure their own lives, especially before the 1870 Married Women's Property Act, surviving life assurance materials list many women. Cross-referencing these records with other traces of their lives is more difficult as they are, on the whole, less likely to appear in sources like newspapers. We know much less about Mary Ann Warner than we do about her husband Robert, for example, though she established the firm's thirteenth policy for £500 in its first month. Chapter 7 discusses some of Sceptre's women policyholders, but here we consider one early temperance life assured by the UKT.

Temperance lives: Betsy Ann Griffin (1814–1906)

Elizabeth (Betsy) Ann Warne was the oldest of seven children born to Edmund and Eliza Warne in St Neot, Cornwall, in 1814. Her father became an itinerant preacher with the Bible Christians through William Bryant (later O'Bryan), who founded that denomination in Devon in 1815. The memoir that Eliza Warne wrote and published after Edmund's death in 1828 has much to say about her husband's faith and missionary travels around Cornwall, but little about their eldest daughter Betsy, or indeed temperance.[107] In 1834 Betsy married Richard Palk Griffin (1792–1883) in Padstow.[108] Richard and his two brothers had been silk ribbon manufacturers in Coventry and later in London between 1817 and 1822.[109] Richard and Betsy's daughter Hannah was born later in 1834; James Thorne, by then the leader of the Bible Christians and a close friend of the family, baptised Betsy and Richard's first son Samuel at their home in 1835.[110] Samuel died just over a year later, though Samuel Nathanial Richard Palk Griffin, usually known as Richard, was born in 1856.

The family appears to have been comfortably off, employing a domestic servant in later life. Richard, variously described as 'gentleman', 'landed proprietor' and 'retired lace manufacturer', sought a UKT agency in June of 1841.[111] The following month, both Richard and Betsy Ann were issued policies, Betsy assuring her life for £100 and Richard his life for £52 2s. 6d.[112] Richard was active in Cornish temperance at this time, with a correspondent to the *Teetotal Times and Essayist* reporting that 'all Cornwall is now alive to the deeply interesting question of temperance. Many disjointed societies have acquired new life and activity, and others are quickened'.[113] In the 1861 Census, Richard was described as 'landed proprietor and Methodist Local Preacher'; in 1881, aged eighty-nine, as 'insurance agent'.[114] When Richard died in 1893 he was buried as a Bible Christian.[115] While it's not clear why he had come to Cornwall, he had certainly taken up his wife's faith and was presumably preaching in it into his sixties.

Betsy Ann would have claimed Richard's policy on his death, if it had not been surrendered or sold on, but she was not the recipient of his estate, valued at £298, which went to their only surviving child, Richard junior, Hannah having died in 1872.[116] Betsy gave up Rose Hill Cottage on the High Street for Richard, who had been practising as a surgeon in Padstow since 1885; he married Beatrice Hawken in 1886, with their daughter, also Beatrice, arriving in 1889. He was declared bankrupt in 1899, described as sick and unable to work and died in September 1905.[117] Betsy Ann died at the end of 1906, leaving a substantial sum, over £1,000, to her daughter-in-law Beatrice.[118]

We know a little of the life of Betsy Ann Griffin, then, through the recording of births, marriages and deaths and the actions of the men in her family. Betsy outlived them all, though, passing her estate on to Beatrice and her granddaughter. And while it is hard to know if her husband's UKT policy contributed to that estate, or what her other assets were, the money would presumably have been very welcome to Beatrice Griffin, who had been widowed at forty. There is an echo here of Betsy's mother's memoir of her husband, Edmund Warne. While Eliza Warne wrote it for the edification of other Bible Christians, it was sold to benefit her materially, as a widow in her early thirties with seven children. In his preface to Eliza's memoir, the Bible Christian leader James Thorne wrote:

> While I indulge the hope that this memoir will be rendered a spiritual blessing to its readers, I cannot but remind them that the more extensively it is circulated the more benefit will accrue to the widow, which is a most desirable object, and the more so, because it is declared in the word of inspiration to be one of the marks of our being religious, that we should 'visit the fatherless and widows in their afflictions'.[119]

The widow and orphan were also often evoked in life assurance literature, as firms warned men to consider what would happen to their families after their death. Betsy's life is in part a story of early deaths and of the passing of wealth from generation to generation, one with both spiritual and material lessons. The Bible Christians were closely associated with Cornish temperance, particularly after 1841, when Wesleyans were forbidden from allowing their chapels to be used for temperance meetings, but there is no reference to Betsy's own beliefs beyond her identification as a Bible Christian.[120] Like Samuel Bowly and John Laverock, Betsy Griffin's life combined worldly security with religious belief, but while the UKT's archives allow us to pick out ordinary lives like Griffin's, we know next to nothing about her faith or her own thoughts on temperance, and little about the source of her prosperity.

Conclusion: Ordinary temperance lives

The records of temperance life assurance offices allow us to explore temperance institutions and lives that were in many ways deeply ordinary, unremarkable, unspectacular or mundane. The 'ordinary' may not be the same thing as 'everyday life', though, as – following the influential work of Michel de Certeau – the everyday has often been presented as a world of hidden creativity, an alternative to another, more 'official' grid of surveillance and power.[121] An agent filling up a form, a doctor examining an applicant or a teetotaler attending a tea meeting – these were genuinely everyday activities, but they do not have the romantic or resistant appeal of de Certeau's 'tactical' operations, and they were very different to a rally, a speech in parliament or the breaking up of a saloon. 'Usual', 'commonplace' or 'routine' are better matches.

The UKT and its rivals operated much as other assurance firms did, and the lives they assured were not always clearly connected to temperance, let alone to its more visible, political manifestations. Even Samuel Bowly, who had campaigned for both the repeal of the corn laws and for abolition, was not a particularly active worker for the Alliance's parliamentary agitation. Rather than seeing the UK Alliance as the *culmination* of early Victorian temperance efforts, their translation into a movement dedicated to parliamentary reform, perhaps it was – at least for individuals like Bowly – an *additional* kind of temperance work to be put alongside moral suasion, temperance savings and other work.

Temperance may well have been an important part of the everyday life of individuals who assured with these firms, like John Laverock and Betsy Ann Griffin, and they might have been happy for the Alliance to speak in their name, or for their lives to contribute to comparisons of life expectancy, but they are not recorded as active workers. Their choice of the UKT as an assurance office might have had more to do with its respectability, its refusal to judge them for their abstinence or its appeal to modestly prosperous families. They might have been swayed by local nonconformist communities or by charismatic travelling agents like James Teare, who preached temperance and life assurance from Lancashire to Cornwall on behalf of the UKT (Chapter 5); they might have assured with the UKT because they were 'reformed drunkards' no other company would touch. Temperance might figure in these decisions and relationships in different ways, but it is also possible that it was a small, perhaps unconsidered, part of these lives, not least because these relationships were also financial ones, associated with a wider set of meanings of security, aspiration and care. In this way spiritual and material considerations merged into one another.

Something similar seems to have characterized the business of temperance life assurance in general. The more successful British temperance life offices had close connections with the wider movement through their directors and patrons, and through their recruitment of teetotalers as agents and policyholders. This was particularly true of the UKT – which had an early advantage in this regard – and of Scottish Temperance, Sceptre and Whittington. Other firms may well have opened an Abstainers' section because the directors saw a commercial opportunity as temperance grew and a new market opened up. The actuarial imaginary is not fussy about the things it assures, after all.

The radical character of temperance changed as it grew and became more ordinary. In his address to the UKT's members' meeting in 1918, the company's chairman Thomas P. Whittaker responded to criticism of the UKT's enthusiasm for War Loans, issued to fund the British war effort. By 1917 the firm held over £2.5 million worth of these loans – a quarter of its total invested funds – making it one of the largest British investors in war funds.[122] By the end of the war, these loans constituted about 30 per cent of the UKT's total funds of more than £11 million.[123] Whittaker argued that 'if the offices had got the money or could obtain it from their bankers in order to take up War Bonds, they would as patriots feel bound to do so'.[124] Whittaker's patriotism was a long way from Wilfrid Lawson's criticism of imperial wars in Southern Africa, or the UKT's Robert Charleton, who travelled to Russia to try to prevent the Crimean War.[125] It is also a long way from the positions of other temperance figures in 1918. We will see in Chapter 2 that conscientious objectors to the war were supported by temperance societies in Lancashire and Yorkshire; radical and socialist strands of temperance survived. Still, even in extraordinary times, temperance life assurance could be very ordinary, whether this took the form of investment in War Loans as a form of banal nationalism, or as simply getting on with business.

The UKT and other temperance life assurance firms started the post-war period with a boom in new policies and healthy returns on their invested funds. As temperance life assurance became more ordinary, it grew closer to mainstream actuarial practice. While it was still being sold well into the interwar period, temperance life assurance was now just part of British business, a specialized product for a particular market segment of abstainers. Of course, none of this could have been predicted from the UKT's origins in 1840, as we will see in Chapter 3, which returns to the experiment conducted by Warner and his friends. In Chapter 2 we consider the *place* of this ordinary temperance. British temperance possessed a particular geography, clustered and concentrated in particular regions, cities and towns, and life assurance networks mapped themselves onto those distributions in complicated ways, sometimes reflecting and sometimes troubled by them. Chapter 2 considers these geographies as forms of ordinary temperance materialized in space.

Notes

1. *Wanganui Chronicle* (NZ), 16 November 1892, 2.
2. Longmate, *The Water Drinkers*; Harrison, *Drink*; Anthony E. Dingle, *The Campaign for Prohibition in Victorian England: The United Kingdom Alliance 1872–1895* (London: Croom Helm, 1980); Lilian Lewis Shiman, *Crusade against Drink in Victorian England* (London: Macmillan, 1988); David M. Fahey, *Temperance Societies in Late Victorian and Edwardian England* (Newcastle upon Tyne: Cambridge Scholars, 2020); Annemarie McAllister, 'Picturing the Demon Drink: How Children Were Shown Temperance Principles in the Band of Hope', *Visual Resources* 28, 4 (2012), 309–23, and 'Giant Alcohol: A Worthy Opponent for the Children of the Band of Hope', *Drugs: Education, Prevention and Policy* 22, 2 (2015), 103–10; Stephanie Olsen, *Juvenile Nation: Youth, Emotions and the Making of the Modern British Citizen, 1880–1914* (New York: Bloomsbury Academic, 2014).
3. Harry Gene Levine, 'The Committee of Fifty and the Origins of Alcohol Control', *Journal of Drug Issues* 13 (1983), 95.
4. Mark Lawrence Schrad, *The Political Power of Bad Ideas: Networks, Institutions, and the Global Prohibition Wave* (Oxford: Oxford University Press, 2010), 6.
5. Harrison, *Drink*, 36.

6. Ibid., 367.
7. Joseph Rowntree and Arthur Sherwell, *The Temperance Problem and Social Reform* (London: Hodder and Stoughton, 1899). For studies of the Gothenberg system see James Kneale, 'Good, Homely, Troublesome or Improving? Historical Geographies of Drinking Places, c. 1850–1950', *Geography Compass* 15 (2021), e12557.15; and Dan Malleck, *Try to Control Yourself: The Regulation of Public Drinking in Post-Prohibition Ontario, 1927–44* (Vancouver: University of British Columbia Press, 2012).
8. Harrison, *Drink*, 382.
9. John Greenaway, 'The "Improved" Public House, 1870–1950: The Key to Civilised Drinking or the Primrose Path to Drunkenness?', *Addiction* 93 (1998), 173–81; David W. Gutzke, *Pubs and Progressives: Reinventing the Public House in England, 1896–1960* (DeKalb: Northern Illinois University Press, 2005); Emily Cole, *The Urban and Suburban Public House in Inter-war England, 1918–1939*, 3 vols (London: Historic England, 2015); Fiona Fisher and Rebecca Preston, 'Light, Airy and Open: The Design and Use of the Suburban Public-House Garden in England between the Wars', *Studies in the History of Gardens & Designed Landscapes* 39 (2019), 5–21; Robert Duncan, *Pubs and Patriots: The Drink Crisis in Britain during World War One* (Liverpool: Liverpool University Press, 2013).
10. David M. Fahey, 'Temperance and the Liberal Party: Lord Peel's Report, 1899', *Journal of British Studies* 10 (1971), 149.
11. Virginia Berridge, *Demons: Our Changing Attitudes to Alcohol, Tobacco, and Drugs* (Oxford: Oxford University Press, 2013), 46.
12. Henry Yeomans, *Alcohol and Moral Regulation: Public Attitudes, Spirited Measures and Victorian Hangovers* (Bristol: Policy Press, 2014), 72.
13. Ibid., 89.
14. Berridge, *Demons*, 48.
15. For example, Robert D. Storch, 'The Plague of the Blue Locusts: Police Reform and Popular Resistance in Northern England 1840–1857', *International Review of Social History* 20 (1975), 61–90, and 'The Policeman as Domestic Missionary: Urban Discipline and Popular Culture in Northern England, 1850–1880', *Journal of Social History* 9, 4 (1976), 481–509.
16. Antonio Gramsci, 'Rationalisation of Production and Work', in *Selections from the Prison Notebooks of Antonio Gramsci*, edited and translated by Quintin Hoare and Geoffrey Nowell Smith (New York: International Publishers, 1971), 386.
17. Berridge, *Demons*, 43.
18. Olsen, 'From Parish to Palace', 239.
19. RA VIC/MAIN/QVJ (W) 6th July 1841 (Princess Beatrice's copies). Queen Victoria's Journals. Retrieved 27 March 2017.
20. Harrison, *Drink*, 92.
21. Stephen G. Jones, 'Labour, Society and the Drink Question in Britain, 1918–1939', *Historical Journal* 30, 1 (1987), 105. See Brian Harrison, 'Teetotal Chartism', *History* 58, 193 (1973), 193–217.
22. Albert Edward Musson, *Trade Union and Social History* (London: Frank Cass, 1974), 196. For more on Finch, see R. B. Rose, 'John Finch, 1784–1857: A Liverpool Disciple of Robert Owen', *Transactions of the Historic Society of Lancashire and Cheshire* 109 (1957), 172.
23. Rosemary Mitchell, 'Brewster, Patrick (1788–1859)', in *Oxford Dictionary of National Biography* (Oxford University Press, 2004) (www.oxforddnb.com/view/article/3374,

accessed 5 December 2013). Clare Midgley, *Women against Slavery: The British Campaigns, 1780–1870* (London: Routledge, 1995), 84.
24. John F. Quinn, *Father Mathew's Crusade: Temperance in Nineteenth-Century Ireland and Irish America* (Amherst: University of Massachusetts Press, 2002); Paul A. Townend, *Father Mathew: Temperance and Irish Identity* (Dublin: Irish Academic Press, 2002).
25. Meetings, 28 December 1840 and 1 March 1841, Minutes of the Standing Committee 1, MS FL436, Aviva Archives; *Bristol Temperance Herald* 4, 9 (1840), 70; *Bristol Temperance Herald*, 41001/WTL/J/1/4, Bristol Record Office; James Gregory, *Of Victorians and Vegetarians: The Vegetarian Movement in Nineteenth-Century Britain* (London: Tauris, 2007) and '"Zealously Affected in a Good Thing": The Publishing Career and Life of William Horsell (1807–1863)' (online, 2013), 1 and n6.
26. Alistair Durie, 'Almost Twins by Birth: Hydropathy, Temperance and the Scottish Churches 1840–1914', *Scottish Church History Society* 32 (2002), 143. For David Urquhart's argument that the Turkish Bath could cure intemperance see Charlotte Jones, 'An Historical Geography of the Turkish Bath in Victorian Britain', PhD thesis, University College London, 2017.
27. Invitation to memorial stone ceremony, London Temperance Hospital, 1879, Time capsule, Museum of London Archaeological Service.
28. 'Sir Wilfrid Lawson on the Drink Traffic', *Leeds Mercury*, 9 May 1879, 7.
29. 'Samuel Bowly', *Friends' Quarterly Examiner* 18 (1884), 149, Library of the Society of Friends.
30. Clare Midgley, 'Slave Sugar Boycotts, Female Activism and the Domestic Base of British Anti-slavery Culture', *Slavery & Abolition* 17, 3 (1996), 137–62.
31. Frederick Sessions, *The Life Story of Samuel Bowly: A Champion of Freedom, Progress and Temperance* (London: Friends Tract Association, 1903), 20, 289/3, Library of the Society of Friends.
32. Ibid.
33. 'Editor', 'Samuel Bowly', 153.
34. Harrison, *Dictionary of Temperance Biography*, 13.
35. *Leicester Chronicle and the Leicestershire Mercury*, 27 May 1882, 8.
36. James Dawson Burns, *Temperance History. A Consecutive History of the Rise, Development, and Extension of the Temperance Reform. Volume 1. 1826–1842* (London: National Temperance Publication Depot, 1889), 125.
37. 'Editor', 'Samuel Bowly', 153.
38. 'Three Temperance Stalwarts', *Friends' Quarterly Examiner* 65 [n.s.], 16 October 1925, 913.
39. Maria Taylor, *Memorials of Samuel Bowly, Born March 23, 1802, Died March 23, 1884* (Gloucester: Privately published, 1884), Library of the Society of Friends.
40. UKT prospectus, 2.
41. Taylor, *Memorials.*
42. Dawson Burns, company history, 60.
43. Sessions, *Samuel Bowly*, 11.
44. 'Temperance Savings', *Manchester Guardian*, 25 September 1839, 4; Alcoholism ephemera box 1, EPH 568, 14, Wellcome Library.
45. Duncan M. Ross, '"Penny Banks" in Glasgow, 1850–1914', *Financial History Review* 9, 1 (2002), 21–39, and 'Savings Bank Depositors in a Crisis: Glasgow 1847 and 1857', *Financial History Review* 20, 2 (2013), 183–208.

46. Anthony E. Dingle, 'Drink and Working-Class Living Standards in Britain, 1870–1914', *Economic History Review* [2nd series] 25 (1972), 608–22.
47. Ross, 'Penny Banks', 39.
48. Linda Perriton and Josephine Maltby, 'Working-Class Households and Savings in England, 1850–1880', *Enterprise and Society* 16, 2 (2015), 413–45.
49. Seymour J Price, *From Queen to Queen: The Centenary Story of the Temperance Permanent Building Society 1854–1954* (London: Franey, 1954), 12.
50. Judy Slinn, 'Shaen, William (1821–1887)', in *Oxford Dictionary of National Biography* (Oxford University Press, 2004) (www.oxforddnb.com/view/article/50082, accessed 13 October 2013).
51. Price, *From Queen to Queen*, 12, 15; Anon., 'Proceedings of the Statistical Society', *Journal of the Statistical Society of London* 28, 4 (1865), 538.
52. Price, *From Queen to Queen*, 82.
53. P. H. J. H. Gosden, *The Friendly Societies in England, 1815–1875* (Manchester: Manchester University Press, 1961); Simon Cordery, *British Friendly Societies, 1750–1914* (New York: Palgrave, 2003); Daniel Weinbren, 'The Good Samaritan, Friendly Societies and the Gift Economy', *Social History* 31, 3 (2006).
54. Henry Mudge, *Exposure of Odd Fellowship* (London: Whittaker and Son; Bodmin: Liddell and Son, 1845).
55. Francis G. P. Neison, *Contributions to Vital Statistics*, 3rd edition (London: Simpkin, Marshall, 1857) Penelope Ismay, 'Between Providence and Risk: Odd Fellows, Benevolence and the Social Limits of Actuarial Science, 1820s–1880s', *Past & Present* 226 (2015), 145.
56. Woolley and Johnson, *Temperance Progress*, 106.
57. James D. Ivy, 'Sons of Temperance', in *Alcohol and Temperance in Modern History: An International Encyclopedia*, edited by Jack S. Blocker, Jr, David M. Fahey and Ian R. Tyrrell, vol. 2 (Santa Barbara: ABC-CLIO, 2003), 572–4.
58. 'Temperance Sections in Life Offices', *The Spectator* 15, 5 (1 November 1875), 613, 614.
59. *The Times*, 22 April 1920, 24.
60. Joanna Slaughter, 'How UK Provident Tempted Providence', *The Observer*, 13 April 1986, 35.
61. 1841 Census (Class: HO107; Piece 521; Folio: 45; Page 34; GSU roll: 1114).
62. England & Wales Non-conformist and Non-parochial Registers (Class: RG4; Piece: 2443, #32), Bank Street Chapel (Wesleyan), Warrington.
63. *The Third Report of the Wesleyan Methodist Missionary Auxiliary Society, for the Liverpool District, for 1819* (1820), viii.
64. *Pigot and Co.'s National Commercial Directory for 1828–9* (London: J. Pigot, 1828–9), 464; *The Manchester Magazine*, 1838, 23.
65. Meeting, 26 April 1841 and 19 July 1841, Minutes of the Standing Committee 1; Aviva Archives; 'Awful Sudden Death', *Manchester Courier and Lancashire General Advertiser*, 28 August 1841, 5.
66. 1841 Census (Class: HO107; Piece: 521; Folio: 45; Page: 34; GSU roll: 1114).
67. Meeting 30 August 1841, Minutes of the Standing Committee 1; Board Meeting, 3 September 1841 and 4 March 1842, UKT Minute Book 1; Aviva Archives; England & Wales Civil Registration Death Index, July–September 1841, Lancashire (vol. 20), 591.
68. 1851 Census (Class: HO107; Piece: 2203; Folio: 34; Page: 5; GSU roll: 15).
69. 'Local and General', *Leeds Mercury*, 24 December 1869, 1.
70. 'Copy of Returns. The Manchester and Liverpool District Banking Company', *Derby Mercury*, 20 February 1867, 2; 'Re James Laverock, Deceased', *The Standard*, 17

January 1872, 4; 'Woollen, Drapery, Tailoring, and General Business', *Manchester Guardian*, 19 August 1871, 10.

71. Death of Ellen Laverock, October–December 1874, age eighty-five, Warrington, England and Wales Civil Register Death Index, Lancashire (vol. 8c), 140.
72. *First Report of the United Kingdom Total Abstinence Life Association to the Annual Meeting of Members*, 31 December 1841, 1; UKT annual reports and balance sheets 1840–1910.
73. Winskill, *Temperance Movement*, vol. 1, 65, 69, 130.
74. Alfred T. Bowser, 'Temperance Sections in Life Offices', *The Spectator* 15, 5 (1 November 1875).
75. David M. Fahey, 'Pope, Samuel (1826–1901)', in *Alcohol and Temperance in Modern History: An International Encyclopedia*, vol. 2, 486; *Hampshire Advertiser*, 10 August 1872, 7.
76. Board Meeting, 6 February 1865, Sceptre Minute Book 1, CLC/B/005/SC01/05/01/001, London Archives.
77. Woolley and Johnson, *Temperance Progress*, 381.
78. Board Meeting, 14 September 1866, Sceptre Minute Book 1, London Archives.
79. Burns, *Vital Statistics*, 7; *Manchester Guardian*, 24 February 1890, 4; 'Insurance Notes', *Financial Times*, 24 March 1893, 2.
80. *Manchester Guardian*, 17 February 1911, 3.
81. *The Times*, 23 May 1917, 2; *The Times*, 21 July 1917, 11; Advert, *The Observer*, 20 January 1918, 5; Eagle Star Abstainers' Section Prospectus, second edition, 1 January 1918, CLC/B/005/SC04/01/03/001, London Archives.
82. *The Observer*, 16 May 1920, 2.
83. Woolley and Johnson, *Temperance Progress*, 384.
84. Advertisement, *The Insurance Register 1889*, 175.
85. 'Emperor Life and Fire Assurance Society', *The Standard*, 26 November 1864, 7; 'High Court of Justice', *The Times*, 29 March 1886, 3.
86. Advertisement, *The National Temperance League Annual for 1882* (London: National Temperance Depot, 1882), 496; Burns, *Vital Statistics*, 6; see Alborn, *Regulated Lives*, 67–9.
87. 'Small Incomes and Life and Old Age Assurance', *Cheshire Observer*, 19 February 1876, 7.
88. Dawson Burns, *Vital Statistics*, 7.
89. Gordon Jackson and Charles Munn, 'Trade, Industry and Commerce', in *Glasgow. Volume II: 1830–1912*, edited by W. Hamish Fraser and Irene Maver (Manchester: Manchester University Press, 1996), 88.
90. Mamie Magnusson, *A Length of Days: The Scottish Mutual Assurance Society 1883–1983* (London: Henry Melland, 1983), 25–6.
91. Quoted in Magnusson, *Length of Days*, 16.
92. 'The Scottish Temperance Life Assurance Company', *Evening Telegraph*, 2 March 1888, 2; 'Scottish Temperance Life Assurance', *Financial Times*, 23 February 1899, 2; 'Reports and Notices', *The Economist*, 2 March 1918, 411.
93. Advertisement, *Isle of Man Times and General Advertiser*, 2 February 1884, 8.
94. E. C. Hill, letter to the *Bristol Mercury and Daily Post*, 18 October 1893, 3.
95. *The Insurance Register 1883*, 130; *The Insurance Register 1894*, 159; Advertisement, *The Good Templars' Watchword*, December 24, 1888, ii; Advertisements, *The Insurance Register 1903*, 172.

96. Steven Spencer, '"The Fatal Gaze of This Moral Basilisk": The Salvation Army's War on Drink in Victorian Britain', *Social History of Alcohol and Drugs* 33, 2 (2019), 230–56.
97. Thomas Whittaker, *Life's Battles in Temperance Armour*, 3rd edition (London: Hodder and Stoughton, 1888), 317.
98. Charles A. Jenney, *Report on Insurance Business in the United States at the Eleventh Census: 1890. Part 1: Fire, Marine and Inland Insurance* (Washington, DC: Department of the Interior, Census Office, 1894), 283–316; Lisa M. F. Andersen, *The Politics of Prohibition* (Cambridge: Cambridge University Press, 2013), 193 and fn 8, 194.
99. Woolley and Johnson, *Temperance Progress*, 384; 'The Equitable's New Class for Abstainers', *New York Times*, 9 June 1901, 14.
100. Andersen, *Politics*, 194–8, 196, 197.
101. 'Life Assurance: Influence of the T&G', *Brisbane Courier*, 10 October 1931, 18; see Jureidini and White, 'Life Insurance', 203.
102. Alan Henderson, 'Insurance – Early Life Insurance', *Te Ara – The Encyclopedia of New Zealand* (www.teara.govt.nz/en/insurance/page-1, accessed 11 September 2023).
103. New Zealand Government Life Insurance Department, Appendix to the Journals of the House of Representatives, 1894 Session I, H-08, 12.
104. 'Address by the President, Henry Moir. State and National Enterprise', *Transactions, Actuarial Society of America* 21, 63–64 (1920), 1–15.
105. Ann-Kristin Bergquist and Liselotte Eriksson, 'Sober Business: Shared Value Creation between the Insurance Industry and the Temperance Movement', *Business History* 61, 2 (2019), 322–42.
106. Summaries of the Whittington's accounts, policies, shares, investments, etc., 1892–4, compiled in an audit by accountants for the National Life Assurance Society, with related correspondence, National Mutual Life Assurance Society, MS CLC/B/166/MS34412, London Archives.
107. Eliza Warne, *A Memoir of the Life and Ministry of Edmund Warne, Lately an Itinerant Preacher in the Bible Christian Connexion*, revised by James Thorne (Devon: S. Thorne, 1830).
108. England Select Marriages, 158–1973, FHL film no. 1596121, ref id 24.
109. Advertisement, *The Times*, 31 December 1817, 1; *The London Gazette*, 20 April 1822, 662.
110. *England and Wales Non-conformist and Non-parochial Registers*, 1567–1963, no. 272, class number RG 4, Cornwall, Bible Christian, Piece 0108: St Irvan (Bible Christian), 1820–37.
111. Board Meeting, 28 June 1841, UKT Minute Book 1, Aviva Archives; *Pigot and Co.'s Royal National and Commercial Directory, 1844* (London: Slater, 1844), 121; 1851 Census (Class: HO107; Piece: 1905; Folio 316; Page: 15; GSU roll 221057); *Post Office Directory of Cornwall, 1856* (London: Kelly, 1856), 111; 1871 Census (Class: RG10; Piece: 2325; Folio: 64; Page: 5; GSU roll: 838826).
112. Board Meeting 2 July 1841, UKT Minute Book 1, Aviva Archives.
113. Anon., 'Fowey', in *The Teetotal Times and Essayist 1848–1851*, n.d., 59.
114. 1861 Census (Class: RG; Piece: 1540; Folio: 19; Page: 32; GSU roll: 542828); 1881 Census (Class: RG; Piece: 2290; Folio: 12; Page: 2; GSU roll: 1341550).
115. England and Wales Civil Registration Death Index, 1837–1915, Jan–Mar 1883, registration district Bodmin, Cornwall, vol. 5e, p63; FHL film no. 1596121, ref id 40, Buried as a Bible Christian, record 4475704, accessed 18 March 2021.

116. Probate 6 April 1886, England and Wales National Probate Calendar, 1858–1995.
117. 'A Padstow Surgeon's Bankruptcy', *Royal Cornwall Gazette*, 18 May 1899, 6.
118. Probate 31 December 1906, Bodmin, E&W National Probate Calendar, Civil registration death index, estimated birth year at 1814, death registered Oct–Dec 1906, Cornwall, vol. 5c, p. 58.
119. Eliza Warne, *A Memoir*, viii.
120. Winskill, *Temperance Movement*, vol. 2, 54.
121. Michel de Certeau, *The Practice of Everyday Life*, trans. Steven Rendall (Berkeley: University of California Press, 1984), and Nigel Thrift, 'Driving in the City', *Theory, Culture & Society* 21, 4–5 (2004), 41–59.
122. 'The Great War Loan', *Derby Daily Telegraph*, 17 February 1917, 3.
123. *The Times*, 22 April 1920, 24; *The Times*, 27 March 1918, 13.
124. *The Times*, 27 March 1918, 13.
125. Griselda Fox Mason, *Sleigh Ride to Russia* (York: Sessions, 1985), Library of Society of Friends.

2

Temperance towns

Introduction: Mapping ordinary temperance

Historians of drink and temperance in Britain have long recognized that place matters, focusing on sites as different as Banbury, Lincoln and Liverpool.[1] Temperance was unevenly distributed throughout the period covered by this book, with groups forming around particular individuals or encouraged by travelling missionaries and agents. These groups were further influenced by local denominations that could be friendly or hostile to the cause and had to negotiate tensions related to local politics, class and more, as they did in Cornwall and Cardiff.[2] Campaigns for Parliamentary reforms of licensing legislation were organized in London, Manchester or Glasgow and were focused on Westminster, but the abstainers who might have lent their support to those efforts were scattered across Britain.

We have already seen that temperance could take highly individual local forms, uniting personal, religious, social and economic worlds. Betsy Ann Griffin lived in or near Padstow for over seventy years, for example, and her family and faith were firmly embedded in North Cornwall and northwest Devon. Independent and Bible Christian Methodism shaped teetotalism in Griffin's Cornwall and John Laverock's Warrington; Samuel Bowly's activism drew upon and shaped the community of the Society of Friends in Gloucestershire. Bowly probably knew his second wife Louisa not only through Friends' meetings, but through the temperance work of her first husband, Jacob Henry Cotterell.

At the same time the national business of the temperance companies that are the focus of this book took the form of a network of local sites, connected together by travelling representatives, letters, newspaper advertisements and other mobile people and things. The main offices that were the centres of these networks had to work hard to maintain these connections. All of the significant temperance life assurance firms discussed in Chapter 1 were based in London, apart from Scottish Temperance (Glasgow) and the Abstainers and General (Birmingham). This reflected the wider geography of life assurance – the metropolis was the capital of English life assurance, though the Scottish industry was dominated by Edinburgh firms – but it did not match the geography of temperance. The Scottish Temperance office could quite reasonably claim to speak for Scotland, reflecting Glasgow's key position in the movement north of the border, but it was a different story to the south.[3] The concentration of English firms in the metropolis, far from the heartlands of temperance activism, created tensions between different strands of the wider movement, between London – which could be suspicious of or even hostile to temperance, especially total abstinence – and the teetotalers of industrial cities like Manchester or Bradford.

How might we begin to map this ordinary temperance? One response might be to look for those religious communities that offered support to temperance. Mapping Quaker membership through recorded attendance at meetings from both the 1851 religious census and the Friends' own census of attendance in 1904, Elizabeth Ischei concluded that 'in 1851 and in 1904, most Friends were members of large meetings in big industrial cities, though Quakerism was also strongly entrenched, through historical circumstances in a few smaller cities and towns such as Norwich, Banbury, and Kendal'.[4] As Ischei's map suggests (Map 2.1), Robert Warner's networks – religious, social, business – may have reflected the strength of the Society in Hertfordshire and Essex, just as Bowly's were formed in the long-standing Quaker communities of the West Country and West Midlands.

The Quakers remained divided over teetotalism for several decades however, so Ischei's map cannot be taken as a proxy for the geography of mid-century temperance support. Instead, we might map individuals who subscribed to temperance causes, therefore clearly signalling their involvement in the movement, as Martin Purvis did for members of the British and Foreign Temperance Society and the UK Alliance, though he mapped organizations with rather different relationships to moderation and temperance, reducing its value for this study.[5]

Temperance business records present us with another option. The UKT's archives allow for the possibility of mapping teetotal support in 1840, for example, through the lists of agents and medical referees provided in the firm's first prospectus 1840 (Map 2.2).

We will return to this map in Chapter Five, but it is worth considering it briefly here. The map presents us with the firm's own sense of the geography of support for temperance life assurance, showing just how scattered this was in 1840. All maps are snapshots of a moment in time, and the UKT's network of representatives developed quickly after this point, as we will see in Chapter 5, though it remained uneven. The reasons for this pattern require us to consider the role of local places in more detail. This chapter does exactly that, beginning with a tour of perhaps the most recognizable 'temperance town' of this period, Manchester, before turning to smaller and less obvious places where the archives of temperance life assurance companies can provide valuable insights into local communities. A review of historical work on the idea of temperance as a separate world provides some guidance for this.

The chapter then explores the temperance worlds of two rather different places. The first, a cluster of small mill towns in northeast Lancashire, differed from nearby Manchester both in terms of scale and the importance of very local concerns and networks; the strength of Manchester's global connections and its place on the national stage of temperance activism could not be replicated in Sabden or Padiham. The second example, the city of Exeter, is a much less likely temperance centre. By the 1870s representatives of the licensed trade exercised a significant influence over the city's politics through the Conservative Party, who remained in power for most of the

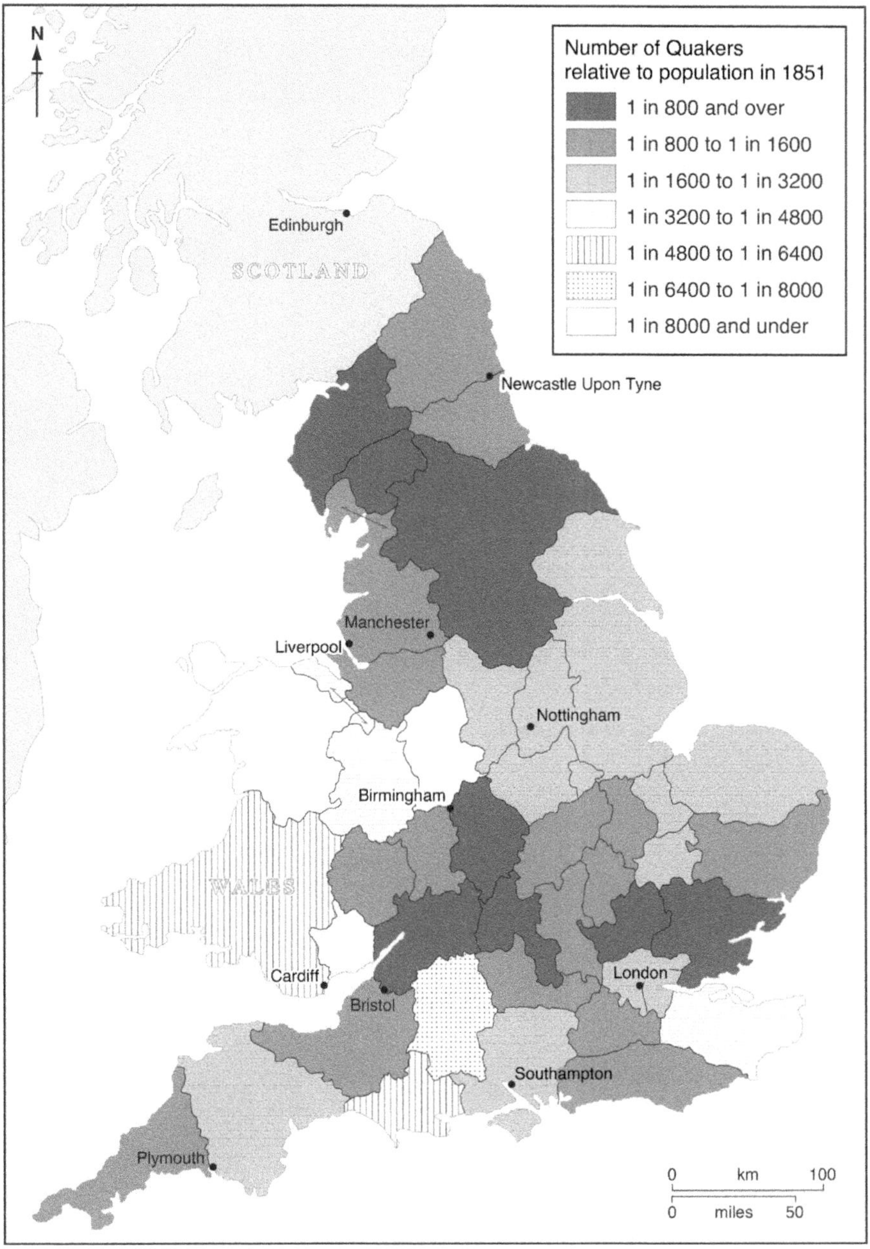

Map 2.1 The distribution of members of the Society of Friends in England and Wales in 1851.

Source: Ischei, *Victorian Quakers*, 170. Redrawn by Miles Irving, UCL Department of Geography.

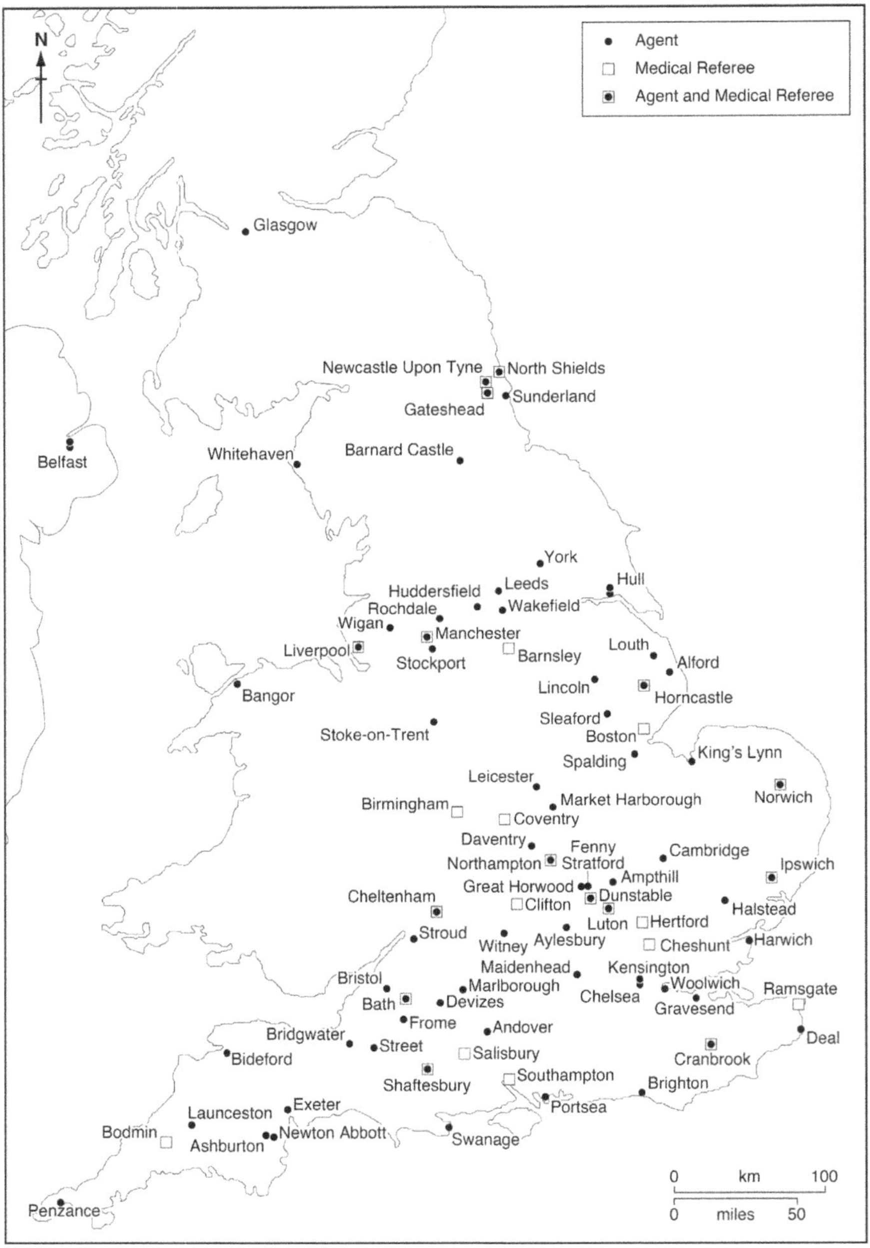

Map 2.2 Agents and medical referees for the UKT, 1840.

Source: Prospectus, 1840. Redrawn by Miles Irving, UCL Department of Geography.

period covered by this book. Despite this, temperance took root here and elsewhere in Devon from the 1830s, and temperance life assurance found agents and policyholders in the county. Our next temperance life, that of Torquay banker and amateur scientist Edward Vivian, explores his own rather awkward place in this conservative county. The chapter concludes by considering the traces of metropolitan temperance business in the form of a small estate in East London built by the Temperance Permanent Building Society from the 1850s, a tiny metropolitan temperance enclave which seems to have been rapidly forgotten.

In considering these temperance towns the chapter will demonstrate the value of temperance businesses as records of ordinary temperance across England, materializing these taken-for-granted, unspectacular forms of teetotal activity in their local contexts to provide a clearer glimpse of these 'alternative worlds'.

A tour of temperance Manchester

While temperance businesses have yet to receive much attention from historians, temperance alternatives to the pub – temperance halls and reading rooms, coffeehouses and temperance hotels – may be the exception. Teetotal 'British Workman's Public Houses' were built in northern towns from the 1860s, and coffee and cocoa taverns and palaces and coffee carts at railway stations were established across the country.[6] Andrew Davison notes that 'by the 1850s it was entirely possible for the teetotal commercial or business traveller to stay at a temperance hotel in any large town in the country, and the great majority of the smaller ones'.[7] These sites tell us something about the role of businesses like these in providing a place for ordinary temperance.

While medical advisors to life assurance firms warned that 'commercial travellers are not desirable risks; their hours are irregular, they have too much temptation to smoke and drink too much, and they suffer from badly-prepared food', teetotal commercial travellers did exist – there are nine in the Sceptre sample, for example.[8] If one of these travellers – perhaps James Smith Raynes, of Burnley, who had been assured with the Sceptre since 1877 – had arrived in Manchester in 1888, *Hawes' Handbook of Temperance Hotels*, published by the National Temperance League, would have offered him a choice of six temperance hotels in the city centre.[9] From the end of 1895 our traveller might have considered patronizing the newly opened Deansgate Temperance Hotel, the construction of which had been funded by the Manchester Temperance Hotels Company Ltd., whose directors included Robert Andrew Allison, the Liberal MP for Eskdale in Cumberland, and John Robert Barlow, the son of Bolton mill owner and philanthropist James Barlow, who was also the treasurer and later the president of the British Temperance League, Bolton's mayor between 1867 and 1869 and a director of the Mutual Fire Insurance and Wesleyan Trust Fire Insurance companies.[10] James and his wife Alice opened a coffee tavern, the Barlow Arms, in Edgworth, which was also listed in *Hawes' Handbook*, and John's older brother Sir Thomas Barlow was the UKT's teetotal medical director from 1876 (Chapter 8). Our teetotal traveller has already shown us some of the possible connections that could be drawn between temperance leisure, philanthropy, insurance and medicine.

The Deansgate Temperance Hotel had a café, dining room, a smoke and coffee lounge, a steam laundry and 120 bedrooms for visitors (Figure 2.1). It hosted meetings discussing temperance as well as topics like women's suffrage.[11] The hotel prospered, paying its shareholders dividends worth 2.5 or 3 per cent, until it was destroyed by enemy action in 1940; the company was wound up in 1942–3.[12] The Manchester Temperance Hotels Company Ltd. could be seen as a form of 'commercial liberal philanthropy' like the building of houses for the working classes, returning a dividend to its investors while providing an 'improved' hotel.[13]

Walking along this busy commercial street, our teetotal traveller might have noted the offices of Scottish Temperance next door to the Deansgate hotel.[14] Andrew Imrie, the Scottish firm's representative in the city since 1891, might well have frequented the Deansgate's café or coffee lounge.[15] The branch office of the UK Temperance and General Provident, the leading temperance insurers of the day and the Scottish office's main rivals, was on Cross Street, less than a ten-minute walk away. From its beginnings, the UKT considered its Manchester office second only to London in importance, 'in consideration of the great size of the town, and of the circumstances of there being two temperance societies there', as the Directors noted in 1841.[16] In its first decade the UKT had difficulty finding Manchester agents; they had initially hoped to use the agent of another temperance society, but could not agree terms.[17] The UKT's Manchester office would later be run by a family of agents: while Benjamin Sugden ran the Cross Street office, John Sugden, the firm's district supervisor for Lancashire, and F. H. Sugden, agency supervisor, had offices in Manchester Chambers on nearby Market Street, alongside Samuel Sugden, who represented the United Temperance Permanent Building and Investment company.[18] The offices of the two most important teetotal friendly societies, the Sons of Temperance and the Rechabites, who collected members' savings to cover illness and burial costs, were less than fifteen minutes' walk from Deansgate on York Street and Red Bank.[19] The Rechabites had begun in the neighbouring city of Salford in 1835, as the Independent Order of Rechabites (Salford Unity). All of these businesses were run by and for members of the temperance movement, and their presence in the heart of Manchester's business district made temperance both ubiquitous and ordinary in that city.

Of course, Manchester might be said to be the capital of British temperance by the end of the nineteenth century, reflecting and concentrating the long history of the movement in Lancashire. The national office of the United Kingdom Alliance for the Suppression of the Traffic in All Intoxicating Liquors was also on Deansgate, and the city was full of temperance societies and cultural institutions. The Central Association for Stopping the Sale of Intoxicating Liquors on Sunday were situated on Brown Street, the Licensing Law Reform Committee on Cross Street and the National Union for the Suppression of Intemperance on Oxford Street. There were also offices for many temperance societies, including the Church of England Temperance Society on Cannon Street, the Lancashire & Cheshire Band of Hope Union, on Portland Street, the Manchester, Salford & District Temperance Union on Cross Street, the National Conservative Temperance Union on St. Ann's Square, the Wesleyan Methodist Temperance and Band of Hope Union and the Women's Christian Temperance

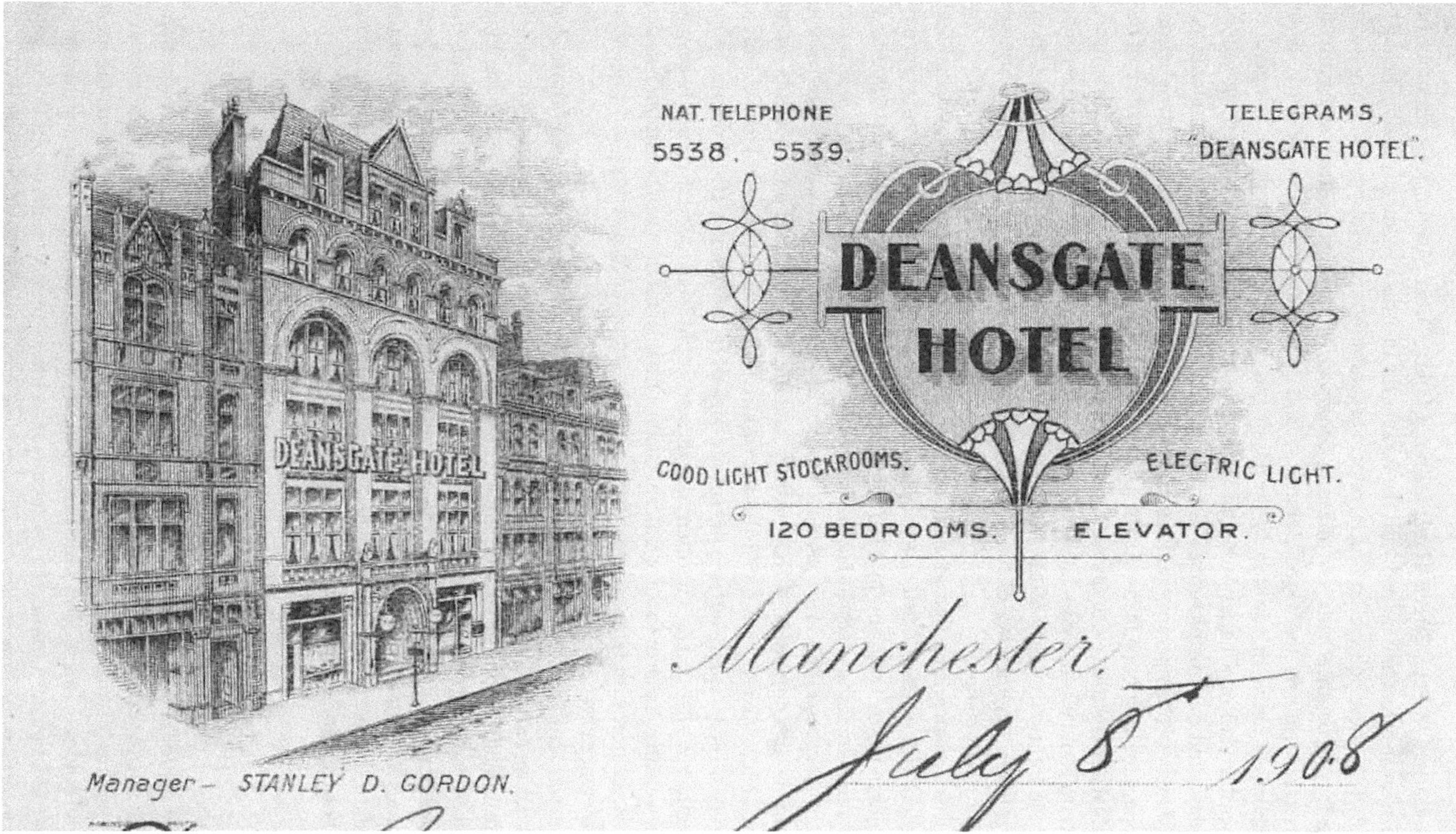

Figure 2.1 The Deansgate Temperance Hotel, 1908.

Source: Author's collection.

Association on Peter Street. The latter ran a Police Court Mission from an office on Brazennose Street and helped with the Retreat for Inebriate Women in Fallowfield.[20]

By 1895 these political and social reform organizations were supported by a network of forty temperance halls and meeting rooms in Manchester, Salford and outlying districts, including the Good Templars' Hall on Dale Street, and by thirty-eight temperance hotels in addition to the Deansgate Hotel.[21] The Brighton Temperance Assembly Hall on Charles Street and the Manchester Temperance Choir on Queen Street round out this picture of the rich associational life of northern temperance.[22] In Manchester temperance and insurance also came together in other places besides temperance assurance firms. As the District Manager of the Manchester office of the Mutual Life Insurance Company of New York at 28 Brown Street, just off Market Street, Edward Neild was not associated with a distinctively temperance office, but he was also the Honorary Secretary of the Manchester and Salford District Temperance Union, as well as a key member of the British Temperance League and the Central Sunday Closing Association.[23]

It is not surprising that Manchester was richly provided with political, social and economic institutions associated with temperance. The city's temperance society was founded in 1830, and by 1836 John Finch estimated that there were 10,000 total abstainers in Manchester and its surrounding districts; while it is hard to confirm this figure, it suggests the wider conglomeration of towns was by far the leading temperance centre in the northwest.[24] The Quakers had their own Manchester Friends' Total Abstinence Society from 1850; the Lancashire and Cheshire Band of Hope Union, begun in 1863, rapidly became the second biggest in the country after London.[25] Our imaginary visitor to late Victorian Manchester would have found it relatively easy to find welcoming places to eat, drink and sleep. Other teetotalers worked in temperance firms, assured with temperance offices, went to temperance meetings and sang with temperance choirs.

It was also possible to find these parallel worlds in other towns, even those that did not share Manchester's industrial, nonconformist and radical histories, and which were sometimes hostile to temperance as a consequence. There was a geographical unevenness to British temperance, but in many cities and towns, large and small, the close interweaving of the social and business worlds of temperance would have been obvious to contemporary observers. By 1918, British temperance was more than just a political cause or a social movement; it was a parallel world with its own institutions and expectations, supported by a varied set of businesses and infrastructures.

Total communities, alternative worlds?

If we are looking for ordinary temperance beyond the struggle to regulate alcoholic drink, then Lilian Lewis Shiman's exploration of the 'total temperance community' and Annemarie McAllister's description of these 'alternative worlds' are perhaps the most useful guides.[26] This section will briefly consider Shiman's example of Birstall alongside other local places illuminated by temperance life assurance material. In doing so it demonstrates the importance of ordinary temperance in a range of different sites.

Shiman traced a 'developing dichotomy between the temperance and the non-temperance world' in the last quarter of the nineteenth century, as teetotalers became 'increasingly isolated from the rest of the population'.[27] Her reconstruction of the temperance life of Birstall, a small woollen town in the West of Yorkshire, provides an excellent example of a temperance world. Originally meeting in local schoolrooms, Birstall's teetotalers soon built their own hall, extending and then rebuilding it as the society grew. The hall hosted guest speakers, meetings of the local Band of Hope, amateur concerts and other weekly and annual events. Some of this activity was political – engaging with arguments presented in temperance journals, or with the local Alliance agent and the campaign for Local Option – but Shiman is also clear that these meetings were 'an integral part of the fabric that united the members', 'instrumental in promoting alliances and marriages among them', and a forum for exchanging news about jobs as well as temperance affairs.[28] However the arrival of Gospel Temperance in 1890 prompted the society to use the hall as a place of worship, a decision that divided local members as it severed connections with other congregations. For some 'the temperance hall became the one centre of their lives', while other local teetotalers chose multiple, overlapping identifications with place and community.[29] This study of Birstall as a small 'temperance town' shows the extent to which it became a 'total temperance community' for some of its inhabitants, while other teetotalers remained within their chapel or church communities, or other social groupings. Still, Birstall was not a dry town, possessing twelve inns and public houses, eight beersellers, two licensed grocers and two brewers in 1881, when its population was under 7,000 people.[30] Teetotal sociality was a key part of the town, but it did not define it, and Birstall's teetotalers were themselves divided on key issues of faith.

Indeed, Shiman shows that in practice it was difficult to keep these worlds apart, even for those who worked for a teetotal firm and lived in a 'prohibition village' like Saltaire or Liverpool's Toxteth Park. It was much easier to find or create specialized spaces in which teetotalers could meet to socialize and discuss temperance issues, including places of worship, temperance halls and other sites. This social infrastructure – defined by Alan Latham and Jack Layton as the 'networks of spaces, facilities, institutions, and groups that create affordances for social connection' – materialized temperance sociality, in enclave form at least.[31] Temperance was only one part of urban life, even in Manchester; the solidly middle-class milieu explored by Simon Gunn does not seem to have touched the city's temperance world at any point, for example.[32]

Annemarie McAllister's paper focuses on the *visibility* of this 'alternative world', 'the public performance of temperance' that was carried on through forms of visual culture like magic lantern shows, print culture and street processions.[33] This chapter will certainly consider some of these highly visible public performances, which might temporarily lay claim to settings normally unwelcoming to temperance, as they did in Exeter. However, we also need to consider the less public, rather taken-for-granted aspects of abstaining in a drinker's world. How might we glimpse temperance activity of a less visible kind? In Birstall, for example, the Sceptre life assurance company assured two men and a woman, a gardener, a cloth fuller and a provision merchant.[34] How visible would their ordinary temperance lives have been?

Temperance lives: Burnley and Pendle

The records of the Sceptre office provide a glimpse into the temperance world of the mill towns of northeast Lancashire. Between 1870 and 1881 fifteen abstainers' policies were established in Clitheroe, Sabden, Padiham, Nelson and Colne, a series of small settlements arrayed around Pendle Hill, with another eight policies in Burnley to the south. This area was part of Blackburn's cloth manufacturing district and was characterized by a high level of women's participation in both the industrial workforce and union activity and by equal pay for men and women.[35] Between them these hamlets and small towns contributed 22 per cent of the 105 lives in the Sceptre sample assured in Lancashire between 1865 and 1881. The cities of Manchester and Salford accounted for only a slightly larger number of policyholders between them, with 25 per cent of the Lancashire lives in the Sceptre sample, clearly illustrating the uneven geography of temperance life assurance.

Sceptre had agents in Liverpool, Blackburn, Preston and smaller Lancashire towns, with the district superintendent's office in Manchester. The firm's agent in Sabden, James Moorhouse (1818–1883), sold eleven of the policies around Pendle Hill and would have been assured with the firm himself. He had been an overlooker at one of the town's mills and seems to have taken up his role as an agent when he retired. James married Dina Denbigh in 1837 and they had two daughters and two sons, all four working as cotton weavers from their teens.[36] He was a Wesleyan, secretary to the chapel at Padiham and a frequent speaker at the circuit's meetings, teas and Sunday schools in his years as an agent.[37] Moorhouse, 'a good leader', was one of several local prominent Wesleyans; a late Victorian historian of local Methodism reported that by 1840 'the Wesleyan might be called the established church at Padiham, as it was by far the largest and most influential congregation in the town'.[38] In 1841 the Methodist Conference forbade Methodists from speaking about temperance in their chapels or circuits, but it seems likely that James continued to combine Methodism and teetotalism in this period. Elsewhere in the area temperance support came from other forms of Methodism, as it had in Warrington and Cornwall; Nelson's Salem Independent Methodist Chapel had been 'the rendezvous of teetotalers in this district' since the 1840s.[39]

The teetotalers who assured with Moorhouse included bleachers, cotton weavers, spinners and overlookers, as well as a grocer, rate collector, painter, quarry foreman and a registrar to the Burial Board. Their fortunes were as mixed as their occupations. The bleacher-turned-weaver George Wilkinson assured his life in 1870, when he was twenty-nine, and probably died 1909–10; by 1908, when he would have been about sixty-seven, his £50 policy had earned £25 in bonuses.[40] Hannah Chatburn of Sabden also established a £50 policy in 1870, and her husband William took out a General policy with the company, but both policies lapsed within five years. When William and Hannah married in 1860, they gave their occupations as 'weaver'.[41] Hannah was one of only two women in this group, the other being Elizabeth Ellen Waterworth, a housekeeper in Burnley, whose policy also lapsed before any bonuses could be earned.

Edward Marsh was more fortunate, living to claim the £100 policy he had established in 1881. Born in Preston in 1857, where his father had been a labourer, Edward worked as a cotton spinner and weaver in Read and Sabden; his wife, Margaret Mary, was also a cotton weaver, their daughter Lena following her mother's profession by 1901, when she was fourteen. In 1911 Edward was a blowroom operative in a mill, a low-status but probably relatively undemanding job for a man in his mid-fifties. Margaret was not working, though both of the surviving children were weavers. Edward received bonuses on his policy until 1913, and the policy was paid in 1916, when he would have been sixty. It seems likely that Edward lived until 1935, when he would have been in his seventies.[42] As these brief sketches suggest, the lives of these Sceptre policyholders had varying outcomes. Of the twenty-three Sceptre policies in the sample established in this area, thirteen were claimed, six lapsed as payments were not kept up, and three were surrendered (sold back to the firm at a discounted rate).

The outcome of the twenty-third policy is not recorded in the ledger. That policy was written for John Haworth, an engine driver at a Sabden mill who assured his life in 1881, when he was twenty-seven. A year later John married a local woman named Lydia Sagar, and by 1891 he was employed as a greengrocer. By the next census he had already retired, though, at the age of forty-five, and the couple were living with Lydia's widowed mother. By 1911 John and Lydia had moved to Poulton Le Fylde, near Blackpool, and when John died in 1917 he left Lydia nearly a thousand pounds in his will.[43] The sudden change in John and Lydia's circumstances might be explained by their marriage, as Lydia's father John Sagar was an important local Wesleyan preacher. A Sabden blacksmith and mechanic, John Sagar helped redevelop the chapel at Nelson, became a circuit steward and laid the foundation of the new chapel and Sunday school in 1872; he preached in these mill towns from the late 1870s and supported Gospel Temperance meetings in the 1880s.[44] He died in 1900, leaving just over £600 to be divided between his son-in-law John Haworth and Robert Hindle, the owner of the town's calico printing works and the largest donor for Sabden's new Chapel. It is not clear how John Sagar earned this money, but it might explain why John Haworth became a greengrocer, perhaps with help from his father-in-law, and why he and Lydia retired immediately after receiving some of Sagar's estate.

The Sceptre ledgers let us see something of this 'temperance world', then, organized at least partly through Wesleyan and Independent Methodist chapels and circuits, bringing together factory workers, shopkeepers and clerks. Temperance is one part of the story, but few of the fourteen local abstainers in the Sceptre sample seem to have been very public participants in their local societies. They might have listened to the speeches given by higher-profile advocates like James Moorhouse or John Sagar, but their temperance seems likely to have been more passive and anonymous than the public displays examined by McAllister. Paying their premiums to Moorhouse may have felt like a version of the teetotal pledge – renewing their commitment to temperance and to the Sceptre office every year or quarter – but this was not a promise that was made publicly. These towns were not 'total temperance worlds' like Shiman's dry model villages, either, though the nearby hamlet of Low Moor, housing workers at Thomas Garnett and Son's yarn and cloth mill, was a model settlement like Saltaire, without 'public-house nor beershop, dramshop, pawnshop, nor tommy-shop'.[45] In

1896, Colne had twenty-two pubs and one temperance hotel for around 21,000 inhabitants; Sabden had a beerhouse, two inns and a beerseller for its 1,550 inhabitants in 1906.[46] Still, temperance would have provided part of the milieu in which people socialized, agreed, argued and married; John Haworth and Lydia Sagar may well have met through the Sabden chapel.

The temperance world made visible by the ledgers and minute books of life assurance firms was ordinary, anonymous, sometimes private. While these teetotalers may have supported the Alliance, argued over Local Option, or campaigned for Sunday Closing, their membership of the wider movement meant much more than this narrowly political sense of temperance. Both more extensive and less dramatic than political activism, this form of ordinary temperance could still be important.

The local setting of these North East Lancashire lives may well have been highly significant. Just thirty miles to the southeast of Burnley, the wool town of Huddersfield would prove to be a significant centre of anti-war activity in the early years of the Great War, due to the town's combination of a long-established nonconformist Liberalism and emergent Labour and socialist movements. Anti-war feeling, manifested in and organized by meetings of trade unionists, members of the Society of Friends, the women's movement, the Independent Labour Party, British Socialist Party and other groups, provided the town with both a significant number of Conscientious Objectors and the networks to support them and oppose the war. Temperance formed part of the 'wider local pre-war ethical and political culture' which produced this opposition.[47] The temperance world of early twentieth-century Huddersfield was supplied with a social infrastructure of halls, hotels and meetings; it was also politically Liberal, producing local councillors and drawing on nonconformist support, particularly from the Society of Friends. Arthur Sherwell, the town's MP between 1906 and 1918, was the author – with Joseph Rowntree – of *The Temperance Question and Social Reform*, as well as several other investigations of temperance, and was opposed to conscription.[48]

Of course, this wider culture clearly contained groups who might not agree on anything beyond opposition to the war, or even on their reasons for that stance. Philip Snowden (1864–1937), Labour's first Chancellor, personified some of these local tensions as his political career crossed the Pennines between Keighley and Blackburn, between the local culture identified by Pearce and that implied by the lives of the area's Sceptre teetotalers. Brought up near Keighley within both Wesleyan Methodism and Liberal Radicalism, Snowden remained a determined teetotaler. His family moved to Nelson when he was fifteen, and he found work in an insurance office in Burnley while immersing himself in Nelson's 'hot-bed of Radicalism'.[49] Keith Laybourn argues that Snowden absorbed a particular version of socialism from the Keighley branch of the Independent Labour Party (ILP), which he joined in 1895, but when he returned to Lancashire to contest the Blackburn constituency in 1900 for the ILP and Social Democratic Foundation (SDF) he found his old Liberal views strengthened in this new context, as he promoted Labour to both working-class Tories and Liberals interested in Radicalism. In the same period he began to support women's suffrage after his marriage to the socialist and feminist Ethel Annakin, and as a result of the strength of women within Lancashire unions.[50]

From the late 1970s through to the 1990s historians and geographers including Jill Liddington and Jill Norris, Patrick Joyce, Linda McDowell and Doreen Massey, and

Carolyn Steedman considered the legacies of the nineteenth-century radicalism that had emerged in this part of Lancashire, its influence on the Labour party at the start of the twentieth century and its consequences for the political landscape revealed by Thatcherism.[51] For these authors the political activity of Burnley and Nelson's women weavers set this area's working-class culture apart from the patriarchal traditions of a town like Preston. For Liddington and Norris temperance also provided a key influence on the form of this culture, though this would cause tensions within radical suffragism: 'in the Lancashire cotton towns and the West Riding wool villages on either side of the Pennines the traditions of Non-conformism and temperance were particularly strong, and gave their ILP branches an atmosphere of self disciplined "high thinking and low living"'.[52] This rich combination of older forms of Liberalism with elements of the labour and suffrage movements created a distinct political culture across the Pennines; the complex relationships and tensions between different individuals and ideologies drew on, challenged, or sustained local interrelations, so that while a broad 'landscape of dissent' is visible across the Lancashire–Yorkshire border over this period, it took highly varied forms in different places.[53]

It is perhaps not surprising that the northern industrial centres of Manchester, Birstall and the towns of northeast Lancashire were temperance towns, though there are many differences between them. Temperance was less visible in the rural south, though there were often local clusters of support and activity, even in cities and counties that could be actively hostile to it, like Exeter, where local elites and working-class conservativism provided a direct challenge to teetotalers in the last quarter of the century.

Exeter, an unlikely temperance city

> Devonshire, if not the most prolific in matter for gratulation and astonishment, in connection with Teetotalism, is at least ... far from the most unproductive or the least interesting county that might have been selected.[54]

Exeter's strength as a woollen manufacturing centre was largely gone by the 1830s, and the 1835 Municipal Corporations Act made little difference to the city's politics, with the Tories retaining control until 1868, when a Liberal mayor and two Liberal MPs were elected.[55] Conservative control was quickly reasserted, partly through the efforts of the drink trade, and would be maintained until 1900. Robert Newton's study of Victorian Exeter suggests that local Conservatives and Liberals shared a common conservatism, though. For Newton the fact that the city's three greatest Victorian leaders were two bishops (Phillpotts and Temple) and a member of county society (Sir Stafford Northcote) clearly demonstrated the continuing importance of the established church and the local aristocracy.[56] The city's Liberals were concentrated in local nonconformist communities, as they were elsewhere, but 'the heroic days of Dissent in the city, and Exeter's own prominence as a Dissenting stronghold, belonged to the eighteenth century'.[57] Allan Brockett suggested that the evangelicalism of Victorian Methodism 'was alien to the middle-class merchants who had formed the backbone of old-style Dissent in Exeter'. Despite this, the varied strands of Methodism made up the second largest denomination in 1851 when considered together.[58]

A city which provided little support for Reform does not seem like fertile ground for teetotalism. Exeter's first temperance society was formed in 1834, though, in connection with the moderationist British and Foreign Temperance Society. Teetotalism was adopted in the following year, and James Teare, the teetotal missionary and agent for the UKT, visited in 1837, further swelling the society's numbers.[59] J. W. Havill's Temperance Star Coffee and Reading Rooms opened next to the Corn Exchange Hall on Fore Street, the city's main road, in 1840.[60] Early support for temperance came from two Anglican vicars, rather than local nonconformists like the Methodists.[61] Arguments over moderation and total abstinence left their scars, as they did everywhere, but by 1841 the society had been reorganized, Devon's first Rechabite Tent had been opened in the city, and speakers from Exeter were travelling to nearby towns like Ashburton and Exmouth to promote teetotalism.[62]

The energy demonstrated by Exeter's society probably explains why the city was included in the UKT's first prospectus, issued in 1840. John Bale, an accountant and solicitor's clerk, served as the office's agent in the city for nearly twenty years, also acting as a travelling agent and lecturer in the county, and eventually as district superintendent.[63] Bale was probably a Wesleyan and had close links to the Exeter Rechabite District, making him a natural fit for this role with its emphasis on temperance, finance and the collective sharing of risk. The decision of the Exeter District Rechabite Tent to deposit £21 with the UKT as part of the office's banking service in December 1841 seems likely to have been organized by Bale.[64] It's not clear how dedicated his own teetotalism was, though. After taking out several policies in his own name, in 1848 Bale asked to switch from the Abstainers' to the newly opened General department; he produced medical evidence to prove that he was in sound health, and this was approved.[65] He may have been more comfortable with moderation, or was perhaps struggling with abstinence, as others did; possibly the freedom offered by the new General section appealed to him.

Bale's moderation does not seem to have harmed his effectiveness as a salesman. Ten years later he told a meeting at the Athenaeum that there were about 200 members in Exeter, collectively contributing £1,000 a year in premiums; in 'the Western counties' he had assured 1,500 people.[66] The UKT had been sending travelling agents into Devon since its first year of business, supporting Bale's efforts to find policyholders in local temperance societies.[67] The UKT had agents in Ashburton, Bideford and Newton Abbott in 1840, and in Plymouth and Devonport by 1841; by 1853 there were agents in another thirteen places in the county.[68]

The teetotal lives assured by these agents could be very modest ones. In 1845 the UKT approved a £10 policy for a Stoke Damerel woman named Jane Carne, whose husband, the stone mason William John Carne, also had a £10 policy; policies of this size could only have been burial insurance.[69] Twenty-five years later the Sceptre also found a market for its teetotal life assurance in the county. The Sceptre sample contains twenty-nine teetotal Devon lives, less than a third of the number established in either Lancashire or Yorkshire in this period, which were issued to a typically mixed cross-section of people: a tailor's cutter and a draper in Exeter; a gasfitter and an elderly porter and his wife in Barnstaple; and a minister, a tailor's cutter, a master baker and a shoemaker in South Molton. In Teignmouth the farmworker turned Primitive Methodist Minister Henry Alcock and his wife Fanny both established £50 policies, but surrendered them before moving on to a circuit in Sherborne, Dorset in 1871.[70] At Buden Park, Shebbear, the farmer Thomas Hocking established a £100 endowment for his six-year-old daughter Mary Elizabeth Grace Hocking in 1881 to collect when she reached twenty-one; Shebbear was the birthplace of the Bible Christians, and it seems likely that the Hockings were members, like the Griffins (Chapter 1).

Exeter's teetotal community developed its own social infrastructure. Magic lantern entertainments were offered at temperance teas in the city in the 1860s, and by the late 1870s the city boasted a Temperance Hall on Friar's Walk, three temperance hotels and two British Workman Temperance Clubs or coffee taverns.[71] Despite this, the last three decades of the century were very challenging for Exeter teetotalers. The loss of both Parliamentary seats to the Liberals in 1868 galvanized the city's Conservative Association, which turned to local licensed victuallers to take on the day-to-day business of Conservative organizing, keen as they were to resist licensing reform as well as Liberal threats to Church and Union. By 1870 '"the trade" had taken up the entrenched position from which it exercised a decisive influence on local politics until the twentieth century', further strengthened by opposition to the Liberals' 1872 Licensing Act.[72] Harding, Richards and Thomas's brewery at St Anne's Well played a particularly significant role. W. J. Richards was chair of the Conservative Working Men's Union between 1868 and 1886, and Joseph Harding and Henry Drew Thomas were mayors of Exeter in 1871–2 and 1877–8 respectively. In the year that Thomas was mayor, the other two partners served on the council as aldermen, and Samuel Jones – a wine, spirit, ale and porter merchant – was elected Sherriff. Critics in the city condemned this 'open jobbery'.[73]

Attacks on temperance were part of a wider conservative reaction. 'Exeter elections remained rough, disorderly and drunken' right through to the twentieth century, and so did political meetings. In 1872 a meeting on the licensing question broke up when the chair, the Liberal teetotaler Bishop Frederick Temple, was hit in the face with a bag of flour; the trouble was started by 'toughs' led by Harding and Richards's employees. Six years later Harding and Richards's men were also accused of breaking up a meeting discussing disestablishment, singing 'John Barleycorn' and cheering their Conservative MPs; in 1882 a meeting on Sunday Closing, again chaired by Bishop Temple, was broken up by youths throwing pepper and stink bombs. Captain Bent, the superintendent of police and former chair of the Conservative Association in one of the city's wards, was also present at that last meeting; he did not intervene to assist the bishop.[74] It's significant that local Conservative hatred of temperance was so strong that it overcame the deference usually shown to the Church; Temple would become the Archbishop of Canterbury in 1896, after all.

Temperance life continued, despite this opposition. An anniversary tea meeting of Exeter's society at the hall on Friar's Walk in 1871 attracted only a moderate attendance of about a hundred, but the election of the Independent Methodist Reverend John J. Jones to the School Board was taken as an encouraging sign.[75] Though the Society's grand procession and picnic was 'miserably dampened' by heavy rain in July 1873, with the spectacle of crying children carrying banners through the mud exciting the sympathy rather than admiration of onlookers, the strength and diversity of local organizations was still apparent. Local Good Templars were strongly represented, with the Bovey Tracey brass band and Exmouth fife and drum band leading the procession; after the rain let up there were running races and an archery competition.[76] The report read at the Society's 1880 meeting counted 350 members. There had been nearly 200 meetings on temperance at the temperance hall; the Band of Hope, which met three times a week, included more than 400 children. Bishop Temple, chairing, said 'it was a satisfaction to know that they were not really suffering defeat in spite of all the forces arrayed against them – (cheers) – and that though they might still be very far from having done what they desired to do, yet they were steadily gaining ground'.[77]

Exeter's temperance groups persevered, despite 'the forces arrayed against them'. This regular participation in temperance sociality in a setting where this was a minority activity without strong local links to Reform or radicalism was another form of ordinary temperance, but it seems likely that it would have been strongly meaningful to the men, women and children who established policies, attended meetings, or took part in juvenile foot races. Our next temperance life explores some of the meanings of this ordinary temperance further.

Temperance lives: Edward Vivian (1808–1893)

Edward Vivian was another Liberal out of place in Conservative Devon. A cousin of Richard Hussey, Baron Vivian, Edward was born in Bushey, Hertfordshire, where his father was rector, and was educated at Oxford, where he became friends with Gladstone.[78] Visiting the tiny Devon resort town of Torquay on a yachting holiday, he was so taken with it that he took up residence there around 1829–30. His first wife Harriet Bacon died in 1832, two years after their marriage, and he married Emma Catherine Johnson in 1834. Edward joined the board of the Torquay Bank, became the proprietor of Torquay's newspaper and editor of the local *Directory* and helped found the town's museum. In time he would serve as Justice of the Peace, town commissioner, vice-president of the Local Board of Health and governor of the Torbay Infirmary and Dispensary.[79] By mid-century he had become part of Torquay's narrow political elite, controlled by his banking partner William Kitson on behalf of the town's Conservative landowners; in 1853, ten of the twelve members of the Board of Health – including Vivian – were accused of being 'elected by the Kitson influence'.[80]

As a gentleman, Vivian was wealthy enough to be able to indulge his interests in science, the arts and improvement in general. As one local newspaper put it, 'The learned gentleman is an apt moral teacher, and is always unwilling that opportunities should pass unimproved'.[81] Exploring the prehistory of Kent's Cavern with Torquay's natural history society, he lectured the Geological Society of London and sat on the British Association committee founded to study the site with Charles Lyell, William Pengelly and others. An active member of the Devonshire Association for the Advancement of Science, Literature and Art, Edward published meteorological measurements of Torquay's mild climate, including some taken from a balloon flight; he grew prize-winning dahlias, bred prize-wining fowl and had subtropical plants imported for his

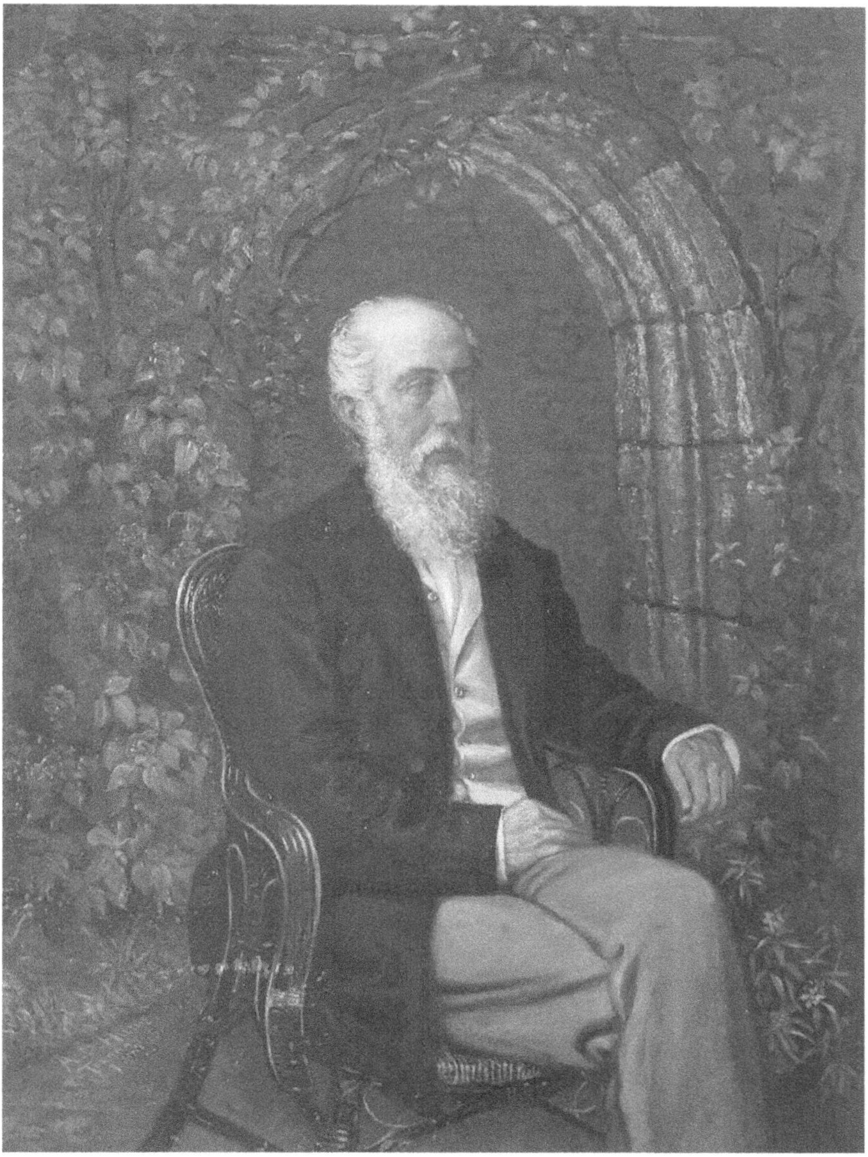

Figure 2.2 Edward Vivian, by A. B. Hume.

Source: Courtesy of Torquay Museum.

gardens.[82] Vivian was also a keen artist and supporter of the town's new School of Science and Art, inviting Ruskin to present its prizes.[83] Finally, he was interested in questions of political economy, presenting a paper on vital statistics to the British Association for the Advancement of Science's Economic Science and Statistics section from 1860 until the 1880s, to Edwin Chadwick, the economist William Newmarch, and the eugenicist Francis Galton. These vital statistics were drawn from the UKT's experience, demonstrating the difference in mortality shown by the Abstainers' and General sections.[84]

Vivian had been a director of the UKT since 1846 and 'one of the largest assurers in the Institution', assuring his life for £2000.[85] His teetotalism was apparently a response to personal ill-health, possibly on the recommendation of his medical advisor in Exeter, Dr Robert Hayward Lucas, who was appointed as one of the UKT's medical referees in February 1841.[86] An active member of the Western Temperance League and the Alliance from the 1860s, Vivian discussed the Permissive Bill with Lord Shaftesbury and chaired temperance speakers – Bishop Temple, Neal Dow, John B. Gough, Samuel Bowly – at local events and entertained them at his home.[87] Wilfrid Lawson, the Alliance's Parliamentary spokesman, was a frequent correspondent, and the tone of Lawson's letters suggests the two were good friends.[88]

Vivian's progressive instincts seem to have been genuine, though his political initiatives had little real success. He had an early brush with Exeter's rough-and-ready political world in 1841, as one of the 'Rads' who organized a meeting urging Melbourne's government to reform monopolies and promote free trade. The gathering was taken over by a much larger group of Tories who instead petitioned Parliament to resist these reforms.[89] Vivian tried to arrange work in industrial Manchester for Devon's unemployed farm workers at the time of the Swing Riots, travelled to Ireland to meet Daniel O'Connell and rented some of his own land to members of the local Chartist Association in 1848. In 1865 Vivian stood for the parliamentary seat at St. Ives and was identified as 'an out and out Liberal' by the Conservative *Royal Cornwall Gazette*, which celebrated his defeat as a rejection of temperance and religious freedom, which Vivian supported for Catholics and nonconformists.[90] Vivian stood for St Ives again in 1868, but withdrew from the contest.[91] Late Victorian temperance retained some progressive potential, but was defined and divided by the great controversies and movements of its day – religious and educational freedom, women's suffrage, Ireland. When his old friend Gladstone visited Torquay in 1889, for example, Vivian snubbed him over Home Rule.[92]

Vivian's final radical moment came when he intervened in the 'Battle of Torquay' in 1888. The town prosecuted the Salvation Army for marching on a Sunday, which it had banned under the Torquay and Harbour District Act, as part of the fierce and sometimes violent opposition Salvationists encountered.[93] The arrest of dozens of Salvationists, many of them local labourers and fishermen, and their insistence on serving their sentences to highlight the injustice of the situation, soon became a national scandal. The offending clause was repealed and the right of Salvationists to march – in Torquay or anywhere in the UK – was confirmed. Vivian became involved in this 'Battle' as Torquay's senior magistrate, refusing to sit on the bench while the Bill was used in this way, while the other magistrates prosecuted Salvationists on behalf of the landed families who controlled Torquay.[94]

Edward Vivian died in 1893, aged eighty-five. His estate was worth more than £23,000, but obituarists also noted his contributions to the town 'in the days when the town most required leading'.[95] As a member of the Anglican gentry, Vivian enjoyed a rather different life to Warner and Bowly, his fellow UKT directors. He was also a different kind of capitalist, seemingly less entrepreneurial than either man. His liberalism was more pronounced than Warner's, but perhaps less radical – or less effective, politically – than Bowly's. Some of these differences may well have reflected his awkward place in a county that was suspicious of – and sometimes outwardly hostile to – temperance.

Conclusion: 'A regular Maine-law estate' in East London

Temperance business archives can help us find 'temperance communities' or 'alternative worlds' of the kind described by Shiman and McAllister in Manchester, Northeast Lancashire, Exeter and Torquay, though these networks were made up of individuals whose temperance lives could be visible or private, radical or conservative. It would have been quite possible for a visitor to miss these signs of temperance life, though, even in Manchester, as these businesses and societies became better established. One good example of this, presented to conclude the chapter, is the small temperance enclave built by the Temperance Permanent Building Society (TPBS) in East London, between the 1850s and 1870s.

The TPBS was established to allow its members to borrow their pooled funds in order to build houses, but for the first two decades of its existence it was also able to act as a developer in its own right. Other banks and building societies built houses, like the Birkbeck Land and Building Societies, which built in Acton, Beckenham, Enfield, Mill Hill, Archway and other locations in suburban London from the 1850s.[96] The TPBS bought land near Forest Gate, Stratford, East London, in the same decade, dividing it into 121 plots along six new roads. Progress seems to have been halting and piecemeal, as it was for some of the Birkbeck estates, but by February 1858 all but one plot had been disposed of. The 1869 Ordnance Survey map shows a few new buildings in the northeastern corner of the estate, though Janson Road was still only a few dozen yards in length. The buildings constructed on the estate included cottages with gardens, brick-built three-bedroom villas and several shops including a grocers with a shop parlour, drawing room, kitchens, four large bedrooms and stabling.[97]

Unlike the Birkbeck Building Society, which built taverns on some of its London estates, the TPBS planned for a *temperance* estate. The TPBS held a 'demonstration' on the land it had purchased for the estate in August 1858. William Janson presided, and 150 members and supporters took tea, coffee, cake, shrimp and watercress in a 'spacious marquee'. William Tweedie spoke in his capacity as a director of the firm, remarking 'that their estate was a regular Maine-law estate, as no house for the manufacture or sale of intoxicating drinks would, on any account, be allowed to be built on the premises'.[98] In 1851 the US state of Maine had prohibited the sale and manufacture of alcoholic drink; the UK Alliance aimed to introduce something similar to British licensing districts. The development of an estate of 121 houses without a pub was, for Tweedie, another way of creating an alcohol-free enclave. The TPBS also hoped that this estate would also create new property owners, and thus voters; the report of the firm's fourth Annual General Meeting in 1858 noted that the Directors took pleasure 'in stating their belief that the votes thus created are in the hands of the persons who will use them in advancing the cause of temperance, and other movements tending to improve the condition of the masses of the community'.[99]

The estate's six streets were named after prominent teetotalers, some associated with the firm, and these can be found on the right and in the centre of Map 2.3. Cruikshank Road was named after the TPBS's trustee George Cruikshank, the artist famous for his illustrated temperance series *The Bottle* (1847) and *The Drunkard's Children* (1848), as well as the painting *The Worship of Bacchus* (1863). Heyworth and Trevelyan Road commemorate Lawrence Heyworth, MP, and W. C. Trevelyan, respectively president and vice-president of the TPBS. Buckingham Road seems likely to be named after James Silk Buckingham, chair of an important early parliamentary inquiry into intemperance, patron of the UKT and a proponent of temperance saving schemes.[100] Janson Road marks William Janson, Quaker banker and founding UKT director; Gough Road probably referred to John B. Gough, the popular American teetotal speaker and author.

However, the houses presumably quickly lost their original associations with temperance as they were sold on or rented out; once the covenants' restrictions expired, they could even be converted into pubs. The rapid disappearance of these temperance connections can be seen in a tragic case concerning the Feast family, residents of one of the cottages on Cruikshank Road. In 1871 neighbours noticed that the Feast children, aged ten and four, appeared to be fending for themselves. Investigating, they found William, a forty-year-old clerk at Bishopsgate Station for the Great Eastern Railway, lying dead in the house, having apparently bled to death at least a week earlier from a wound in his temple. His wife Jane was discovered in bed, unconscious and near death. The neighbours sent for a doctor, who diagnosed Jane as suffering from delirium tremens. She died the following day, from exhaustion and starvation. It was reported that William's brother had brought him £140 a fortnight ago, his share of a bequest; 'the unfortunate man and his wife appear to have at once entered upon a career of absolute and utter drunkenness', as one newspaper put it, reporting that very little money had been found in the house. At the inquest the coroner heard that Jane had told the workhouse surgeon that William had fallen and cut his head on the fender, but that she had been unable to move him or get help. She also admitted to drinking heavily, as much as 30 shillings worth in a day, a revelation which caused a sensation at the inquest. Neighbours said these sprees were common, with the Feasts staying home until their money ran out, on one occasion for six weeks; they had assumed that this was 'only another Feast drinking bout', and so had been slow to investigate. The jury were unable to say if William's death was an accident; the children were taken into the care of the workhouse.[101]

This tragic case is very much the antithesis of the idea underpinning temperance savings. Instead of investing the money saved from drinking in order to amass a significant sum for future security, a sudden windfall spent on drink had led to death and the workhouse. The Feast story sounds like a temperance tale; in fact, it almost reads like an acting-out of parts of Cruikshank's *The Bottle*.[102] Newspapers reported that Feast 'had been dismissed for drunkenness five times', much as the father is discharged for drinking in the second plate of Cruikshank's series; the inquest jury might have wondered whether William's death was the result of 'brutal violence', the

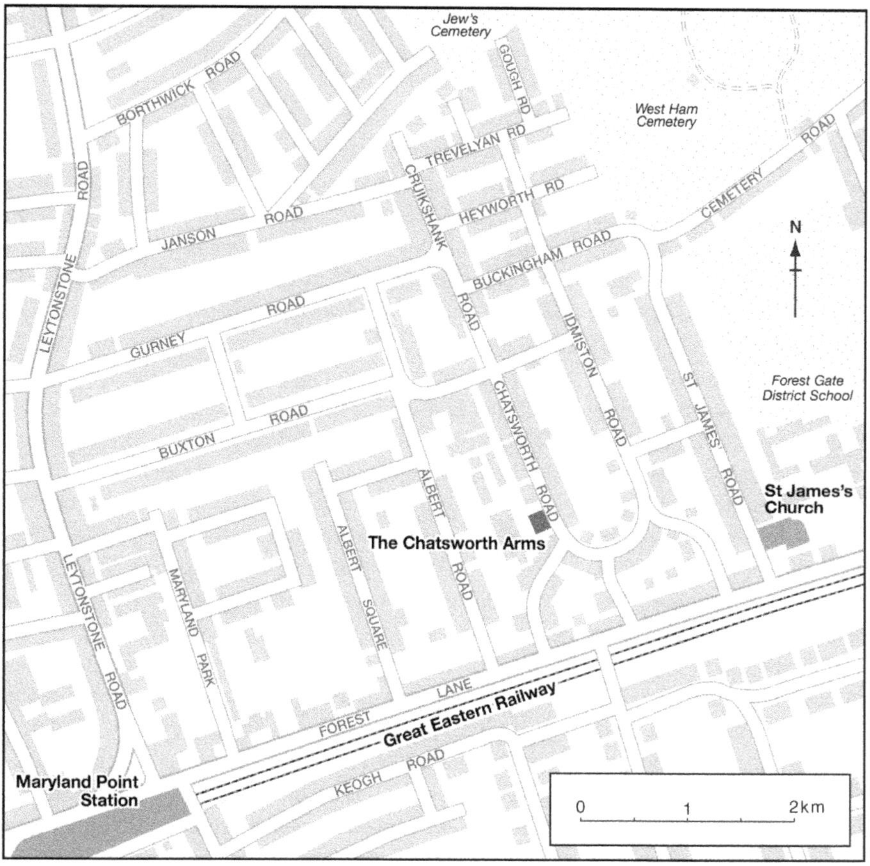

Map 2.3 The Temperance and Permanent Building Society estate, Forest Gate.

Source: Crown Copyright and Landmark Information Group Limited (2025). All rights reserved. Redrawn by Miles Irving, UCL Department of Geography from the Ordnance Survey 25″ map, 1896.

theme of the sixth plate, rather than an accident.[103] But while Cruikshank was still alive, and still famous, when the Feasts drank themselves to death, none of the reports of the Feast case note the unhappy irony of the family's address. It seems likely that the fact that these roads had been built by the collected savings of teetotalers only a decade or so earlier had already been forgotten.

The Feast case also tells us something about the place of drink in this neighbourhood. The census, conducted three months earlier, shows that the Feasts' neighbours were in lower-middle-class and working-class occupations, with some wealthier families in the larger villas; there were many clerks – some employed, like William, by railway companies – but also farm labourers, carpenters and machinists.[104] Despite the apparent respectability of the area, the Feasts' sprees were obviously not particularly noteworthy, and their neighbours seem to have been unwilling to get involved in a private tragedy until it became clear that the children were not being cared for. While domestic drinking might remain hidden from observers, it could also be tolerated when it was discovered, treated as a private matter that only became a public issue when a crime was committed.[105]

The census, and the details of the Feast's drinking, also made it clear that this 'Maine-law estate' could not keep alcoholic drink at bay. The head of the household next door to the Feasts was a brewer's servant – the owners of these houses were unlikely to police the occupations of their tenants. And while there was no pub on the estate, the Chatsworth Arms on Chatsworth Road was a few minutes' walk from the Feasts' cottage and may have been where the eldest child, Jane, was sent for 'six-pennyworths of rum', as she told the coroner.[106] A newspaper reported that Jane told a neighbour, 'Mother, has made a pocket in my jacket to hide the gin-bottle in.'[107] While the coroner instructed the jury to disregard the ten-year-old's confused testimony, the inquest also heard that her mother had been unable to walk, suggesting that her daughter was bringing her drink after William had died. The sensational reporting of the Feast's story drew on familiar figures long associated with arguments about drink and temperance: the 'child messenger', the focus of temperance concern well into the twentieth century, and the 'secret drinker', often a woman, who drank in private.[108] The reporting of Jane and William's deaths brought together a rich complex of ideas about drinking, respectability, privacy, shame and secrecy, seemingly without prompting any discussion of the temperance associations of their address.

Beyond the street names there is nothing visible in this part of East London today to suggest that temperance finance had built this estate of houses; there is an off licence on Cruikshank Road. Temperance enclaves took different forms between 1840 and 1918, from dry model towns and the Pennine 'landscape of dissent' to the TPBS's Stratford estate, which quickly became invisible as London grew. Temperance business archives allow these more ephemeral traces of temperance lives to be found, sometimes in unexpected places, and in this way also suggest that temperance might itself be something that flowed and ebbed, or survived alongside other currents in Victorian and Edwardian social life, rather than a campaign that came to an abrupt stop.

Notes

1. Brian Harrison and Barry Trinder, *Drink and Sobriety in an Early Victorian Country Town: Banbury 1830–1860* (Harlow: Longmans, 1969); J. M. Vieira Paisana, 'Tipplers, Drunkards and Backsliders: The Temperance Movement in England 1830–72, Including a Case Study of Lincoln', PhD thesis, Universidade do Minho, Braga, 2002; David Beckingham, *The Licensed City: Regulating Drink in Liverpool* (Liverpool: Liverpool University Press, 2017).
2. For Cornwall, see Adrian R. Bailey, David C. Harvey and Catherine Brace, 'Disciplining Youthful Methodist Bodies in Nineteenth-Century Cornwall', *Annals of the Association of American Geographers* 97, 1 (2007), 142–57, and David C. Harvey, Catherine Brace and Adrian R. Bailey, 'Parading the Cornish Subject: Methodist Sunday Schools in West Cornwall, c. 1830–1930', *Journal of Historical Geography* 33, 1 (2007), 24–44. For Cardiff, see Martin Daunton, *Coal Metropolis. Cardiff 1870–1914* (Leicester: Leicester University Press, 1977).

3. Elspeth King, *Scotland Sober and Free: The Temperance Movement, 1829–1979* (Glasgow: Glasgow Museums and Art Galleries, 1979).
4. Ischei, *Victorian Quakers*, 169.
5. Martin Purvis, 'Popular Institutions', in *Atlas of Industrializing Britain, 1780–1914*, edited by John Langton and R. J. Morris (London: Routledge, 1986), 194.
6. Mcallister, *Demon Drink*, n.p.
7. Andrew Davison, '"Try the Alternative": The Built Heritage of the Temperance Movement', *Brewery History* 123 (2006), 101; and see Peter T. Winskill, *The Temperance Movement and Its Workers: A Record of Social, Moral, Religious, and Political Progress*, vol. 3 (London: Blackie, 1892), 211–14.
8. Francis De Havilland Hall, *The Medical Examination for Life Insurance. With Remarks on the Selection of an Office*, third edition (Bristol: John Wright, 1903), 77.
9. Policy 11281, Sceptre Life Association Limited Policy Ledger 4, SC04/01/04, London Archives; C. W. Hawes, *Hawes' Handbook of Temperance Hotels 1888*, new edition (London: National Temperance Publication Depot, 1888), 14.
10. Shareholders' report of fourth annual general meeting, 20 March 1896, MS M618/1/1, Shareholders' report of fifth annual general meeting, 19 March 1897, MS M618/1/2, The Manchester Temperance Hotels Company Ltd., Manchester County Record Office; Winskill, *Temperance Movement*, vol. 3, 15; for the Barlow family see Francesca Moore, '"A Band of Public-Spirited Women": Middle-Class Female Philanthropy and Citizenship in Bolton, Lancashire before 1918', *Transactions of the Institute of British Geographers* 41 (2016), 149–62.
11. 'Women's Suffrage Meeting in Manchester', *Manchester Guardian*, 15 April 1896, 10.
12. *Manchester Guardian*, 10 November 1924, 13; 'Legal Notices', *Manchester Guardian*, 25 November 1942, 1; Advertisement, *Manchester Guardian*, 4 April 1943, 3.
13. Richard Dennis, 'The Geography of Victorian Values: Philanthropic Housing in London, 1840–1900', *Journal of Historical Geography* 15, 1 (1989), 40–54.
14. *Slater's Manchester Salford and Suburban Directory for 1903. Part 1: Topography and Street Directory* (London: Slater, 1903), 272.
15. R. B. Caverly and George Nugent Bankes, *Leading Insurance Men of the British Empire* (London: Index Publishing, 1892), 349.
16. Board meeting, 2 June 1841, UKT Minute Book 1, Aviva Archives.
17. See Board meetings, 6 August and 3 September 1841, UKT Minute Book 1, Aviva Archives.
18. *Slater's Manchester Directory, 1903*, 138.
19. *Slater's Manchester Salford and Suburban Directory for 1895. Part 2: Trades, Institutions, Streets, etc.* (London: Slater, 1895), 334, 110.
20. *Slater's Manchester Directory, 1895. Part 2*, 333–4.
21. Ibid., 334.
22. Ibid., 343.
23. Caverly and Bankes, *Leading Insurance Men*, 398.
24. Winskill, *The Temperance Movement*, vol. 2, 21.
25. Winskill, *The Temperance Movement*, vol. 3, 46; vol. 2, 199.
26. Shiman, *Crusade against Drink*, 156–69; Annemarie McAllister, 'The Alternative World of the Proud Non-Drinker: Nineteenth-Century Public Displays of Temperance', *Social History of Medicine and Drugs* 28, 2 (2014), 161–79.
27. Shiman, *Crusade against Drink*, 156.
28. Ibid., 164.
29. Ibid., 166.

30. *Kelly's Directory of the West Riding of Yorkshire, 1881. Part 1* (London: Kelly, 1881), 106–7; *Census of England and Wales, 1881, Preliminary report, and tables of the population and houses enumerated in England and Wales, and in the Islands in British Seas on 4th April 1881*, BPP 1881 XCVI [C.2955], 14.
31. Alan Latham and Jack Layton, 'Social Infrastructure and the Public Life of Cities: Studying Urban Sociality and Public Spaces', *Geography Compass* 13, e12444 (2019), 3.
32. Simon Gunn, *The Public Culture of the Victorian Middle Class* (Manchester: Manchester University Press, 2007).
33. McAllister, 'Alternative World', 163.
34. Sceptre sample.
35. Sonya O. Rose, *Limited Livelihoods: Gender and Class in Nineteenth Century England* (London: Routledge, 1992), 156–7.
36. England Births and Christenings, 1538–1975 (Film: 0093667-0093669), England Marriages, 1538–1973; 1871 Census (Class: RG10; Piece: 4153; Folio: 5; Page: 3; GSU roll: 18); England & Wales Death Index, 1837–2005 (vol. 8e; p. 188).
37. 'Padiham', *Blackburn Standard and North East Lancashire Advertiser*, 30 December 1876, 8; 24 April 1880, 8; 2 July 1881, 3; 29 July 1882, 3.
38. Benjamin Moore, *History of Wesleyan Methodism in Burnley and East Lancashire* (Burnley: Gazette Printing Works, 1899), 179, 178.
39. Winskill, *Temperance Movement*, vol. 3, 238.
40. Sceptre Life Association Limited Policy Ledger 2, LMA.
41. Register: Marriages 1858–80 (Page 24, Entry 48. Source: LDS Film 1471099).
42. 1881 Census (Class: RG11; Piece: 4159; Folio: 27; Page: 23; GSU roll: 783); 1891 Census (Class: RG12; Piece: 3375; Folio: 102; Page: 18; GSU roll: 92); 1901 Census (Class: RG13; Piece: 3876; Folio: 124; Page: 7; GSU roll: 34); 1911 Census (Class: RG14; Piece: 24876; Folio: 27; GSU roll: 71); England & Wales Death Index, 1837–2005.
43. Sceptre Life Association Limited Policy Ledger 5, London Archive; Register: Marriages 1849–1900 (Page 33, Entry 65. Source: LDS Film 1471152); 1891 Census (Class: RG12; Piece: 3389; Folio: 32; Page: 6; GSU roll: 46); 1901 Census (Class: RG13; Piece: 3898; Folio: 40; Page: 19; GSU roll: 139); 1911 Census (Class: RG14; Piece: 25470; GSU roll: 110); England & Wales Index of Wills and Probates, 1853–1943.
44. Moore, *History*, 196–200; *Blackburn Standard: Darwen Observer, and North-East Lancashire Advertiser*: 'Clitheroe', 10 March 1877, 6; 'The Darwen Observer', 4 May 1878, 8; 'Padiham', 29 July 1882, 3; 'District News', 2 December 1882, 3; 'Mission at Rishton', 22 June 1889, 7.
45. Thomas Whittaker, *Brighter England and the Way to It* (London: Hodder and Stoughton, 1891), 129.
46. P. Barrett, *Barrett's Trade Directory of Blackburn and District of 1896* (Preston: P. Barrett, 1896), 484–5, 490.
47. Cyril Pearce and Helen Durham, 'Patterns of Dissent in Britain during the First World War', *War & Society* 34, 2 (2015), 142.
48. Cyril Pearce, *Comrades in Conscience: The Story of an English Community's Opposition to the Great War*, second edition (London: Francis Boutle, 2014); David Fahey, 'Arthur Sherwell (1863–1942): Temperance Reformer and Liberal MP', *Social Science Review* 98, 2 (2002), n.p.

49. Philip Snowden, *An Autobiography. Volume I, 1864–1919* (London: Ivor Nicholson and Watson, 1934), 40.
50. Keith Laybourn, *Philip Snowden: A Biography 1864–1937* (Aldershot: Temple Smith, 1988), 9–10, 44–8.
51. Jill Liddington and J. Norris, *One Hand Tied behind Us: The Rise of the Women's Suffrage Movement* (London: Virago, 1978); Patrick Joyce, *Work, Society and Politics: The Culture of the Factory in Later Victorian England* (Brighton: Harvester Press, 1980); Linda McDowell and Doreen Massey, 'A Woman's Place?', in *Geography Matters! A Reader*, edited by Doreen Massey and John Allen (Cambridge: Cambridge University Press, 1984), 128–47; Jane Mark-Lawson, Mike Savage and Alan Warde, 'Gender and Local Politics: Struggles over Welfare Policies', in *Localities, Class and Gender*, edited by The Lancaster Regionalism Group (Pion: London, 1985), 195–215; Carolyn Steedman, *Landscape for a Good Woman: A Story of Two Lives* (New Brunswick: Rutgers University Press, 1997).
52. Liddington and Norris, *One Hand Tied behind Us*, 240.
53. Cyril Pearce, 'A Landscape of Dissent: Topography and Identity in Three Pennine Valleys', *Landscapes* 3, 2 (2002).
54. *History of Teetotalism in Devonshire* (Devonport: W. Hunt and J. Pasco, 1841), iii.
55. Asa Briggs, *Victorian Cities*, third edition (Berkeley: University of California Press, 1993), 371–2.
56. Robert Newton, *Victorian Exeter, 1837–1914* (Leicester: Leicester University Press, 1968), xiv
57. B. Le Messurier, *A History of the Mint Methodist Church, Exeter* (Exeter: Trustees, Mint Methodist Church, 1962), 22.
58. Allan Brockett, *Nonconformity in Exeter, 1650–1875* (Manchester: Manchester University Press, 1962), 200, 232.
59. Anon., *History*, 79, 82.
60. Advertisement, *Bristol Temperance Herald* IV, 1 (January 1840), 8.
61. Anon., *History*, 81.
62. Ibid., 88, 38.
63. *Woolmer's Exeter and Plymouth Gazette*, 22 January 1853, 4; *Trewman's Exeter Flying Post or Plymouth and Cornish Advertiser*, 3 March 1853, 3 and 11 March 1858, 4.
64. Anon., *History*, 88; Meeting, 20 December 1841, Minutes of the Standing Committee 1, Aviva Archives.
65. Board meeting, 5 May 1848, UKT Minute Book 1, Aviva Archives.
66. *Trewman's Exeter Flying Post*, 18 March 1858, 8.
67. Board meeting, 6 May 1841, and Annual Report, 2 January 1844, UKT Minute Book 1, Aviva Archives.
68. *Trewman's Exeter Flying Post*, 27 January 1853, 1.
69. Board meeting, 5 December 1845, UKT Minute Book 1, January 1841–April 1849, Aviva Archives.
70. Sceptre Life Association Limited Policy Ledgers 2, 4 and 5, London Archives; My Primitive Methodists, www.myprimitivemethodists.org.uk/content/people-2/primitive_methodist_ministers/a-2/alcock-henry-josiah-b1838.
71. John Plunkett and Jill A. Sullivan, 'Fetes, Bazaars and Conversaziones: Science, Entertainment and Local Civic Elites', in *Popular Exhibitions, Science and Showmanship, 1840–1910*, edited by Joe Kember, John Plunkett and Jill A. Sullivan (Pittsburgh: University of Pittsburgh Press, 2015), 46; *Whites' History, Gazetteer & Directory of Devon, 1878–79* (White: London, 1878–9), 390, 415.

72. Newton, *Exeter*, 179.
73. Ibid., 202.
74. Ibid., 108, 201, 319, 192, 202–4.
75. 'Exeter Temperance Society', *Western Times*, 4 April 1871, 2.
76. 'Temperance Demonstration', *Western Times*, 15 July 1873, 5.
77. 'Exeter Provident Temperance Society', *Trewman's Exeter Flying Post*, 4 February 1880, 7.
78. *Cornwall Royal Gazette, Falmouth Packet and Plymouth Journal*, 16 September 1842, 3; W. Harpley, 'Edward Vivian, M.A.', *Transactions of the Devonshire Association for the Advancement of Science, Literature and Art* 25 (1893).
79. Harpley, *Woolmer's Exeter and Plymouth Gazette*, 17 January 1857, 7.
80. 'Torquay. Poultry Exhibition', *Western Times*, 22 January 1853, 7.
81. Ibid.
82. *Western Times*, 14 November 1846, 6.
83. *Woolmer's Exeter and Plymouth Gazette*, 17 July 1841, 1; Edward Vivian Letters, January 1882, HPH115 AR 3217, Torquay Museum.
84. *Morning Post*, 2 July 1860, 3; *The Standard*, 24 September 1883, 3.
85. Board meeting, 11 December 1846 and Annual Report, 1 January 1847, 2, UKT Minute Book 1, Aviva Archives.
86. Meeting, 8 February 1842, Minutes of the Standing Committee 1, Aviva Archives.
87. *Daily News*, 9 April 1861, 2; Edward Vivian Letters, 14 February 1889, HP G76 AR 3324.
88. See, for example, Edward Vivian Letters, December 1883, HP L16 (xii) AR 3305.
89. *Woolmer's Exeter and Plymouth Gazette*, 29 May 1841, 3; *Western Times*, 29 May 1841, 1.
90. *The Standard*, 30 December 1844, 1; *Leeds Mercury*, 28 February 1852, 1; *Western Times*, 7 January 1854, 7; *Royal Cornwall Gazette, Falmouth Packet, and General Advertiser*, 14 July 1865, 7; 16 June 1865, 5; and 18 August 1865, 6.
91. *The Times*, 2 July 1868, 5.
92. *Bury and Norwich Post, and Suffolk Standard*, 18 June 1889, 7.
93. Victor Bailey, 'In Darkest England and the Way Out', *International Review of Social History* 92 (1984), 133–71; Victor Bailey, 'Salvation Army Riots, the "Skeleton Army" and Legal Authority in the Provincial Town', in *Order and Disorder in Modern Britain: Essays on Riot, Crime, Policing and Punishment* (London: Breviary Stuft, 2014), 16–33.
94. See James Kneale, 'The Battle of Torquay: The Late Victorian Resort as Social Experiment', in *Coastal Cultures of the Long Nineteenth Century*, edited by Matthew Ingleby and Matthew Kerr (Edinburgh: University of Edinburgh Press, 2018), 79–97.
95. *Royal Cornwall Gazette Falmouth Packet, Cornish Weekly News, & General Advertiser*, December 14, 1893, 4; *Trewman's Exeter Flying Post*, 1 April 1893, 8.
96. Richard Clarke, 'Self-Help, Saving and Suburbanization: The Birkbeck Freehold Land and Building Societies, Their Bank, and the London Mechanics' Institute 1851–1911', *London Journal* 40, 2 (2015), 123–46.
97. Adverts, *Daily Telegraph*, 18 July 1864, 7; *Daily Telegraph*, 12 May 1870, 10; *The Times*, 9 April 1884, 16.
98. 'Stratford & West Ham', *Essex Standard*, 25 August 1858, 2.
99. Cited in Price, *From Queen to Queen*, 33.

100. *Newcastle Courant*, 20 May 1842, 2.
101. 'Supposed Murder At Ilford', *The Standard*, 10 July 1871, 6; 'Supposed Murder At Ilford', *Bath Chronicle and Weekly Gazette*, 13 July 1871, 7; 'Shocking Death of a Man and His Wife at Forest Gate', *Chelmsford Chronicle*, 14 July 1871, 8; 'Accidents and Offences', *John Bull*, 15 July 1871, 14.
102. George Cruikshank, *The Bottle. In Eight Plates* (London: Spottiswoode and Shaw, 1847), Wellcome Collection.
103. 'Accidents and Offences', *John Bull.*
104. 1871 Census (Class: RG10; Piece: 1629; Folio: 74; Page: 25; GSU roll: 133).
105. James Kneale, 'The Place of Drink: Temperance and the Public, 1856–1914', *Social and Cultural Geography* 2, 1 (2001), 43–59.
106. 'Shocking', *Chelmsford Chronicle.*
107. 'Accidents and Offences', *John Bull.*
108. Amelia Bonea, Melissa Dickson, Sally Shuttleworth and Jennifer Wallis, 'The Woman Secret Drinker in the Late Nineteenth-Century Press', in *Anxious Times: Medicine and Modernity in Nineteenth-Century Britain* (Pittsburgh, PA: Pittsburgh University Press, 2019), 119–48; David Beckingham, 'Private Spirits, Public Lives: Sober Citizenship, Shame and Secret Drinking in Victorian Britain', *Journal of Victorian Culture* 26, 3 (2021), 419–34; Dias-Lewandowska and Lock, 'Women, Home, and Alcohol'.

Part 2

Temperance Life Insurance as Speculative Venture and Social Experiment, 1840–50

3

Experiments: Thin and watery and mentally cranked

Introduction

The first section of this book examined the place of the UKT and other temperance life assurance firms within British temperance, tracing its radical and commercial imperatives and locating insurance businesses, employees and policyholders in their local contexts. The most important English firms – the UKT, Sceptre and Whittington – were well established by the end of the century, by which point the principle of giving preferential treatment to abstainers because of their longevity was no longer controversial within life assurance across the Anglophone world.

When the UKT's founders looked back at its history forty or fifty years after the office opened, however, their memories were largely of the difficulties the firm experienced in its first decade. Theodore Compton, the UKT's first secretary, recalled the problems caused by 'the inveterate jealousies of the two London temperance societies'.[1] By this Compton meant the divisions within the New British and Foreign Temperance Society (NB&FTS) which had led to the formation of the British and Foreign Society for the Suppression of Intemperance (B&FSSI) as a breakaway grouping. In 1840 Henry Neave Rickman wrote to Robert Warner to say that the B&FSSI could not support the UKT because assuring teetotalers who had previously been 'habitual drunkards' could only mean that 'the project will be ruinous ultimately'. Rickman also made it clear that the row over short and long pledges had made it impossible for the B&FSSI to work with the UKT; when William Janson, one of the UKT's founders, had lost the role of treasurer of the NB&FTS in 1839 as a consequence of this argument, it had been Rickman who had informed Janson of this.[2] He reiterated his criticisms of the UKT's 'premature' and 'unsafe' scheme at a public meeting intended to promote the office, saying he hoped the founders 'might not involve themselves and others by *proving experimentally* that his fears were groundless'.[3] Differences of principle, and perhaps personality, put the UKT at odds with other temperance institutions, making it a risky experiment.

Compton remembered other problems. The UKT had been 'publicly denounced by a preacher, who held that all provision for the future was contrary to the Gospel, and that Christians ought to have nothing to do with life assurance', and when around £1,500 of the UKT's surplus funds went missing after having been 'placed in the hands of a party supposed to be abundantly safe', Compton and the directors had to cover this loss themselves. Perhaps not surprisingly, in 'the panic and the troublous [*sic*] times of 1848 … Mr. Janson often came to the office and talked to me about giving it up'. Compton did eventually resign in 1851, later noting that the firm had become so successful that 'it can now vote its directors annually more than it paid its first secretary for ten years of anxious and responsible toil'. Compton congratulated his friend Robert Warner, who had 'stuck to his ship' through these 'troubled waters' and could now 'enjoy sailing with a steady breeze and under a sunny sky'.[4] Warner remembered additional problems, however: the forcing out of founding director James Ellis, and 'the meeting in the Chapel in London Wall to determine whether the Institution was to be continued or broken up', probably before the decision was taken to open the General section in 1847. 'To be, or not to be, was the question', Warner remembered, 'and we only succeeded by a very few votes', including those of Mrs Warner and her cook, who travelled into London to vote with other members.[5]

Compton and Warner remembered the UKT's first years as a difficult trial. Unreliable directors undermined the company's security and reputation at the centre of its burgeoning network, while other teetotalers cast doubt on the firm's financial stability, its commitment to assuring 'reclaimed drunkards' and its claims to Christian piety. These issues, specific to the first temperance assurance company, were compounded by a set of tensions endemic to life assurance in general, identified very clearly by Timothy Alborn:

> Many different walks of life needed to come together to develop a market and deliver life insurance to that market. It would be a mistake to imagine that such a heterogeneous mix of people could work together seamlessly … Directors preached profits, actuaries preached caution, branch secretaries preached energy, and salesmen preached whatever they thought would convince a prospective customer to buy insurance.[6]

These actors followed their own, sometimes competing, logics. Directorial promotion of the firm might come up against actuarial caution; commissions on sales incentivized agents to 'push' policies, potentially admitting poor lives into the firm. Applicants for life assurance might also be dishonest about their health or their family history, leading to what is known as 'adverse selection', where the sick are more likely to seek life assurance than the healthy. As the US physician Jonathan Adams Allen put it in his handbook for medical examiners in 1867, 'Too often the applicant is induced to apply for assurance, by selfconsciousness of his indulgence in some pernicious method of excitement, which he knows tends to shorten life, but which he vaguely believes he can abandon or control before it is too late … Very few will voluntarily admit either intemperance, gluttony, or other generally recognized vice'.[7]

These difficulties were compounded by distance. A large, national firm could not expect applicants to visit the London office, so local agents and medical referees had to act on the board's behalf; directors had to manage a large number of people scattered across Britain and beyond, connected by letters, forms, trains and steamships. The examination of applicants at a distance required firms to standardize the process by which decisions are made, creating shared communities of practice. 'The drive for rigor and standardization', notes Theodore Porter, 'arose in response to a world in which local knowledge had become inadequate'.[8] The mutual surveillance of agents, directors, medical referees and policyholders could be done at a distance, through the circulation of standardized measures of health, promising 'mechanical objectivity'. This required work, but it also brought new possibilities; as Susan Shapiro notes, 'agents bridge the social and physical distances that otherwise limit social exchange. Agents incite and facilitate collective forms of action'.[9] Chapter 4 will examine the ways in which the UKT achieved this through building a network of people and material things.

This network was also designed to create trust in the firm and its ability to organize its affairs and protect its members. The legal principle of *uberrima fides* (utmost good faith) is meant to ensure that assurance firms and customers can trust one another; trust makes insurance possible. However, Luis Lobo-Guerrero suggests it makes more sense to see trust as something that *emerges from* networks, 'not a given but an outcome of the insurance relationship. It is actively and continuously produced through the faithful interaction between client and insurer and its effect is a reputation that could be considered as capital for future insurance transactions'.[10] Trust is not a singular, external thing, rather Foucauldian 'orders of trust' are produced locally within particular sets of relationships. Life assurance firms attempt to compel applicants to be truthful about their health; applicants look to regulators to force firms to tell the truth about their products; and both look to other agents – particularly courts – to produce binding truthful outcomes in case of disagreement.

Tensions between different elements of the market for temperance life assurance were also compounded by the nature of assurance as a speculative enterprise – 'insurance produces new anxieties and uncertainties; it is a risk in and of itself', as Kate Booth and Andrew Harwood remind us – and in this case by the novelty that was teetotalism.[11] The practices of mutual surveillance and mechanical objectivity described above were built into the UKT's business in order to create trust and support the market it was building. As James Taylor noted with reference to nineteenth-century joint stock companies, few investors had 'direct knowledge of, or contact with, boards of directors. Reputation and appearance were thus crucial to a company's success'.[12] The mechanisms developed to build trust – the publication of balance sheets, increased scrutiny by auditors and the financial press – emphasized public accountability. The UKT was concerned for its reputation, as we will see. However, it could also count on the support and assistance of sympathetic teetotalers, who might informally monitor agents, doctors, or assured lives, some of whom would have been fellow members of their local temperance societies. At the same time, the business's effectiveness and reputation could suffer from the problems associated with the ongoing rivalries and disagreements within this temperance world.

This chapter explores the course the UKT's speculative experiment took in its first decade, considering the precarious context of London's assurance firms in the 1830s and 1840s. Given that other life assurance companies were suspicious of the UKT, seeing its directors as 'wild enthusiasts and teetotal fanatics', it seems likely that the firm seemed shakier than most.[13] Having explored the UKT's problems with two of its directors, the chapter then goes on to see how it took action to deal with problems of fraud at the margins of the firm's business, the charges made by the influential minister Joseph Barker and the lives of Barker and a drunken Baronet. We turn first to the financial instability of the early Victorian period and the marginal nature of temperance insurance within an already uncertain sector and city.

'Wild enthusiasts' in the city of unlimited paper

In December 1840, just as the UKT was advertising its founding, the Independent West Middlesex Fire and Life office collapsed, its directors absconding with nearly a quarter of a million pounds of investors' money after only four years of business. The firm fitted out lavish offices on Baker Street, promised low premiums for policyholders and generous commission rates for agents and listed highly respectable gentlemen directors and patrons on its advertising materials – who turned out to be entirely fictitious. The fraud, which inspired Dickens's 'Anglo-Bengalee Disinterested Loan and Life Assurance Company' in *Martin Chuzzlewit* (1843–4), turned on what James Taylor calls the 'simulation of solidity and respectability'.[14] It led to closer scrutiny from government, the press and the life assurance industry, a parliamentary enquiry and the (ineffective) Joint Stock Companies Act 1844.[15] The market seemed oversaturated; remembering this period two decades later, Theodore Compton suggested, 'Life Offices were now set on foot faster than the public were prepared to follow them.'[16] Indeed only fifty of the eighty firms established between 1841 and 1850 survived until 1900.[17] There were other significant failures thirty years later, with the collapse of the Albert (1869) and the European (1871), which had both absorbed dozens of other offices; their failure 'cast a pall over British life insurance for another decade'.[18] And while the Life Assurance Companies Act 1870 provided stronger regulation, much closer scrutiny of firms and controls on marketing, further closures meant that life assurance would be associated with sudden failure for another decade.[19]

These crises took place against a wider backdrop of national financial uncertainty. Repeated cycles of speculation and panic caused regular bank failures and economic depression in Britain in 1836–7, 1846–7, 1856–7, 1866, 1878 and 1890, despite the apparent prosperity of the mid-Victorian period.[20] Some of those later crashes affected institutions very similar to the UKT and its rivals. The collapse of the Liberator Building Society in 1892, and the subsequent flight, extradition and trial of its director, Jabez Balfour, dragged his company's fraud and recklessness into the public eye.[21] The Balfour family had close connections to many important temperance institutions, including the UKT. James Dawson Burns, the author of the firm's unpublished company history, was Jabez Balfour's brother-in-law and one of the Liberator's directors, and Jabez Balfour's life was assured by the UKT, as we will see in Chapter 7. The Birkbeck Bank, established to support exactly the same kind of aspirational lower-middle- and working-class customers the UKT courted, experienced 'runs' on its funds in 1892 because of the collapse of the Liberator, and again in 1910, eventually failing in 1911.[22]

The financialization of Victorian culture brought a heightened awareness of and anxiety about the uncertainties of financial capital.[23] As the fungibility of money converted material things into numbers, and speculation then allowed those numbers to grow in value without any associated production of material things, others besides Marx and Engels noted that all that was solid in Victorian life threatened to melt into air. Garrett Ziegler has argued that the financial journalist John Hollingshead's 1857 essay 'The City of Unlimited Paper' linked anxieties about the dangerous insubstantiality and volatility of finance to the emptying out and rebuilding of the City of London in the middle years of the century. The City was 'continually transformed in response to the reordering of the institutional forms of banking in the national space economy of the nineteenth century', as Ian S. Black puts it.[24] The UKT sought a new place for its offices within this changing landscape, moving in 1854 to a reassuringly solid building at the end of London Bridge designed to communicate the firm's stability to its neighbours in the City of London (Chapter 6). As Liz McFall and Francis Dodsworth explain,

> Standard devices for laying claim to the strength of a company were references to the eminence of the board of directors, the number of policies held, the financial resources of the company and its antiquity ... A grand office, preferably one located close to the financial or legal heart of the City, was proof of the real basis of these statements, locating their propaganda in the real and tangible, rather than the inflated and ethereal.[25]

In its first decade, though, the UKT was threatened both from within, by the troubled finances of its own directors and agents, and perhaps by the 'reformed drunkard', and from without, by temperance criticism. The chapter takes each of these issues in turn.

Private feelings and public duty: James Ellis and James Day

The UKT could not afford to give the impression that it was anything other than a respectable business, so the financial failure of two of the firm's guarantors in 1841 and 1845 could well have been fatal for the firm, given that the fortunes of these respectable gentlemen were meant to secure the firm against financial disaster. These stories demonstrate the importance of networks of news and of reputation.

James Ellis was a founding director of the UKT, held one of the first three policies it issued and chaired the first board meeting in January 1841.[26] Between 1838 and 1840 he was a director and sub-treasurer of the NB&FTS and secretary of the Society's South London Auxiliary.[27] He would have sat on the NB&FTS executive committee with Janson and Warner and was clearly a trusted friend; early meetings discussing the founding of the UKT were held at Ellis's home in South London.[28] Within a year of those first meetings, however, Ellis was no longer a director, disappearing from the firm's records.

Robert Warner later remembered that Edward Fox, Compton's assistant, returned from 'the straw plait country' – probably Bedfordshire – in the summer of 1841 to report 'that he could do no business there while Mr Ellis was on the board, he being an uncertificated bankrupt from that part of the country'.[29] It was the same in the northwest; Fox had found support for the office in Manchester, Liverpool and Warrington, but 'a considerable amount of suspicion existed, and many enquiries are made respecting the nature and amount of the guarantee fund'.[30] In October Fox reported 'statements which had been made in his hearing, injurious to the Association, and involving the reputation of a gentleman on the Directors [*sic*]'. Compton told Ellis to resign from the board, as 'much prejudice exists against Mr Ellis, and that he did in 1829 or in 1825, make a declaration of insolvency'; confidence in the directors was felt to be 'essential to the stability of the public company'. Ellis had recovered from that insolvency, but in 1838 debts forced him to dissolve partnerships with Sarah Ellis and John Ellis, both drapers from Ampthill, Bedfordshire.[31] Compton expressed regret, but had 'faith that in matters where the property interests of members are concerned, private feelings *must* give way to public duty'. This was ratified by the board in November 1841.[32]

Ellis was one of the guarantors of the firm's finances, with liability for up to £5,000, and potential policyholders who knew about his earlier insolvency might well wonder if the UKT could not guarantee its own future, let alone theirs.[33] Ellis's reputation was at risk not only from the published reports of his bankruptcy and insolvency but also from gossip within business networks in the northwest and Bedfordshire. Ultimately his commitment to temperance was less important than his reputation as a businessman.

A similar situation arose four years later. One of the early directors of the UKT, James Day was present at the first full board meeting in January 1841 alongside Baker, Ellis and Warner, and it seems likely that he was also associated with the NB&FTS. His house at Richmond-upon-Thames hosted one of the London temperance meetings of the NB&FTS in its *Intelligencer* in 1839; in 1841 James was seventy, and his wife Sarah was seventy-five.[34] Day sat on the general board and the standing committee though his main role seems to have been acting as a trustee alongside Janson and Warner, securing the UKT's finances.

In February of 1844 the UKT advanced a £1,000 loan to Day, at 5 per cent interest; Warner also borrowed £1,000 in this board meeting, at the same rates, so this might not have been an unusual arrangement.[35] By September, however, the board had recalled Day's loan, and by October a lien was placed on his Richmond estate until the debt was repaid; in November the firm discussed taking their case to the Court of Chancery. Day filed for bankruptcy at the end of December, and a special meeting of the board was called to secure the institution's interests.[36] Less than a fortnight later Day died, after a short illness. The details of Day's bankruptcy are not discussed in the firm's records and the case seems to have received little attention, which the UKT must have been grateful for. The UKT recovered only some of the £1,708 he owed the firm, and the sum left for the directors to cover seems to have been significant – William Janson's share of the liability, paid in November 1846, came to £268 18s. Shares were sold and an additional guarantee fund was set up to cover any future demands on the UKT's funds made by Day's creditors.[37]

In the first five years of the UKT's life, one of the firm's guarantors had had to resign because of his past insolvency, while another died leaving the firm with substantial debts. Ellis and Day threatened the trust that was necessary for the firm to prosper and the finances of the firm and its fellow directors. As we will see in the next section, the problem of respectability also haunted the process of appointing agents.

Fraud at the margins: Limerick and Ipswich

The UKT experienced a churn of agents in its first years. At the end of 1840, for example, the grocer William Murgatroyd, the president of the Hull and East Riding Total Abstinence Society, was appointed the agent for Hull. Three months later the board noted that Murgatroyd had been declared bankrupt, immediately dismissing him from the agency.[38] That was easy to handle, but two cases of what seem to have been deliberate fraud proved more complicated.

The first, later described as an attempt at 'gross fraud', involved the firm's Limerick agent Patrick Lynch, who was appointed agent for the counties of Limerick, Clare, Kerry and Tipperary in 1841. In 1842 Lynch sent in a proposal from John Quilligan, who wished to assure his life for £300; less than a year later Lynch notified the office of Quilligan's death, informing the directors that the nominated beneficiary was a man named Stephen Roche. Policyholders, not agents, nominated their beneficiaries, and Roche should have been named *before* Quilligan's death; these irregularities prompted the board to send Compton to Limerick to investigate. On his return a month later, Compton reported that Lynch had issued only two other policies, for men named Ryan and O'Connell; unfortunately, these policies had 'been irregularly assigned to Mr Roche and P. O'Brien'. The UKT refused to accept Roche's claim on Quilligan's life and Roche's and O'Brien's other nominations, cancelling Ryan's and O'Connell's policies. In June 1843 the board placed an advertisement in the Limerick newspapers confirming Lynch was no longer acting as their agent. Threats of legal action and pleas for arbitration were ignored, Compton claiming to have 'abundant evidence' of fraud, and that seems to have been the end of Roche's claim and Lynch's agency.[39]

There is little more to be said about the Limerick case, but it prompted a visit from Compton, forcing him to miss a month of meetings, and it left the UKT wary of expanding into Ireland. They had appointed an agent in Belfast in 1840 and several more across the country in 1841–2, and Compton spoke in Cork to promote the company in December 1841.[40] In 1846, however, T. Parkes of the Temperance Society at Carlingford was told that 'at present the Board is not disposed to appoint agencies in Ireland' when he enquired about becoming an agent for the UKT.[41]

There were fraudulent agents closer to home, too. Ipswich had been introduced to total abstinence in 1836, and the UKT added it to its network with Richard Dykes Alexander, Joseph Mumford Burton and John Barker listed on the 1840 prospectus as country director, agent and medical referee respectively.[42] Alexander, a Quaker, banker, founder of the local Ragged School and keen photographer, was later described as 'one of the fathers in the Temperance cause' locally, opening a Temperance Hall in 1840 and publishing the monthly *Temperance Recorder* and the *Ipswich Temperance Tracts*.[43] Burton was an agent for a friendly society, a bookseller, stationer and printer; Barker, a surgeon, also promoted the UKT as an agent.[44]

Burton resigned his agency two months later, however, and was replaced by Isaac James Franklin in April 1841. Isaac was twenty-five in that census year; his occupation was not recorded though his father, also Isaac, was a clerk. In October Isaac was listed as the nominee for Richard Simmons's newly established policy for £600, but in June of 1842 the standing committee 'resolved that I. J. Franklin of Ipswich be discharged from the Agency'.[45] Two days later Compton, who had been in the town promoting the UKT, told the board that

> he had learned at Ipswich, that the Agent, Franklin, had attempted to defraud the Institution by insuring a bad life by impersonating the party by another man who was examined in lieu of the assured by the Medl. Referee. That he had made further enquiries since his return and found the assertion amply confirmed. Letters were read from the assured, Richard Simmons, declaring that he had never insured and had never been examined, and from J. Whittaker, who has seen Simmons, alleging similar facts.[46]

It seems likely that Franklin brought someone else to the referee's practice; Simmons was unaware of the deception. Compton returned to Ipswich with the firm's solicitor, Charles Gatliff, and 'having satisfied themselves of Franklin's guilt, had called upon him to give up the policy'. Franklin made a full confession, signing a £15 promissory note to cover expenses and asking the board not to prosecute. The board discussed the case 'with regard to the expediency of prosecuting [Franklin] for his fraudulent conspiracy', asking their local medical referee, John Barker, to visit Simmons 'and to obtain satisfactory evidence whether he is or is not the identical person he examined for the assurance'. By the end of June a new agent, John Sawer, had been appointed.[47]

Just as in the Limerick case, the best way to monitor, investigate and discipline individuals within the firm's networks was for Compton, the board's representative, to travel from the centre to the margins. In the Ipswich case it seems likely that someone else must have tipped Compton off about the fraud, presumably as he travelled through East Anglia speaking to local temperance societies. Both Franklin and Simmons would have had to be members of their local teetotal society to work for or join the UKT, and someone might have cast doubt on their membership. The UKT made quick use of its employees to negate the potential loss of £600, but it seems clear that the firm was only able to respond because its networks included individuals and societies that were effectively doing some of its work for it. However, in the case of Joseph Barker, who condemned the UKT as un-Christian swindlers, the firm's teetotal networks threatened to undermine its reputation.

'A mere swindling concern': Joseph Barker's libel

In September 1842 the UKT received an anonymous letter, 'stating that the *Christian Investigator*, a pamphlet said to be edited by Jos. Barker, of Gateshead, contained a libel upon the association'. In January this popular but heterodox preacher had published a piece on insurance in which he said: 'I would caution my readers against the Teetotal Life Insurance Association. Life Insurance Associations are all anti-Christian, whether teetotal or anti-teetotal, dissenting or conforming, and I hope the friends will be on their guard against them. The Teetotal Insurance Association is less worthy of regard than the rest. It is, in my judgement, a mere swindling concern.'[48] Barker asked, 'How can the managers tell who is teetotal and who is not? They can do no such thing', declaring 'I have no insurance office but God's own and I am well content. God's promises can never fail. I would advise all my friends to insure themselves with God, and to leave all other insurances, so called, to perish'.[49]

This echoed two established criticisms of life assurance: that companies could not accurately assess an applicant's health or habits, and that it was impious to put faith in actuarial statistics rather than God's providence.[50] In fact Barker was certain of the impiety of *all* attempts to save, stating, 'No one surely can imagine that hoarding money in Banks and Insurance Offices, in Benefit Societies, or Beneficent Funds, is laying up treasures in heaven … it is impossible for a man to do both. The man therefore who lays up for himself treasures on earth, must give up all hopes of having treasures in heaven.'[51]

God did not care for your earthly wealth. 'If you put it in Banks, the Banks may break; if you put it in Railways, the shares may become worthless … If you lodge it in Benefit Societies, they may fail, and even Insurances themselves are not secure.'[52] Barker criticized ministers who 'require stipulated salaries, and worldly securities. Their trust for the future is in Banks and Bonds, in Life Insurances and Beneficent Funds. They are anxious and distrustful; they shrink from the very thought of trusting in the providence of God'.[53] And for Barker life assurance companies, friendly societies and burial clubs were iniquitous because they did not help those most in need; 'Men are wanted that can *pay in*, and none must have relief who are not able to purchase it.'[54] Barker's criticisms were significant because they came from a man influential within nonconformist temperance circles. In fact, as Barker was preaching across the north of England in the first years of the UKT's life, for example in Bradford's temperance hall in November 1841, he might well have expressed these sentiments to exactly the people the firm was hoping to recruit.[55]

The UKT took the anonymous note very seriously; Compton wrote to the publisher threatening legal proceedings unless this libel was swiftly retracted. Two letters on the subject were read at the next meeting of the standing committee. The first was from James Backhouse of York (1794–1869), the Quaker missionary and botanist and cousin of Jonathan Backhouse of Darlington (1779–1842), one of the UKT's early patrons. Backhouse's letter contained further details of Barker's allegations from a Leeds man named Varley. The other letter was from Barker himself, who offered to publish 'some evasive remarks' – as the committee minuted it – rather than a retraction; the board instructed their solicitor to begin proceedings.[56]

Two weeks later the firm's agent in Bradford, George Halliday, wrote to say that as 'Barker's libel has done great injury' to the firm, he would have to resign if steps were not taken. The firm's counsel, Benjamin Rotch, thought a prosecution would be successful and 'might be of great service in advertising the institution', but he estimated that the expenses might amount to £120. Rotch thought a prosecution might not be necessary, 'as Barker was evidently a fanatic … and moreover the paper was about to become defunct'. In November the UKT placed advertisements in Bradford and Gateshead newspapers and in the *Temperance Advocate*, announcing that their counsel's opinion on Barker's libel 'is now in the hands of the Northern agents', presumably so those concerned could consult it for reassurance. This seems to have worked.[57]

Joseph Barker's dismissal of the UKT united older suspicions of insurance as un-Christian with radical criticisms of its failure to support those most in need. This episode may well have sown mistrust amongst potential policyholders, particularly in northern nonconformist communities. The UKT's connections with temperance workers in Bradford, York and Leeds – with Backhouse, Varley, Halliday and the author of the note sent in September – brought the issue to their attention. Unlike the Franklin case, though, these connections could work both ways; Halliday's threat to quit his agency reflected his rival obligations to the UKT and to Bradford's teetotalers.

The life of Joseph Barker, which we consider next, presents another opportunity to examine the radical roots of some aspects of temperance, but also to compare this with the more pragmatic, commercial attitudes of some of the directors of the UKT.

Temperance lives: Joseph Barker (1806–1875)

The son of a Yorkshire handloom weaver, Barker became a Wesleyan lay preacher before joining the Methodist New Connexion ministry. Winskill thought Barker was 'one of the first ministers in the country to adopt and publicly advocate [teetotal] principles' at Sheffield. He then became closely involved in the growing teetotal activity of Lancashire and neighbouring counties, and 'a tower of strength to the infant cause', as Winskill put it. Barker co-edited the *Star of Temperance* newspaper with the Reverend Francis Beardsall and – with Beardsall, Joseph Livesey, Dr Ralph Barnes Grindrod and others – was part of the group that met to discuss the formation of the British Temperance Association in 1835. He served on that society's committee and supported temperance efforts in Liverpool and North Wales. Thomas Whittaker, who moved in similar circles, described Barker as enjoying 'the esteem of the Christian world' when they met in 1837.[58]

However, Barker's heterodox views led to him being expelled from the New Connexion in 1841, by which point he was preaching on the Gateshead circuit, where Whittaker described him as 'almost idolized by the people. The pitmen and ironworkers drank in his words, and sat at his feet with joy and gladness'.[59] Winskill described the New Connexion as 'plunged into a state of great agitation by one who had been a very popular minister amongst them' by his expulsion, so much so that over 4,000 members were said to have followed him out of the Connexion.[60] His new church of 'Barkerites' in Newcastle upon Tyne gradually dwindled, but Barker's views continued to be disseminated in print. Having previously lectured against Owenite socialism, by 1846 Barker adopted radical views – republicanism, the nationalization of land, the confiscation of Church of England property and an independent Ireland – and was arrested for seditious libel after acting as a delegate to the 1848 Chartist convention, though the charges were dropped. Barker had supported the anti-slavery movement since the late 1820s, meeting Lloyd Garrison and Frederick Douglass in 1846, and his involvement grew after he emigrated to the United States in 1851. In the process, however, he lost his Christian faith, seeing the Bible 'as a proslavery document'.[61] This did not endear him to his Ohio neighbours, and he returned to England in 1860, where he slowly found his way back to Methodism.[62]

Winskill felt that Barker's turn to heresy and freethinking was the consequence of his persecution by 'the ministerial advocates of moderation' and 'influential members and officials of the denomination who were engaged in the liquor traffic'. For his part, Whittaker did not know whether Barker's freethinking was due to 'pride of intellect, or mortified ambition, or moral blindness', but he knew it had harmed the movement: 'Those who had followed and idolized him as a teacher of Christian truth seemed in thousands to turn from it as by common consent with him, and as amongst these there were many of our active teetotallers, religion and temperance suffered equally alike. Those two interests were put back for years.'[63]

Betty Fladeland suggests that Barker 'made extravagant claims for whatever his current cause or philosophy might be. Then, when he again became dissatisfied, his discouragement led to equally exaggerated attacks on whomever or whatever he blamed'. However, while he lost and refound his faith, and discovered Chartism, republicanism, abolition and other radical causes along the way, Barker's support for temperance never wavered. Thomas Whittaker met him again in Brooklyn in 1875, not long before Barker's death. Barker told Whittaker he regretted losing his faith, and congratulated Whittaker on doing only one thing – teetotalism – but doing it well. Whittaker reported Barker as saying, 'I have tried too much and done too little, and now the time of my departure is at hand, and it is too late to redeem much of the past.'[64]

Barker's life provides another reminder that temperance could form part of a wider set of unorthodox or radical ideas. It also reminds us that the UKT did not seek to challenge Barker on *theological* grounds, as other temperance organizations might well have done; instead, they focused on his accusation that they were swindlers and threatened to sue him for libel. As we will see in later chapters, the UKT was a commercial as well as a religious organization, and was quite capable of choosing secular means to promote temperance.

Reclaimed drunkards and other 'poor lives'

Directors, agents and external critics caused problems for the UKT in its early years, but the lives of the men and women the firm assured were also of concern. There were not enough of them, for a start, and new applicants were increasingly taking out smaller policies. After a strong first year, buoyed by the policies of patrons and influential teetotalers, the average sum assured for new policies in 1842 was only £68; while this rose to nearly £100 in 1845, it then fell again in 1846, the year in which the firm began to discuss how to secure its future (Table 3.1). It may also have been significant that the proportion of new policies issued for less than £100 reached 58 per cent in 1846; in fact, 28.3 per cent of new policies issued in 1846 were for less than £20.

The opening of the General section saw the average value of policies increase by over two-thirds between 1846 and 1847, as wealthier moderate drinkers joined the institution; moderate drinkers could not be assured for policies under £25.[65] The numbers of policies issued rose dramatically from 1848, while the proportion of policies established for under £100 fell. As the firm expanded smaller policies became a dwindling part of their business, though a Working Men's Section offered 'industrial'

Table 3.1 New policies established with the UKT, 1841–50

Year	Policies issued	Total sum assured, new policies (£)	New policy average value (£)	% of new policies under £100	% of new policies over £200
1841	255	31,185	122	25.5	28.2
1842	320	21,880	68	47.5	15.0
1843	344	29,045	84	42.7	11.9
1844	454	40,467	89	43.6	9.5
1845	490	48,010	98	48.9	13.3
1846	491	43,150	88	58.0	13.6
1847	273	40,576	149	30.4	26.7
1848	540	73,420	136	31.7	17.8
1849	910	145,305	160	27.0	26.8
1850	789	170,161	216	21.5	27.6

Source: 'Investments for the Working Classes', *Edinburgh Review* 95, 194 (1852), 416.

life assurance policies from £5 to £20 in return for weekly penny premiums between 1853 and 1875, in competition with specialist offices like the Prudential, Refuge and Pearl.[66] Details of these policies were not always reported, but the average size of new working men's policies ranged from just under £15 to just under £17 between 1859 and 1875; one surviving 1861 policy card in the firm's archives shows the sum assured as only £11 11s. 9d. Over the same period the average size of the firm's other policies had risen from £150 to £244.[67]

The small size – £10, £25 or £50 – of some of the earlier abstainers' policies suggests that the firm's intended market of teetotalers was made up of less affluent men and women. A significant number were established by women, many (but not all) assuring with their husbands. It seems likely that the smallest policies were seen as a form of burial insurance, Julie-Marie Strange concluding that in late Victorian Britain, 'even for those with relatively low earnings, burial insurance (also referred to as "life insurance") was a cheap investment'. Late Victorian and Edwardian assurers – from the Plasterer's Union and the Prudential to friendly societies like the Oddfellows, the Foresters and the teetotal Sons of Temperance – paid £10 or £12 for breadwinners' funerals, or between £15 and £20 for both spouses, though this would probably not cover the cost of the funeral.[68] It seems likely that a £10 or £25 policy established with the UKT in the 1840s would have been a similar investment.

The fear that Henry Rickman had identified in 1840, that the firm would attract 'reclaimed drunkards', ensured that the firm kept a close eye on their assured lives. As Alborn notes, firms could guard against 'bad' lives through surveillance by medical examiners and others at the point of sale, or by refusing to pay when policies were claimed. We will say more about these checks in later chapters, but the second strategy advertised the firm's prudence, creating trust. The case of a man named Thomas Wood provides a good example. Wood was probably assured in 1843, given his policy number, and died in 1847 or 1848, the firm receiving a claim for his £50 policy in January 1848. Noting that 'The certificate of abstinence was lacking', the firm made enquiries;

a report from their travelling agent, J. A. Smith, was received 'respecting the alleged intemperance of Thomas Wood deceased' and the claim was refused on account of Wood's drunkenness. Smith was given a guinea for his inquiries. Once again doubts at the centre were confirmed by an agent on the ground, probably with assistance from Wood's local temperance society, which would have been responsible for producing that certificate of abstinence.[69] Disciplining bad risks could provide good marketing material. At the fifth annual members' meeting in 1846 the directors reported a recent case: 'A female had assured her life for £50, and had subsequently fallen into intemperate habits. This being discovered, she was informed that the assurance was void. The policy was surrendered, and her last payment returned. Within a few weeks, she died.'[70]

It was not always easy to catch 'bad lives' when they first applied for assurance, however. Our final life in this chapter comes from a later period and was certainly not a temperance, or even a temperate, one. However, it shows what firms were trying to avoid and how some of the mechanisms already discussed allowed trust to be made and broken.

Temperance lives: Sir Richard Mansel Mansel (1850–1892)

Sir Richard Mansel Mansel was born in London in 1850, the son of Courtenay and Eliza Mansel, with one older brother and five sisters; the family's baronetcy was established in the reign of James I, and they owned substantial estates in England and Wales.[71] Despite this Richard died bankrupt at the age of forty-one, supported by the earnings his much younger second wife made on the music hall stage. Richard's life – noble, wealthy, scandal-ridden and decidedly intemperate – is rather different from those presented so far, but it offers an excellent example of the kind of life that assurance offices were trying to avoid.

In 1885 Mansel established a policy with the National Life Assurance, the firm that would later absorb the Whittington. He was re-examined in 1888, the medical officer tersely noting, '[He] shows signs of free alcoholic indulgence – bloated face, tremulous hands, dull in conversation. Should not have accepted him had we seen him at first. Accepted in 1885, on Dr Ogle's report for the Eagle, with 10 years. This amount will not cover the risk at present.'[72] The National had apparently been reassured by Dr Ogle's 1885 report for the Eagle office, which accepted him with an additional ten years, meaning that Richard, then thirty-five, would have been charged the premiums for a man of forty-five. The National's medical officer was certain those higher premiums would not cover the substantial claim that would follow Richard's early death. He was right to be concerned; Richard would be dead within four years.

Richard's life was already associated with drink and scandal. A court case over his father's will in 1875 shone an unflattering light on Richard's 'unwholesome and unhealthy life' as well as his father's consumption of whisky and morphia. This might have worried Richard's assurers – Pollock and Chisholm's *Handbook* for medical examiners noted that 'intemperance runs in families, who not only inherit the feebleness and nervous constitution which drunken parents transmit, but that peculiar temperament which flies to stimulants'.[73] Two years later, the London life assurance office charged Richard with obtaining his policy under false pretences because he had not told them that he had been declined by five other firms when he completed the National's proposal form. The fifth question asked for details of all of the applications made to other offices, and whether they were declined, or accepted with or without an increased premium. The Master of the Rolls reminded Richard that insurance relies on 'the utmost degree of good faith, *uberrima fides*' and found for the office, terminating Richard's policy.[74]

In 1878 Richard inherited his father's estates after challenging his brother's claim, marrying Maude Margaretta Bowen shortly after. Their son Courtenay was born in 1880.[75] Richard became Baronet Mansel in 1883, but within months had begun bankruptcy proceedings, with debts estimated at more than £50,000.[76] In the same year Maude and Richard divorced. Richard's estates near Wimbledon and Carmarthen were sold or mortgaged in 1885, the same year that he established his policy with the National.[77] Life assurance policies could act as security for a debt or loan, and Richard may have been trying to reassure his creditors, as the beneficiary would receive the policy when Richard died.

By May 1890 it had been established that Richard's assets more than covered his debts, and the following year Richard married again, this time to Ada Alice Lea, a music hall performer. Ada was born in Bethnal Green in 1866; her mother was a professional singer and teacher of music, and Ada was already a variety artist at ten. It was later said that she was a schoolmate of Lottie Collins, of 'Ta-ra-ra Boom-de-ay' fame. Under her stage name – 'Lily Ernest' – she performed as a singer, comedienne and actress, touring as Vesta Tilley's stand-in, though Ada was most famous as a skipping-rope dancer.[78] This was the era of the 'Gaiety Girl', and Ada's marriage was discussed alongside other performers who had married aristocrats, though she was clearly a principal performer in the music halls, rather than a supporting female player in musical comedies.[79] One publican's newspaper published an appreciative profile, with an illustration of 'My Lady of the Halls' dominating the front page.[80] It was reported that the new Lady Mansel was earning £40 a week at the Trocadero Music Hall; Richard, on the other hand, had begun insolvency hearings. His liabilities amounted to over £9,500, including £5,000 from his brief and ill-fated management of the Empire Theatre, Leicester Square.[81]

Richard moved to Brighton in 1892, developed pneumonia and died on the 3rd of June, aged forty-one. His father's will had been fought over by his children, and now Richard's was contested by his teenage son, Courtenay, though it turned out there was little left to divide between the heirs.[82] Ada went back to the stage. She toured the United States, sued a Liverpool hall for libel and fell afoul of Social Purity complaints in London before buying the Tivoli music hall in Bristol in 1899, but was bankrupt by 1912.[83] Her marriage to Richard brought unwanted attention, particularly in the United States. The 'Marquise De Fontency', Frederick Cunliffe-Owen, an English society journalist whose columns were syndicated in US newspapers, told his readers that Sir Richard had been 'a bankrupt and a drunkard', and 'a drunken spendthrift, whose extravagance resulted in the loss of the ancestral home of the family', while Ada

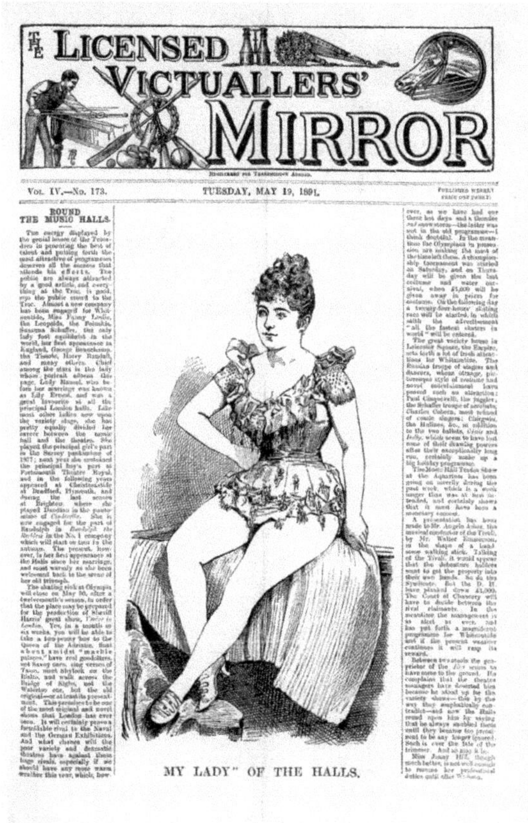

THE LICENSED VICTUALLERS' MIRROR

VOL. IV.—NO. 173. TUESDAY, MAY 19, 1891.

ROUND THE MUSIC HALLS.

"MY LADY" OF THE HALLS.

Figure 3.1 'Lily Ernest' (Ada Alice Lea).

Source: *Licensed Victuallers' Mirror*, 19 May 1891, 229. Content provided by THE BRITISH LIBRARY BOARD. ALL RIGHTS RESERVED. With thanks to The British Newspaper Archive (www.britishnewspaperarchive.co.uk).

had supported Richard and his son financially.[84] Ada died in Lambeth in March 1916 and was buried in Streatham Park Cemetery.[85]

Sir Richard Mansel's life was very different to those of the teetotalers we have considered so far; his was the kind of life most firms wanted to avoid. The National did not sell abstainer's policies until it took over the Whittington in 1891, but by the 1880s few firms wanted to insure 'free drinkers'. Richard presumably needed to keep his creditors happy and was prepared to lie to London Assurance to establish a policy and to then fool Dr Ogle, which brought him policies from the Eagle and the National. The legal principle of *uberrima fides* had saved the London office, but the National, Eagle and perhaps other firms probably had to pay up when Richard died. Trust had to be *established*, by medical examiners and directors and through the courts – Richard was in court, on and off, for seventeen years of his short life. Publicity was also effective, though in this case Richard served as a warning against immoderation. Nothing like a temperance life, Richard still provided an example of what could go wrong if an office trusted someone with an apparently sound reputation as a wealthy peer of the realm.

Conclusions: Networks of trust

Returning to the questions raised at the start of the chapter, it is clear that trust in the UKT in its first decade of business was not simply a matter of reputation and respectability, considered as the *external* conditions that made the firm's business possible, but something actively *made* within the network. For Çalişkan and Callon, the problem with many conceptualizations of trust is that 'it is used as an undifferentiated explanation of coordination that black-boxes maintenance operations and socio-technical devices'.[86] The elements that *make* trust should be our focus, in other words.

Historians have tended to focus on public respectability and reputation, and these were certainly important issues for the UKT. When Joseph Barker was challenged by the firm, for example, he 'confessed he knew nothing of the office, but that two of its patrons were about two of the most respectable men in the country'.[87] Speaking in 1845 at a meeting in York chaired by James Backhouse, just as the UKT was considering legal action against James Day, the firm's travelling agent James McKenna said that 'the strictest and most unreserved confidence might be placed in any life assurance institution based on sound principles and having honourable men as directors'.[88] And again, while it was struggling to work out how to cover Day's debts, the UKT ran an advertisement for 'funeral money' policies for as little as £10, with payments from sixpence per month, asking 'will you join an institution formed and supported by those manifest friends of the cause, the Eatons, the Alexanders, the Bowlys, the Heyworths, and a host of others, whose names, whose fortunes, and whose philanthropy are the guarantee of your security?'[89] Alexander, Bowly and Heyworth have already been mentioned in this chapter or the preceding chapters; Joseph Eaton was a wealthy Bristol iron manufacturer, another Quaker active in the campaign against slavery and a financial supporter of temperance.[90] Other patrons included James Silk Buckingham, Richard Tapper Cadbury, John Dunlop and Sir Culling Eardley Smith, though the popular Irish temperance leader Father Mathew twice declined to take on this role.[91] These directors and patrons were all influential teetotalers, and most were also wealthy men.

However, publicity could undermine respectability. Ellis's insolvency and Day's bankruptcy were made public through the *London Gazette*, one of the official mechanisms designed to generate trust in business, and Ellis's earlier business failures were also the talk of the North West and the 'straw plait country', this gossip presumably circulating through informal networks. When Compton told Ellis that the board's private feelings for him had to yield to their public duty to the firm's ordinary members, he drew a distinction between the public face of the firm and the dense social ties that bound its directors together as private individuals in overlapping networks of temperance and business.

Publicness was only one part of the solution to the distrust created by firms like the Independent West Middlesex, however, because most of the UKT's potential customers did not meet the firm's directors but contacted their local agents and medical referees, who might well have been strangers to them. The twenty-first-century policyholders interviewed by Booth and Harwood complained that their ties to insurers are weak, 'connected by strung-out, stretched-out ties to companies of the globalising ether'.[92] The UKT's solution to the mid-nineteenth-century version of this problem was to work through temperance organizations and individuals within the directors' social networks. Prospective policyholders and agents had to be members of their local temperance societies and would know each other through those connections. These were closer social ties than these applicants would have had with the firm's distant patrons or directors; even the local country directors would have been gentlemen of a much higher social class than the modest men and women who made up the bulk of the firm's early members. Trust in the UKT emerged out of members' networked relations with local agents, medical referees and other members of temperance societies, congregations, businesses and institutions. These social connections were also maintained through material things like letters and forms, as well as the medical instruments which became increasingly important for referees as they sought to convert applicants into quantities and qualities that could be understood at the London office.

Remembering Çalişkan and Callon's suspicion of the black box of trust, this section concludes by considering the challenges detailed in this chapter to see how the firm worked to produce trust and minimize distrust through its procedures, directing an *agencement* of people, objects and ideas necessary for this new market to work. The discovery that James Ellis had suffered earlier insolvency led the board to dismiss him; James Day's debts were partly recovered through the courts, with directors paying the remainder between them. The board created a new guarantee fund after the first case and set up an additional fund to cover future liabilities that might come to light from Day's bankruptcy. In both cases these actions made financial or legal sense, but they were also performative in the sense that they acted out the care and prudence that were necessary after the Independent West Middlesex fraud. Compton's investigation of the Limerick fraud followed a procedural problem noted in the London office. Travelling to Limerick and making enquiries locally allowed Compton to declare this a fraud; the firm refused the claim, severed their connection with Lynch and cancelled his agency's other policies. In Ipswich Compton again turned up suggestions of fraud as he met local temperance societies, ending the UKT's relationship with Franklin, the local agent. The claims of policyholders who had concealed their intemperance from the firm were refused because their policies had not been established in good faith, in line with existing insurance practice and the governing legal principle of *uberrima fides* (utmost good faith), though of course some intemperate applicants did slip through the net.

In each of these cases swift action was taken to sever connections with directors, agents and policyholders, and these decisions were often publicized in newspapers and temperance journals. However, the threat of legal action was required as an additional sanction in Limerick and Ipswich; it seems likely that Barker would have ended up in court had he persisted in libelling the firm, and firms did resort to the courts to defend their refusal to pay claims, as we will see in Chapter 7. Courts are more than just another public arena in which claims are made and heard, of course; they *coerce confessions* from participants, as Lobo-Guerrero points out, making 'orders of truth' for particular arrangements of people and things, with binding consequences for those involved, like Richard Mansel.[93]

Susan Shapiro noted, 'One of the ironies of trust is that we frequently protect it and respond to its failures by bestowing even more trust', creating second- and third-order trustees when the first order fails. She saw this 'inflationary spiral of escalating trust relationships' as a problem.[94] Certainly contemporary insurance is dogged with mistrust, but in the 1840s the UKT created sufficient trust in its business to allow it to build a market. Here Shapiro's 'inflationary spiral' looks more like the UKT successfully tinkering with its *agencement*, adding additional elements to oversee the firm when elements of the network broke or faltered: guarantees and guarantee funds; sections for drinkers and abstainers, with strict rules on transfers between them; more trustworthy agents and directors; newspaper adverts and notices; the *London Gazette* as an official record of business failure; and always, as a final measure, the courts as a site for compelling witnesses to confess, where binding truths and trusts are produced.

At its ninth Annual Meeting in January 1850, the UKT was happy to report that mortality remained under 1 per cent, 'notwithstanding the ravages of the cholera' – lower than the general UK mortality rate and around half that of other offices. Dr Jabez Burns moved a vote of thanks to the directors for their 'integrity and zeal'.[95] Integrity and zeal were crucial to the success of this experimental venture, as we will see in the next two chapters, but were enmeshed in social networks where close ties and personal reputation were more important than trust in a distant, abstract institution. James Day, James Ellis, Joseph Barker and the frauds in Limerick and Ipswich cast doubt on the integrity of individuals, and thus on the firm as a whole; the zeal of the board, as capitalists and teetotalers, threatened the prudence expected of a serious life office in the decade following the collapse of the Independent West Middlesex.

This was not a question, then, of trust in institutions being substituted for trust within relationships with known individuals. The UKT depended on dense networks of association – temperance societies, business relationships and personal friendships – but these were also often *distant* relations, mediated by print, forms and letters. These materials had to circulate effectively through the firm's networks, working as mutable mobiles from the firm's centre of calculation – its London office (Chapter 4). At the same time the firm's representatives could also be highly mobile (Chapter 5). The firm's success in managing this emerging *agencement*, and the trust it produced in the process, were not the result of decisive actions by the UKT's directors, inspired by 'one man's bright idea', either, though Warner and the others did take the credit for the successful working of this machinery.

Chapter 4 considers the role of numbers and calculation in the establishment of this market, and Chapter 5 looks to the building of the network through which these numbers travelled.

Notes

1. Theodore Compton, 'Early Days of the Temperance Provident Institution', reprinted from 'The Temperance Record', 30 June 1881, Single printed sheet, MS FL367, Aviva Archive.

2. Copy of letter sent by H. Rickman to Robert Warner, December 1840, MS FL357, Aviva Archives; Winskill, *Temperance Movement*, vol. 1, 231; vol. 2, 144.
3. 'United Kingdom Total Abstinence Life Association', *British & Foreign Temperance Intelligencer* 5, 21 February 1841, 59, emphasis added.
4. Compton, 'Early Days'.
5. Robert Warner, letter to Thomas Cash, 27 January 1896, MS FL368, Aviva Archives; Burns, Manuscript company history, 1896.
6. Alborn, *Regulated Lives*, 77.
7. Jonathan Adams Allen, *Medical Examinations for Life Insurance*, first edition (Chicago: Horton and Leonard, 1867), 10, 9.
8. Porter, *Trust in Numbers*, 93.
9. Susan P. Shapiro, 'The Social Control of Impersonal Trust', *American Journal of Sociology* 93, 3 (1987), 626.
10. Luis Lobo-Guerrero, 'Uberrima Fides, Foucault and the Security of Uncertainty', *International Journal for the Semiotics of Law* 26 (2013), 24.
11. Kate Booth and Andrew Harwood, 'Insurance as Catastrophe: A Geography of House and Contents Insurance in Bushfire-Prone Places', *Geoforum* 69 (2016), 44–52, 50.
12. James Taylor, 'Numbers, Character and Trust in Early Victorian Britain: The Independent West Middlesex Fire and Life Assurance Company Fraud', in *Statistics and the Public Sphere: Statistics and the People in Modern Britain, c.1800–2000*, edited by Tom Crook and Glen O'Hara (New York: Routledge, 2001), 186.
13. Peter T. Winskill, *The Comprehensive History of the Rise and Progress of the Temperance Reformation from the Earliest Period to September 1881* (Warrington: P.T. Winskill, 1881), 249.
14. Taylor, 'Numbers', 198, and see Liz McFall and Francis Dodsworth, 'Fabricating the Market: The Promotion of Life Assurance in the Long Nineteenth-Century', *Journal of Historical Sociology* 22 (2009), 30–54.
15. Alborn, *Regulated Lives*, 54–9.
16. Theodore Compton, 'The Temperance Provident Institution. Copied from the Weekly Record of Nov 8th, 1862', MS FL361, Aviva Archives.
17. Alborn, *Regulated Lives*, 55.
18. Hugh A. L. Cockerell and Edwin Green, *The British Insurance Business: History and Archives* (Sheffield: Sheffield Academic Press, 1994), 106; Alborn, *Regulated Lives*, 60–3, 62.
19. Alborn, *Regulated Lives*, 67–9.
20. Poovey, 'Economics and Finance'.
21. David McKie, *Jabez. The Rise and Fall of a Victorian Rogue* (London: Atlantic Books, 2004).
22. Clarke, 'Self-Help'.
23. Patrick Brantlinger, *Fictions of State: Culture and Credit in Britain, 1694–1994* (Ithaca, NY: Cornell University Press, 1996); Mary Poovey, *Making a Social Body: British Cultural Formation, 1830–1864* (Chicago: University of Chicago Press, 1995).
24. John Hollingshead, 'The City of Unlimited Paper', *Household Words*, 12 December 1857; Garrett Ziegler, 'The City of London, Real and Unreal', *Victorian Studies* 49, 3 (2007), 431–55; Ian S. Black, 'Spaces of Capital: Bank Office Building in the City of London, 1830–1870', *Journal of Historical Geography* 26, 3 (2000), 353.
25. McFall and Dodsworth, 'Fabricating the Market'.
26. *Good Templars' Watchword* 15, 779 (24 December 1888), 623, Aviva Archives; Board Meeting, 14 January 1841, UKT Minute Book 1, Aviva Archives.

27. Advert, *Temperance Intelligencer* 2, 87 (7 July 1838), 224; *Journal of the New British and Foreign Temperance Society* 2, 1 (4 June 1840); Advert, *Morning Chronicle*, 20 July 1839, 1.
28. Compton, 'Early Days'; 1841 Census (Class: HO107; Piece: 1086; Folio: 21; Page: 35; GSU roll: 1345); Meeting, 13 November 1840, Minutes of the Standing Committee 1, Aviva Archives.
29. Letter from Robert Warner to Thomas Cash, 2, Aviva Archives.
30. Meeting, 13 September 1841, Minutes of the Standing Committee 1, Aviva Archives.
31. *Morning Post*, 7 March 1838, 7; *Perry's Bankrupt Gazette*, 17 March 1838, 7.
32. Meeting, 11 October 1841, Minutes of the Standing Committee 1, original emphasis; Board meeting, 5 November 1841, UKT Minute Book 1, Aviva Archives.
33. Board meeting, 6 May 1841 and 2 June 1841, UKT Minute Book 1, Aviva Archives.
34. See, for example, *Livesey's Preston Temperance Advocate 1836–37 & Temperance Intelligencer 1838–40* 3, 139 (1839), 264; 1841 Census (Class: HO107; Piece: 1075; Folio: 9; Page: 11; GSU roll: 3079).
35. Board meeting, 2 February 1844, UKT Minute Book 1, Aviva Archives.
36. Board meetings, 6 September 1844, 4 October 1844, 1 November 1844, 8 November 1844, 15 November 1844; Petition filed for bankruptcy, *London Gazette*, 31 December 1844, 5374; Special Board Meeting, 29 November 1844, UKT Minute Book 1, Aviva Archives.
37. *Morning Chronicle*, 10 January 1845, 8; Board meetings, 16 December 1844, 20 December 1844, 15 August 1845, Special Board Meetings, 20 November 1846, 1 February 1847, Aviva Archives.
38. 'Hull Rechabite Festival', *Northern Star*, 14 September 1839, 2; Meeting, 31 December 1840, Minutes of the Standing Committee 1, Board Meeting, 4 March 1841, Minute Book 1, Aviva Archives; 'Assignments', *Perry's Bankrupt Gazette* 13, 659 (28 November 1840), 7.
39. Special Board meeting, 16 September 1846, UKT Minute Book 1; Meetings, 1 November 1841, 20 December 1841, 27 December 1841, 14 February 1842, Minutes of the Standing Committee 1; Board meetings, 3 March 1843, 7 April 1843, 15 April 1843, 5 May 1843, UKT Minute Book 1; Meeting, 9 June 1843, Minutes of the Standing Committee 2, MS FL437; Board meeting, 30 June 1843, UKT Minute Book 1; Meetings, 8 December 1843; 12 January 1844, Minutes of the Standing Committee 2, Aviva Archives.
40. 'Princes Street Total Abstinence Society', *Cork Examiner*, 10 December 1841, 1.
41. Board meeting, 2 October 1846, UKT Minute Book 1, Aviva Archives.
42. Prospectus, 'The United Kingdom Total Abstinence Life Association'.
43. Suffolk Record Office, *Ipswich Remembered 2: Photographs of Victorian and Edwardian Ipswich* (Ipswich: Suffolk Record Office, 1979); and Edwin R. Ransome, 'Bygone Ipswich Friends', *Friends' Quarterly Examiner* 42 (1908), 311–12, both Library of the Society of Friends; Winskill, *Temperance Movement*, vol. 1, 259.
44. Burton and Barker, *Pigot's Directory of Suffolk* (London: Pigot, 1839, 558); 1841 Census (Class: HO107; Piece: 1043; Folio: 30; Page: 15; GSU roll: 3438); Meetings, 21 December 1840, 28 December 1840, 1 March 1841, Minutes of the Standing Committee 1, Aviva Archives.
45. Meetings, 1 March 1841, 19 April 1841, 18 June 1842, Minutes of the Standing Committee 2, Aviva Archives.
46. Meeting, 20 June 1842, Minutes of the Standing Committee 2, Aviva Archives.

47. Meeting, 27 June 1842, Minutes of the Standing Committee 2, Board meeting, 1 July 1842, UKT Minute Book 1, Aviva Archives; *Bury and Norwich Post, and East Anglian*, 29 June 1842, 2.
48. 'Teetotal Life Insurances, &c. &c', *Christian Investigator and Evangelical Reformer* I, 2 (22 January 1842), 336.
49. Ibid.
50. Clark, *Betting on Lives.*
51. 'The Use of Property', *Christian Investigator and Evangelical Reformer* 13, 1 (8 January 1842), 404.
52. Ibid.
53. 'On Preaching', *Christian Investigator and Evangelical Reformer*, 25 December 1841, 346–50, 348.
54. 'Questions and Answers on the Use of Property', *Christian Investigator and Evangelical Reformer*, 22 January 1842, 234, emphasis added.
55. 'Intelligence', *Christian Investigator and Evangelical Reformer*, 25 December 1841, 352.
56. Meetings, 26 September 1842, 3 October 1842, Minutes of the Standing Committee 2; Board meeting, 7 October 1842, UKT Minute Book 1, Aviva Archives.
57. Meeting, 17 October 1842, Minutes of the Standing Committee 2; Board meeting, 5 November 1842, UKT Minute Book 1; Meeting, 14 November 1842, Minutes of the Standing Committee 2, Aviva Archives.
58. Eileen Groth Lyon, 'Barker, Joseph (1806–1875)', *Oxford Dictionary of National Biography* (Oxford University Press, 2004), www.oxforddnb.com/view/article/1406, accessed 6 December 2016; Winskill, *Temperance Movement*, vol. 3, 236; vol. I, 209, 143, 132, 150, 212; Whittaker, *Life's Battles*, 80.
59. Whittaker, *Life's Battles*, 80.
60. Winskill, *Temperance Movement*, vol. 3, 236.
61. Lyon, 'Barker, Joseph'; Betty Fladeland, *Abolitionists and Working-Class Problems in the Age of Industrialisation* (London: Macmillan, 1984), 132, 149.
62. Whittaker, *Life's Battles*, 80.
63. Winskill, *Temperance Movement*, vol. 3, 236; vol. 1, 143; vol. 3, 236; Whittaker, *Life's Battles*, 80.
64. Fladeland, *Abolitionists*, 134; Whittaker, *Life's Battles*, 81.
65. Board meeting, 7 May 1847, UKT Minute Book 1, Aviva Archives.
66. Burns, company history.
67. 1892 (186) Life assurance companies, Statements of account and of life assurance and annuity business, and abstracts of actuarial reports deposited with the Board of Trade, under 'the Life Assurance Companies Act, 1870', during the year ended 31st December 1891, 207; *Morning Chronicle*, 24 May 1859, 6; *Daily Gazette*, 4 June 1873, 2; *Birmingham Daily Post*, 26 May 1875; Working Man's Section Card, Specimen Literature, MS FL387, Aviva Archives.
68. Julie-Marie Strange, *Death, Grief and Poverty in Britain, 1870–1914* (Cambridge: Cambridge University Press, 2005), 112, 116.
69. Board meetings, 7 January 1848, 14 January 1848, 16 April 1849, 4 February 1848, 13 April 1849, UKT Minute Book 1, Aviva Archives.
70. Fifth Annual Meeting 2 January 1846, 2, United Kingdom Temperance & General Provident Institution Annual Reports and Balance Sheets 1840–1910, Aviva Archives.
71. George E. Cokayne, *Complete Baronetage* (Exeter: W. Pollard, 1900), 187–8; Return of Owners of Land 1873, Surrey, 18.
72. National Life Assurance Society, Medical Reports, MS34418, London Archives.

73. James Edward Pollock and James Chisholm, *Medical Handbook of Life Assurance for the Use of Medical and Other officers of Companies*, fourth edition (London: Cassell, 1895), 54–5; 'The Mansel Will Suit', *Western Mail*, 3 March 1877, 3; 'The Local Will Case', *Hampshire Telegraph and Sussex Chronicle*, 7 March 1877, 4.
74. Proposal Form, National Life Assurance Society, MS 34431, London Archives; 'Law Intelligence', *Journal of the Institute of Actuaries & Assurance Magazine* 22, 1 (1879), 21.
75. 'The Mansel Legitimacy Case', *Bristol Mercury*, 25 July 1878, 6; 'Marriages', *The Times*, 7 September 1878, 1.
76. 'The Affairs of Sir Richard Mansel Mansel, Bart', *Manchester Courier and Lancashire General Advertiser*, 7 November 1883, 4.
77. *The Times*, 31 October 1885, 16 and 22 August 1885, 16.
78. Marriage, 2nd quarter 1891, Brighton, England & Wales Marriages 1837–2005, Birth, Marriage, Death & Parish Records, vol. 2B, 417; 1871 Census (Class: RG10; Piece: 483; Folio: 51; Page: 96; GSU roll: 537); 1881 Census (Class: RG11; Piece: 418; Folio: 55; Page: 65; GSU roll: 500); *The Era*, 23 May 1891, 14; *Weekly Mail*, 5 August 1893, 12.
79. Rohan McWilliam, 'The Gaiety Girl and the Matinee Idol: Constructing Celebrity, Glamour and Sexuality in the West End of London, 1890–1914', *Transactions of the Royal Historical Society* 1 (2023), 69–93.
80. See, for example, *The Era*, 9 January 1892, 2 and 18 April 1891, 16; 'Round the Music Halls', *Licensed Victuallers' Mirror*, 19 May 1891, 229.
81. *Lloyd's Weekly Newspaper*, 2 August 1891, 16; 'The Insolvency of Sir Richard Mansel', *The Cambrian*, 31 July 1891, 3.
82. 'Nye and Another v. Mansel', *The Times*, 14 February 1894, 14; England & Wales Government Probate Death Index 1858–2019, Civil Deaths and Burials.
83. 'Notes of the Stage', *New York Times*, 18 June 1893, 12; *Morning Post*, 28 March 1895, 6; 'The Social Purity Party's Objection to Music-Hall Licences', *Illustrated Police News*, 24 October 1896, 6; *South Wales Daily Post*, 10 November 1899, 2; 1911 Census (Class: RG14; Piece: 21394; GSU roll: 102).
84. Marquise De Fontency, 'Behind the Scenes', *Daily Picayune*, 5 March 1894, 6, and 'Another Scotch Marriage Romance', *New York Tribune*, 26 November 1906, 7.
85. First quarter of 1916, b 1867, aged 49, vol. 1D, 448, England & Wales Deaths 1837–2007, Civil Deaths & Burials.
86. Çalişkan and Callon, 'Economization, Part 2', 21.
87. Board meeting, 5 November 1842, UKT Minute Book 1, Aviva Archives.
88. 'Temperance Provident Institution', *York Herald*, 6 December 1845, 6.
89. 'Funeral Funds', Advertisement, *Temperance Gazette* 1 (January 1846), 7.
90. Arthur G. Barker, *The Temperance Century in the West* (Bristol: T. O. Elworthy and Son, 1937); Harrison, *Dictionary of Temperance Biography*, 42, 62.
91. Meetings, 9 November 1840, 27 November 1840, 8 February 1841, Minutes of the Standing Committee 1, Aviva Archives.
92. Booth and Harwood, 'Insurance as Catastrophe', 50.
93. Lobo-Guerrero, 'Uberrima Fides'.
94. Shapiro, 'The Social Control of Impersonal Trust', 649, 652.
95. Advertisement, *Morning Chronicle*, 18 January 1850, 1.

4

Statistics and forms: Those that don't drink don't die so fast

Introduction: From facts to forms

Writing in 1862, James Dawson Burns suggested:

> There are some who have a foolish, fetish sort of faith in statistics, and there are some who have as foolish a dislike and suspicion of them. Since they are simply facts, or supposed facts, arithmetically expressed, their credibility can neither fall below nor rise above the level of the evidence on which they rest.[1]

Burns used the mortality experience of the UKT to support his argument about the 'vital statistics of temperance' in 1883; like other Victorian statisticians, Burns was prepared to show his working – to explain how his figures were derived, how the firm's lives were selected, how representative they were (and of what) and so on. The statistics associated with temperance life assurance often attracted critical attention, though that attention demanded time and effort, as well as statistical and perhaps actuarial training.

The 'simple' facts Burns traded in were also abstractions of the lives of people assured by these firms. Turning the health and prospects of an applicant for life assurance into facts, some of which were 'arithmetically expressed' as numbers, also took time and effort, including the work of many intermediaries. Some of those intermediaries were material things – medical instruments, as time went on, but particularly paper documents, including the many forms that applicants, doctors and others had to complete to send on to the main office, which acted as a Latourian 'centre of calculation', a site where risks were assessed and decisions taken. As Michael Zakim noted, 'the age of capital … was overrun with scribbling men, who serviced an economy that rested on an explosion of new information industries specializing in credit, insurance, communications, prices, and professional training … Facts-on-paper consequently replaced facts-on-the-ground as the determinant operative reality in an increasingly fungible economy'.[2] Historians of scientific knowledge have shown that 'knowledge formats' like insurance forms do not simply pass on information, however; they shape that information in specific ways while structuring the engagement of people with them. Statistics are always made and mediated through social and material contexts; they take *form* in these contexts.

This chapter concerns the facts and forms associated with temperance life assurance, paying attention to the contexts of their production, circulation and use. It begins with the comparisons made between the firm's sections, considering this as part of a wider interest in 'moral statistics' within the statistical movement. But this account must also examine the making of these facts and the way that the social and material elements that made up these networks were themselves disciplined so that they related to one another in effective ways. The UKT's experience – its statistical records of mortality – was not enough on its own. It needed to be made and used in ways that could find a purchase in the hostile world of Victorian business. 'Facts' had to become forms, stable social and material arrangements. We begin the chapter with the early life of the facts the UKT was producing.

Inciting temperance: Comparisons of mortality

While the UKT made much of the respectability and financial stability of its directors and patrons, as we saw in Chapter 3, after its first decade in business it also began to emphasize the firm's 'experience' as evidence that abstinence was healthier than moderate drinking. The report of 1850's annual meeting noted that the firm's mortality was only 54 per cent of that of other offices, but also acknowledged that this could not be shown to be the result of abstinence alone.[3] By 1860, though, public discussions of the firm were beginning to show that policyholders in the Abstainers' section tended to live longer than those in the General section, later summed up in the 1890s by the claim that 'those who don't drink don't die so fast'.

It was not possible to compare the two sections in this way until 1855, when the firm conducted its first division of profits. Crucially the surplus of £34,854 was divided unevenly between the members of the two sections because while mortality was lower than predicted in both, the Abstainers had far fewer deaths than expected; for every £100 of the bonus allocated, the Abstainer's section received £42 and the General section £37, with endowments receiving £17 and joint lives £4.[4]

Dawson Burns presented the following table (Table 4.1) in his manuscript history of the firm, showing the range of bonuses awarded in each section in the quinquennial divisions between 1855 and 1895:

Table 4.1 Quinquennial bonuses awarded 1855–85, whole-life policies only

Division year	Temperance section	General section
1855	24–75	23–50
1860	35–86	25–59
1865	23–56	17–52
1870	34–84	20–49
1875	35–114	20–64
1880	41–135	26–83
1885	41–128	35–101

Source: Burns, company history, 5.

As Table 4.1 shows, the average amount awarded to members of the Abstainers' section exceeded the General section bonus in every division year in this period. The first division was widely reported – bonuses made for good copy – but it wasn't until 1859 that the two bonuses were publicly compared in a way that highlighted the financial, medical and moral benefits of abstinence.[5] At the eighteenth annual members' meeting in that year, H. H. Gill – 'an old member of the society' – announced that 'one friend, on seeing the difference in the bonus declared between teetotalers and non-teetotalers, took out a policy for £1,000 and signed the pledge'.[6] Later that year the Reverend Francis Bishop, chairing a lecture on life assurance given by Joseph Harrap, the UKT's agent for Leicester (Chapter 5), explained that 'the experience of this institution went to show that abstinence from alcoholic drinks was more favourable to health and longevity than even their moderate use, since the profits of the Temperance section considerably exceeded those of the general section'.[7] Here was a clear financial inducement to abstain; as the Reverend John Burder had put it at a meeting in Bristol the year before, 'the institution was exercising a beneficial influence, because it incited a man to become temperate'.[8] After nearly twenty years of work the UKT could make a strong claim for the benefits of abstinence and for its own ability to turn this into bonuses for its members.

Looking back from the 1890s, Dawson Burns thought that the bonus division of 1855 had been good for members, the firm's reputation and temperance in general:

> A liberal bonus excited general congratulations for its own sake, and the evidence furnished by it of the soundness of the Institution, while the specially large bonus apportioned to the Temperance Section accorded with the Temperance position – that intoxicating liquors are not conducive to health and longevity, but that other things being equal the Abstainer's prospect of life, judged by facts, is not less but greater than that of the moderate drinker.[9]

Sales of policies increased by just under 30 per cent from 1855 to 1856, bringing in a decade of healthy growth (Chapter 1), and the firm's 'experience' was used to bolster claims for the relative healthiness of abstinence from the 1860s. Attention shifted away from the figures who haunted the firm's early years – the 'reclaimed drunkards' who made very poor lives, and the 'wild enthusiasts' who challenged insurantial and medical orthodoxies – towards the tens of thousands of teetotalers and moderate drinkers safely accepted by the firm. And as numbers travelled quickly and effectively through print to build trust wherever the UKT and its supporters worked or advertised, the reproduction and circulation of the UKT's comparative tables of mortality may well have played an important role in countering the problems of trust identified in Chapter 3.

The UKT's experience represented a new kind of knowledge about drinking, as an alternative to moral, religious or medical discussions of temperance during this period. In time this would be used to challenge medical understandings. In 1877, for example, the temperance writer James Alexander Mowatt wrote that

> When Dr George W. Beard asserted, in 'Stimulants and Narcotics', that we have no statistics to prove that teetotalers are healthier, or live longer, than moderate

> drinkers, he only wrote in utter ignorance of the thirty-two years' experience of this Temperance life insurance institution [the UKT], and of the equally satisfactory experience of the [Whittington, Sceptre and other companies] … Here are facts and statistics, as to the mortality of teetotalers and moderate drinkers respectively, which can not be gainsayed [*sic*] nor refuted.[10]

This evidence placed greater emphasis on statistical facts, reflecting a new and wider interest in moral statistics. However, these facts required individuals to be trained to produce, understand and work with these numbers, and for this knowledge to be able to circulate through the firm's networks, in the face of critical attention and argument. The successful arrangement of these elements helped to make a market for temperance life assurance, and perhaps also to produce trust in the claims the firm made for abstinence.

For now, though, we need to return to moral statistics and their relation to questions of intemperance.

Moral statistics, moral geographies

The UKT emerged just as the burgeoning statistical movement was beginning to engage with the drink question. The Manchester and London Statistical Societies were founded in 1833 and 1834 respectively, the British Association's statistical section in 1833, and Adolphe Quetelet's influential *Treatise on Man and the Development of His Faculties* was first published in 1835 and translated into English in 1842. Quetelet had high hopes for the statistical study of the causes of drunkenness, which he hoped 'would endeavour to make known the injuries this pestilence inflicts on society'.[11] Charles Babbage had provided Quetelet with records of drunks arrested and released without charge by the London police, and Quetelet thought that 'if we possessed an extensive set of similar documents, we should find in them the most precious memorials of the manners of the English people'.[12] He also wondered if insights might come from business records, from 'savings banks, assurance societies, and the different institutions which encourage foresight'.[13]

Quetelet's work perfectly illustrates the aims and methods of 'moral statistics'. Vital statistics – demography – was the most obvious focus of the new statistical societies, encouraged by the intensification of biopolitical interest in the health of the race or nation, but the statistical movement was equally interested in 'moral statistics' concerning crime, education and religious activity.[14] Drink and drunkenness were also matters of concern. James Silk Buckingham's 1834 Select Committee on Drunkenness was presented with statistical evidence on the relationship between the number of drinking places and alcohol consumption, and the Reverend John Clay, chaplain of Preston's House of Correction, published five papers on the links between intemperance and criminality in the Statistical Society of London's *Journal* between 1837 and 1857.[15]

In the second half of the century interest in the moral statistics of intemperance was sustained by William Hoyle's calculations of the 'National Drink Bill'. Hoyle was a mill worker who became a mill owner, a self-educated Lancashire teetotaler and vegetarian who published pamphlets and books and presented papers to the Social Science Congress and the British Association. His study of the money spent on alcohol in his home county, its consequences for the Poor and Police Rates and its opportunity costs – the goods it might have bought and houses it might have built – prompted so much discussion that *The Times* asked him to calculate the national 'Drink Bill' annually from 1873.[16]

These moral statistics became 'moral geographies' as statisticians noted the uneven spatial distribution of criminality or drunkenness, mapping them as part of a wider project of 'sanitary science', a form of medical geography concerned with the relationships between disease, local environments and populations.[17] While arguments about drinking retained an emphasis on questions of individual moral responsibility until the turn of the century, sanitary science also engaged with 'environmentalist' explanations: did concentrations of drinking places encourage alcohol consumption, for example?[18] Examining relationships between local environments and the character of their inhabitants, these arguments drew on work by ethnologists and medical geographers who argued for the unity of 'race' and place, work which profoundly shaped Victorian statistics and which would ultimately produce moral geographies informed by eugenicist and white supremacist assumptions.[19] Life assurance was shaped by – and would play its own part in – these discussions.[20]

Early moral geographies of drink are well represented by William Felkin's two papers in the first volume of the *Journal* of the Statistical Society of London (1839). Listing the moral statistics of a weaver's district in Norwich and fifteen courts near Gray's Inn in London, Felkin recorded the number of drinking places as one indicator of local demoralization.[21] A former lace maker who became a lace manufacturer and mayor of Nottingham, Felkin established himself as an authority on British lace and hosiery production after his business failed.[22] Later moral geographies of drink can be found in the attention paid to drinking places in Charles Booth's maps of poverty and in the maps presented to the Peel Commission in the 1890s.[23] These investigations of moral statistics were part of a broader effort to know and manage society, which became part of a civilizing mission in Britain's cities. Cullen notes the London Society was closely associated with 'the charmed circle of the Whig-Liberal intelligentsia who were to dominate the parliamentary enquiries and statistical investigations of the 1830s', and the Manchester Society emerged from 'a tightly-knit reforming section of the commercial and industrial aristocracy of Manchester'.[24]

However, statistics were not powerful in and of themselves, either as the products of a technical, specialist knowledge, or because they were produced and circulated by the powerful. We can see this in the case of a simple moral measure, which compared the population of a district to the number of drinking places it contained in the form of a ratio of 'people to pub'. This measure, which allowed comparisons to be made between 'wetter' and 'drier' districts, appears in evidence presented to Parliamentary Committees from 1817 through to the 1890s and was suggested as a tool for setting limits on the number of licences in a district in 1871 and 1899.[25] In the end this measure failed to become a tool of government policy in Britain, though it was adopted in Massachusetts, the Netherlands, Austria and the Australian colony of Victoria. Other statistical measures were adopted in Britain – the crude death rate (CDR) was used to compare the mortality of British cities and to discipline their corporations, for example.[26] Libby Schweber notes that the *Fifth Annual Report of the Registrar-General* (1843) claimed the life assurance table as a tool for examining comparative mortality, claiming it was 'as indispensable in sanitary inquiries as the barometer or thermometer, and other instruments in physical research'.[27] The ratio of pubs to people might have had a similar influence over licensing policy, had circumstances been different; statistics could become 'instruments', given the right circumstances.

Moral statistics shaped geographical understandings of drink as a social problem in the decades following the UKT's founding, and these ideas continued to be influential well into the twentieth century. Numbers could be taken as 'facts' of the kind Burns and others turned to in their efforts to defend and promote temperance, but they were not always effective. Moral statistics and geographies could fail, despite their sophistication and close association with the powerful. The success of the UKT's own moral statistics – its experience – in terms of making a market and perhaps persuading others of the value of abstinence could not be taken for granted and needs to be explained.

We will see in a moment that the UKT's numbers circulated in contexts that made them useful conduits for temperance arguments, but for now we turn to the chapter's first temperance life, in the form of a director who engaged in moral statistics as part of a wider philanthropic mission.

Temperance lives: Robert Charleton (1809–1872)

Robert Charleton, another founder director of the UKT and Quaker, was keenly interested in the moral statistics of temperance.[28] Born in Bristol, Charleton trained as a land surveyor and agent with Henry Fowler Cotterell, one of the first members of Bath's temperance society and later a country director of the UKT. In 1833 Robert set himself up as a pin manufacturer at Two Mile Hill, near Kingsdown, east of Bristol.[29] The inspector who visited the factory in 1841 for the Royal Commission of Inquiry into Children's Employment described Charleton's 'generous benevolence', for example funding a school for the children in and of his workforce.[30] Charleton's biographers suggested that he tried, like Samuel Bowly, to resist the pull of the commercial world, but 'if his worldly business did not bring him wealth it brought him what was far better, the means to do good to his fellow men, temporally, morally, and spiritually', particularly after Charleton retired from business in 1852.[31] By then Robert had married Catherine Brewster, the daughter of Thomas Fox, Robert's stepmother's brother. Through Catherine's family in Ipswich Robert met R. D. Alexander (Chapter 3), with whom he had already corresponded on the topics of total abstinence and philanthropy.[32] Robert and Catherine had one son, Robert A. Charleton, who was born in 1861, by which point the family had returned from Kingsdown to Ashley Hill in Bristol.[33]

Temperance was one of Robert's early interests. He had been the first to sign the pledge in Bristol, spoke at the first meeting of the New British and Foreign Temperance Society in 1837, was treasurer and president of the Western Temperance League and one of the vice-presidents of the National Temperance Society from its founding in 1842.[34] When Charleton took part in the first teetotal procession of Bristol's Society in 1837, he and other Friends were 'especially selected as objects of derision', followed by a procession featuring a dummy Quaker, 'an inverted coffee-pot, mounted on a pole, and … a miniature coffin'.[35] Robert was also a pacifist – travelling to Russia in 1854 with Joseph Sturge and Henry Pease in an attempt to persuade the Tsar not to go to war with Britain – and an opponent of the Contagious Diseases Acts, as well as an active committee member of (and 'most liberal contributor' to) the British and Foreign Anti-Slavery Society.[36] After becoming a minister, around 1859, Charleton supported mission work in Britain and abroad.[37]

In terms of this chapter, though, it is also significant that Charleton was 'well versed in statistics', once spending most of a seaside holiday involved in 'the careful calculation of the statistics and life tables of different benefit and insurance offices'.[38] Thomas Hudson noted that Charleton's speeches involved 'a judicious selection and collation of facts and figures, and the novel application of these in illustration of his subject'.[39] Temperance arguments were no different. Anna Fox gave several examples of 'the statistical method of dealing with this question which [Charleton] often adopted, whilst never neglecting to enforce its moral and religious aspects'. In 1836 he calculated the cost of drink for Kingswood in terms of unproductivity and crime to be £26,358, which he said would pay for the district's rent, fuel, relief of the poor, education and costs of public worship, with a surplus for a reserve fund. Speaking at Exeter two years later, Charleton said Britain's daily drink bill would pay for the Bristol Suspension Bridge, then under construction, five or six times over, and the amount of grain lost to the manufacture of alcoholic drink would cover 12 million acres of land stretching from Bristol to London.[40] The identification of drink with wasted expenditure and the loss of savings was characteristic of moral statistical arguments.

Robert Charleton died in 1872, five years after Catherine, and his funeral at the Friends' Burial Ground in Bristol was attended by representatives of local and national temperance organizations. In its obituary *The Anti-Slavery Reporter* noted 'his pecuniary means were considerable, and few or none have exemplified more fully the idea of Christian stewardship'.[41] Charleton left £6,000 to twenty-one institutions, more than £1,000 going to national and local temperance organizations.[42]

It seems likely that Robert Charleton's exercises in moral statistics and support for the UKT were part of a wider philanthropic mission. Significantly, in this he closely resembles another UKT founder, Theodore Compton.[43] After working as a clerk in a merchant's firm, Compton became the actuary of the National Provident Society and a Fellow of the Institute of Actuaries.[44] It was not uncommon, as Alborn notes, for actuaries to have risen from modest positions, or to begin their careers with very little actuarial training.[45] Compton knew enough to assist Robert Warner in establishing the UKT, working as the office's secretary before moving to the Albion office in 1851, leaving there in 1858 when the Albion merged with the Eagle. Compton was a Quaker and Liberal and was one of the founders of the Metropolitan Association for Improving the Dwellings of the Industrious Classes.[46] He was also active in temperance, serving as secretary to the National Temperance Society until 1846 and organizing the World's Temperance Convention.[47]

Like Charleton, though, Compton gave up business in his forties, moving to the Mendip village of Winscombe for the sake of his oldest child's health. He studied natural history, taught in the night schools he established in Winscombe, got involved in the local temperance society and painted watercolours. A perceptive journalist for the *Observer* had recognized the potential value of the UKT's experience in its second year of business when he noted that Compton 'was a Fellow of the Statistical Society, who will, we trust, occasionally satisfy our curiosity in regard to the effects of teetotalism on mortality, as proved by the progress of this Institution'.[48] Compton did not engage in public discussion of the firm's experience, though. Temperance life assurance might be assumed to be entirely concerned with questions of rational calculation in the service of profit, on the one hand, and promoting temperance, on the other, but the reluctance of men like Compton and Charleton to put their statistical skills to work might reflect a Quaker rejection of worldly temptation. Whatever the reason, it is striking that the two most statistically minded founders of the UKT both chose philanthropy over business success.

Calculation and experience

Charleton's lecturing style – the 'judicious selection and collation of facts and figures' noted by Hudson – was certainly shared by other temperance activists, visible in examples from Joseph Livesey's *Malt Lecture* (originally presented in 1833) to early twentieth-century lantern slides presenting graphs of statistics. However, these numbers needed to circulate and to arrive in places where they could be understood, where they might form new relations with other social, material things. To assess the effectiveness of these claims we need to return to the contexts in which they were made and circulated. This section considers some of the uses that were made of these numbers as they moved through Victorian society.

The UKT's figures began to circulate more widely after the 1855 division of profits appeared to show a significant difference between the mortality of abstainers and drinkers. It is probably not a coincidence that discussion of the firm's vital statistics at meetings of the British Association for the Advancement of Science began in 1860, once the second division, made earlier that year, had confirmed that the results of 1855 had not been a fluke. This initiative may have been the idea of Edward Vivian (Chapter 2), who presented or discussed papers using the UKT's figures at the Association's meetings in Oxford (1860), Bristol (1875) and Southport, Lancashire (1883).[49] *The Lancet*'s report on the latter was reprinted in *Scientific American*.[50] The lessons drawn from the firm's experience would also be reported as 'Science: Industries. Notes and News' in 1892, between stories about a new India rubber substitute and the discovery of coal deposits in Yorkshire.[51]

The firm also began to use its comparative experience in its advertising in the 1870s. An advertisement in the *Leeds Mercury* reproduced the mortality figures for each section in the five divisions that had been made since 1850, showing that abstainers received a greater return each time.[52] These figures were mentioned in temperance presentations from the end of the 1860s, for example in a Rechabite meeting in North Wales, while the 1876 annual meeting of the Scottish Temperance League annual meeting heard that the UKT's evidence was 'the last link in the chain' in the analysis of 'the real character of alcohol', alongside evidence from medicine and the workhouse.[53]

The UKT's experience began to appear in letter columns as temperance supporters drew upon it to defend abstinence, promoting both the firm and the idea of healthy teetotalism as they did so. In 1872, for example, J. Dyson wrote to the *Sheffield and Rotherham Independent* to challenge the remarks made by Mr Davis, a stipendiary justice, who had claimed 'that the working men of England not only require beer, it was necessary for them, but plenty of it'. Dyson's criticism of this argument rested in part on the UKT's comparative mortality figures.[54] The firm's experience was also used in a letter to the *Preston Chronicle and Lancaster Advertiser* in 1875, replying to a correspondent from Blackburn who claimed that temperance did not encourage longevity.[55] William Stanyon, one of the UKT's agents in Leicester, wrote to the *Leicester Chronicle and the Leicestershire Mercury* several times between 1879 and 1882 to publicize statistics from the annual members' meetings, and James Whyte, the secretary to the UK Alliance, cited the UKT's experience in his letters to the *Manchester Guardian* in support of temperance between 1888 and 1902.[56] As this suggests, references to the UKT's figures were often made in response to discussions of the health-giving properties of alcoholic drink.

These figures were often combined with evidence from other assurance firms, as the UKT's position became less unusual within life assurance. In 1886 Charles R. Drysdale, Senior Physician with the Metropolitan Free Hospital, wrote to the *Morning Post* to discuss his research on alcohol consumption – probably his 1884 publication on drinking and mortality, based on life assurance statistics – which had concluded that drink was not a necessity for life.[57] He also contributed to a debate on the effects of alcohol in the *British Medical Journal* in 1891, again referring to insurance company evidence to support his argument.[58] Other doctors and medical institutions began to draw upon UKT evidence in public talks, as we will see in Chapter 8.

Writing in 1882, one writer summed up the import of this new evidence very effectively, looking back to the foundation of the UKT to capture something of the shift in opinion that the firm had perhaps helped to bring about. Noting that 'within the last fifty years' it had been common for offices to decline teetotalers or charge them extra for their policies, the story suggested that teetotalers had established the UKT 'in self-defence'. The firm's mortality experience and the different bonuses paid to the two sections had helped to 'conclusively demolish the ignorant prejudice that abstinence from spirits is on the average, injurious to health; and in an age when scientific investigation is treated with profound respect, they will carry great weight'.[59]

Beyond newspapers, though, how did this experience circulate to support this 'scientific investigation'?

Cards and lantern slides: Mobile, socio-material facts

As the firm's secretary, Theodore Compton travelled extensively in Britain and Ireland to promote the UKT. The firm's evidence also travelled through print and mobile speakers; these numbers were mobile because the socio-material networks they flowed through were designed to facilitate that movement. Writing about an attempt to develop a market for electric vehicles, Michel Callon noted that 'entities are converted into inscriptions: reports, memoranda, documents, survey results, scientific papers. These are sent out and received back, acted upon and reacted to'.[60] Temperance firms tried to manage the movements of these inscriptions as well as the people it needed to work with them; people and things needed to be displaced and moved to new sites, put into new configurations. Letters, advertisements and other objects stood in for people, though this did not necessarily make this business more 'impersonal', as might be expected. Discussing fire assurance, Miranda Clow argues that 'the graphic objects generated by the fire offices did not imitate one-on-one relationships that pre-dated them; rather, they created brand new possibilities for personal interaction and geographical extent'.[61] In this way 'the actor-world accumulates materials that render it durable', as Callon put it.[62] The materials we consider in this next section were also mobile inscriptions, and they helped carry the UKT's message about comparative mortality further than Compton could have travelled.

The first example, dating from around 1889, shows the mortality experienced in the firm's two sections, relative to the deaths predicted to occur from life tables, for five periods: the four quinquennial periods following 1865, and the years 1886–8 (Figure 4.1). Between 1871 and 1875, for example, 5 per cent more deaths occurred in the General section than might be expected to occur in the general population, while the Abstainers' section experienced only 71 per cent of the expected mortality. From the card's size and price – a hundred for one shilling and sixpence – it seems likely that it was designed to be given out to interested parties, or perhaps slipped into an envelope to be sent to a correspondent. The chart used the UKT's mortality figures and was designed by Dr J. J. Ridge, one of the founders of the British Medical Temperance Association, alongside James Edmunds, the UKT's physician (Chapter 8).

The second example, from 1891, is an advert in the *British Women's Temperance Journal* listing materials available from the Band of Hope Union's London repository, including a set of 'striking diagrams, facts, and opinions' printed on card and 'suitable for enclosing in letters or for general distribution'. A four-page pamphlet drew upon twenty years of the UKT's experience, 'in proof of the fact that the death-rate is greater among moderate drinkers than among abstainers'. It was listed alongside an acrostic summarizing the opinions of medical authorities on the consequences of drinking, and comparative mortality figures from the Registrar General.[63] Elsewhere the advert promoted diagrams and charts showing the effect of alcohol on the body, printed on 30×40 inch cards, as well as lanterns and slides for hire.

A larger version of these cards may have been displayed at the annual soiree of the Bannockburn Total Abstinence Society in 1856, which was graced by 'a beautiful show-card, issued by the United Kingdom Temperance and General Provident Institution, strikingly showing the relation subsisting between temperance and provident habits'.[64] No further details were given, however. In 1887 Dr Lees showed 'a diagram which contrasted the rate of mortality amongst total abstainers as compared with the rate in the case of moderate drinkers' to an audience at the Central Hall, Newcastle; the figures came from Sceptre and the UKT.[65] It also seems likely that UKT figures might have found their way onto the magic lantern slides used by temperance speakers to illustrate their presentations. Several early twentieth-century slides produced by the Friends Temperance Union display graphs of comparative mortality, comparing the

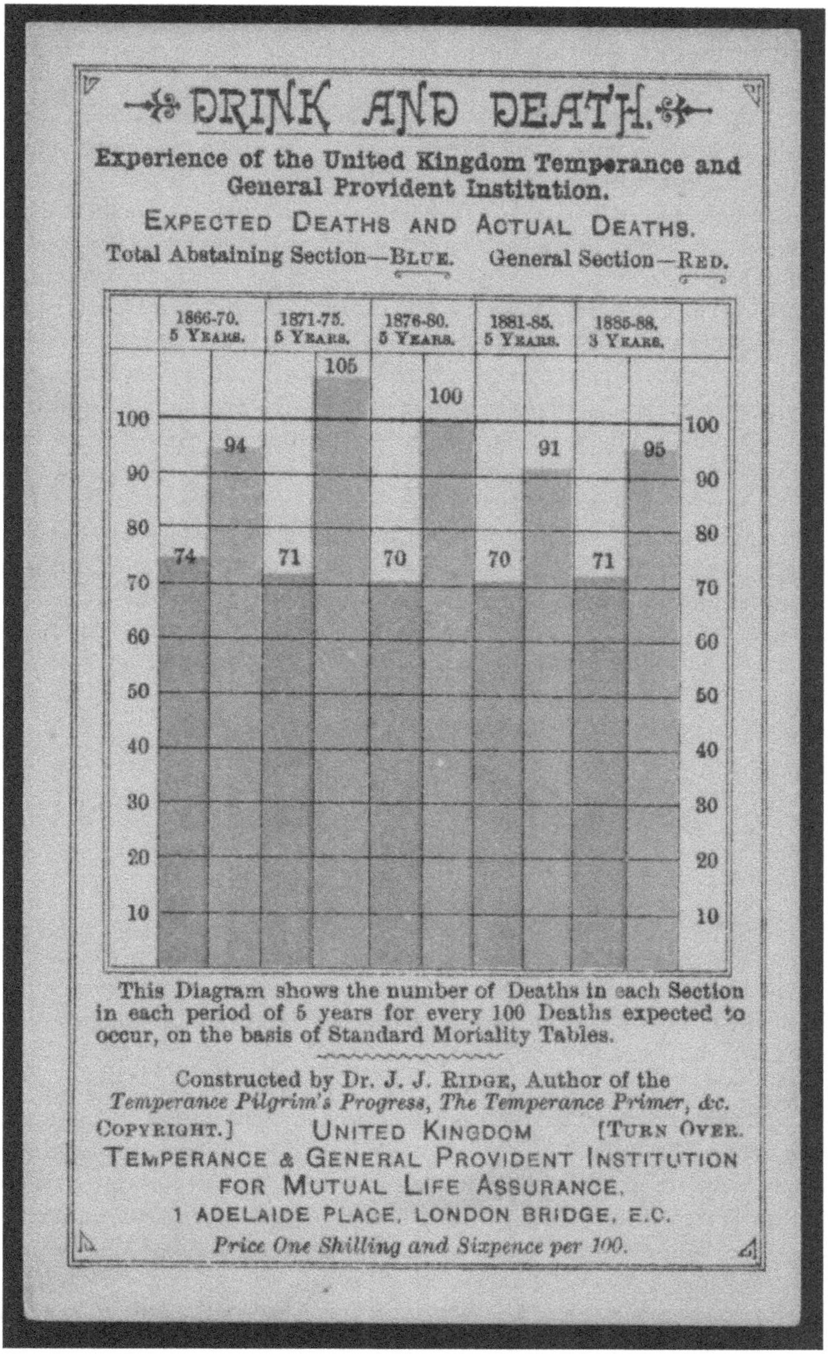

Figure 4.1 'Drink and death' card, UKT, 1889.

Source: Aviva Archive.

life expectancy of publicans and abstainers, for example; these figures might have been drawn from the UKT, though by this point they could have been constructed from the experience of other life assurance firms.[66]

Facts about the relative risks of abstinence and drinking circulated in numerical form beyond the letter columns of newspapers. The mobility and durability of materials like these cards and pamphlets was important, but they would often have been sent to known individuals, or presented as part of a talk, so would have been only one part of a more extensive social and material context. Their audiences would also have been expected to understand how a histogram works, which reminds us that numbers require properly trained presenters and audiences if they are to make sense. These elements had to be correctly arranged for these facts to be effective, and their reception could not be guaranteed. The moderate drinker who found a card showing the comparative mortality of abstainers and drinkers in a letter from a friend might have felt insulted or amused by the implication. The promotion of the UKT's message was an uncertain affair, and these mobile representatives of the firm might well have been met with hostility or bewilderment.

These materialized facts were not as important as the forms that represented the lives these firms assured, though; the translation of real lives into factual information was crucial for the successful operation of this business. And as these companies expanded, the distance between life and office grew and translations had to travel further, which meant the relations between those creating and handling these paper documents had to be carefully controlled. Our next 'life', which concerns a bundle of documents, should make this clear.

Temperance lives: Whittington Policy #18,854 (1885 to present)

Life assurance forms are arguably the most important textual element within these socio-technical arrangements. The archives consulted for this book tend not to include many completed forms, meaning that the lives they assured are often only accessible through other records. However, one bundle of documents survives in the Whittington's archives, created for a man named Henry Thatcher, who lived on the island of Mauritius.[67] The Whittington opened agencies in Amsterdam, Brussels, Paris, Hamburg, Grenada, Jamaica, Trinidad, Sydney, Mauritius and Réunion, and issued prospectuses in French, Dutch and German.[68] Thatcher's is the only complete form in the Whittington collection, but it is particularly interesting because it travelled so far, from the Mauritian capital of Port Louis in the Indian Ocean to the firm's head office on Moorgate Street, London, not far from the UKT's first home. There are several documents in the bundle, including the form itself, and they demonstrate how Henry Thatcher's life was assessed for assurance and what was communicated with the board. These documents can tell us quite a lot about the social-technical network they were part of.

The application form itself, a large document folded four times to fit one long envelope, is in English, and it seems likely that Henry Thatcher answered each of the twelve questions himself. He was a thirty-seven-year-old married lawyer from Port

Louis when he applied to the Whittington's local office for a £300 whole-life policy in April 1885. Henry was born in the north of the island in Rivière du Rempart, amidst sugarcane plantations. He was not a teetotaler. The second document records the premiums he would have to pay: £5 10s. 6d. every six months, which probably included an extra charge for 'tropical residence'.

The medical report records Dr Riviere's opinion that Thatcher's life is 'average', which in life assurance terms means 'entirely acceptable'. The report had two elements: a 'personal report', where Dr Riviere recorded Thatcher's replies to questions about his health, and then a second, longer, report by Riviere himself. The first, signed by Thatcher, would allow the firm to invalidate the policy if it transpired that he had answered untruthfully. It prompted the examiner to record the applicant's previous experience of a range of afflictions: gout, rheumatic fever, insanity, neuralgia, habitual headaches, fits or convulsions, jaundice, liver problems, diabetes, dysentery, haemorrhoids, fistula, dropsy and malaria. Another question asked for possible signs of tuberculosis, a particular concern for life assurance, and later questions asked about parental and sibling health, probing for signs of what were considered to be 'hereditary complaints' like tuberculosis, cancer and insanity.

Riviere's own report suggests a different approach, with the questions prompting the examiner to look for specific warning signs and to record measurements. The applicant's pulse was taken, and the examiner was asked to listen to his heart and percuss his chest, describe the condition of his tongue, check the size of his liver and spleen and so on. Question twenty-one asks the examiner 'do you observe any traces of palsy, epilepsy, insanity, or delirium tremens?' and twenty-four asks whether they 'suspect that the applicant is, or ever has been, of irregular, or intemperate, habits?' based on 'general appearance, or from any particular symptom, or symptoms'. Particular attention was to be given to this question. Riviere's report was to be entirely confidential – in other words, not to be shared with Thatcher – and the form was designed to be posted direct to Alfred T. Bowser, the Whittington's secretary in London.

These forms were supplemented by two 'Rapport D'Un Ami', references provided by the applicant's friends. One was completed by Jules Henri, town clerk and childhood friend of Thatcher; the other referee was E. Dupuy, a local company director. As we will see in a moment, this kind of report had been in use since the early nineteenth century, though firms became increasingly suspicious of them, as friends could not be expected to be impartial. Further confirmation could be sought from the firm's *comité de reference*, headed by the local director, Alfred Lavoquer, who had previously managed the firm's Paris office, and who was mayor of Port Louis in 1882–3 and 1884–5.[69] William Newton, a sugar planter and lawyer for other planters, and Victor Kervern, another lawyer, assisted Lavoquer; the firm's medical directors included the Sorbonne-trained Wilbraham Tollemache Arthur Edwards, the son of a sugar planter.[70]

Through these forms, and the work of Riviere and Lavoquer in Mauritius, and Bowser in London, Henry Thatcher's life could be carefully assessed. As we have seen, agents and medical referees helped firms extend their business beyond London; Thatcher's papers remind us that that extension required people like Thatcher to be converted into numbers and words on paper, becoming mobile, durable references. Most of these forms were completed on Mauritius, before being shipped to London for the board's inspection; they needed to be durable enough to reach that destination, and in Thatcher's case they have survived into the twenty-first century. These papers also provided evidence of a set of relations creating trust, mapping out the responsibility of each actor in the making of this decision. If Thatcher's life turned out to be poor rather than average, did the fault lie with Thatcher, for lying on his application? With Riviere, for missing signs of dissipation or inherited illness? Or perhaps with Lavoquer, for bringing a poor life to the company? Numbers were an important part of this network, as they allowed individual risks to be quantified, but they were only effective because of the networks of people and paper through which they travelled. Converted into numbers in particular knowledge formats – the firms' forms – these manufactured risks were highly mobile, their meanings understood by different actors across the network, and were therefore effective because they ensured that things happened at a distance.

Medical referees as measuring devices

The 'life' of Thatcher's forms provides an opportunity to consider the ways medical referees turned people into 'lives' through the completion of assurance documents. Medical referees became distant tools of the central office, who standardized the examiner's practice to ensure their results were comparable with those collected by other referees. This reduced the importance of the local doctor's own opinions of the risks associated with alcohol, while disseminating, perhaps, an orthodoxy of medical practice within these networks. It did not matter if referees believed that drinking shortened life expectancy, because they had to act as if they did if they were to remain employed by the firm. This increasing standardization came in response to several problems: adverse selection, where unhealthy individuals are more likely to need and apply for life assurance; differences of opinion or professional ability; and medical attendants who acted in their patients' interests, rather than the firm's. These issues affected all life firms, but alcohol consumption presented an additional set of problems. We can see this in a quick survey of the experience of life assurance firms and their medical referees in relation to drinking.

As we saw in the Introduction, in the 1840s mainstream medical opinion tended to assume that moderate drinking, however that might be defined, was far safer than abstinence, drawing on work that had identified alcohol as a food and stimulant; the use of wine or port as a medium for medicines gave alcohol further significance in treatment. Firms had been asking applicants about their alcohol consumption since the beginning of the century, though. When George Nicholls sought life assurance from Norwich Fire and Life in 1809, a friend told the firm that 'he is rather fond of tippling but not to that degree as to injure his health', while his medical attendant said 'I never saw him intoxicated that I can recollect but I have heard that he likes the drink when he can get it, which is but seldom as he has a wife & a large family to maintain'.[71] The firm would probably have been concerned about *immoderate* drinking, assuming that a little tippling was normal and not a source of risk, especially when it rarely lead to intoxication.

The Royal Farmers office took detailed minutes of its cautious assessments of candidates in its records from the early 1840s, possibly because its life assurance business was rather small, and they give us a sense of how the UKT, Sceptre or Whittington might have proceeded, though the office did not sell temperance assurance. A policy on the life of a teetotaler was approved in 1843, for example, subject 'to satisfactory accounts being given as to how long a time the said George Lee has been a Teetotaller and what were his previous habits'; the board may have been concerned that Lee was a 'reformed drunkard'. In the May of the previous year, though, the office had accepted an innkeeper's application without any mention of a medical report.[72] While alcohol consumption exercised directors and medical referees, it was *excessive* behaviour they really feared.

By the 1850s this was beginning to change, helped in part through the dissemination of the developing experience of the UKT, and by the 1870s many doctors seemed happy to accept the argument that abstinence was not dangerous to health and might even be better than moderate drinking. However, handbooks written for medical examiners for life assurance in the 1860s and 1870s continued to be suspicious of teetotalers, even as they warned doctors about excessive drinking. The guides written by the American professor Jonathan Adams Allen encouraged referees to reject 'the habitual drinker of alcoholic spirits', or those who indulged in 'an infrequent debauch', for example, but said nothing about teetotalers, only 'reformed inebriates', who were also undesirable.[73] Again, William Brinton, of the Royal Free and St Thomas's Hospitals, judged teetotalers to be good lives in 1863, not least because of their general prudence and self-restraint, but was clear that 'the reformed drunkard is not a good Life'.[74] In 1921 referees were still being warned to be sceptical of a proposer's claim to moderate drinking, but also that ' "total abstinence" is sometimes a term used when a man has abstained from drink for a month with the idea of becoming insured. It may mean that he has been ordered to abstain', as Thomas David Lister put it.[75]

Some of this uncertainty was due to the slipperiness of the terms used to assess alcohol consumption, particularly 'moderation'.[76] In response medical handbooks for examiners increasingly encouraged doctors to ask for and record detailed accounts of the quantity and type of drinks consumed, and the rhythms and contexts of consumption, differentiating between a shot of whisky consumed between meals, wine accompanying a meal, habitual tippling and the occasional debauch. Francis W. Moinet's 1876 guide prompted the examiner to check if the applicant was of temperate habits; by 1903 F. de Havilland Hall insisted the examiner record the exact amount consumed in a day, what kinds of alcohol were consumed, and when.[77] These issues prompted standardization in examination procedures, codified in the increasingly elaborate forms designed at the centre and sent out to examiners. The consumption of alcohol attracted especial concern and forms instructed referees to look for the traces it left on the applicant's body. As Alborn points out, 'by instructing or reminding doctors what to look for, medical examiners' forms also *routinized* the exam'.[78]

Ray Jureidini and Kevin White suggest 'the clinical examination was the outcome of the interests of insurance companies'; these assessments created the medical examination as we know it.[79] Physicians had been more used to investigating a patient's complaints of ill health than assessing their general health. Theodore Porter notes that the recording of blood pressure became established practice because assurers demanded this information in order to screen applicants for hypertension.[80] Medical directors at the centre sought certainty through measurements of height, weight, chest capacity and pulse, adding blood pressure and urine tests by the end of the century, recruiting 'a teeming assortment of scientific entities in order to defend standard mortality rates against the corrosive tendencies of bureaucratic intrusion and distrust', as Porter put it .[81] Intrusive investigations were replaced by instrumental measurements made by trained doctors and by laboratory testing.[82] The drive for objectivity made expertise less important than consistency; what was needed was 'simple, reliable instruments, that did not depend on refined skills or subtle judgement on the part of medical examiners and that got around the habitual reticence of applicants'.[83]

As Alborn points out, 'a central motivation for [these changes] was to compensate for the problem of transmitting incommunicable knowledge at a distance'.[84] In 1900 Sceptre's board agreed for example that 'the medical officer on a British Gun Boat in the Zambesi District may act as referee if he is duly qualified'.[85] Imperial scale did not necessarily create greater uncertainty, though; at Sceptre's 1904 meeting the board noted 'that notwithstanding the increasing distance from medical selection of the great proportion of the lives the last quinquennium has shown a lower rate of mortality than any of the preceding ones quoted'.[86] The company's surveillance of applicants had not suffered, though its network extended further than ever.

'Speculation on Jabez': Lives for sale

While forms were more mobile than people, the ability of paper documents to stand in for the lives they assured could have strange consequences. Assurance companies could only sell policies to someone with some 'insurable interest' in the life assured, which means they would suffer a loss if that person came to harm. Policies could be sold or transferred to others, who would then acquire an insurable interest in the life assured as the policy became their property, alienated from the life assured, and transferable through the market. This is what happened to the UKT policy established on the life of politician, financier and felon Jabez Spencer Balfour. Jabez's father James was one of the founding directors of the Temperance and Permanent Building Society, his mother Clara Lucas Balfour was a famous temperance writer and lecturer, and Dawson Burns, the UKT's first historian, was his brother-in-law.[87] The Liberator Building Society, which Jabez established in 1868, grew very rapidly, and Jabez became mayor of Croydon, MP for Tamworth and then for Burnley.

Balfour developed a group of companies whose paper assets could be passed back and forth to show a profit to auditors, while the many small sums that came in from ordinary investors helped sustain the group. Jabez fled to Argentina when the fraud was uncovered as the company finally crashed in 1892. Forcibly returned to England, he was sentenced to fourteen years imprisonment in 1895, with bankruptcy proceedings beginning while he was in prison.[88] The scandal caused great distress amongst investors, including many ordinary nonconformists, and created great distrust in temperance business in general, and for the Liberator's directors in particular. Dawson Burns, one of those directors, offered to resign as the UKT's auditor in 1893, presumably because the Alliance demanded his resignation as their metropolitan superintendent in that same year.[89]

In October 1897 the sale of four policies on Balfour's life was advertised as part of his bankruptcy proceedings. One of Balfour's policies was for £500 with the Scottish Amicable, and the other three were for £250 each with the UKT, Economic, and National Provident Institution offices; established in 1868–9, between them the policies had since earned £245 in bonuses.[90] The story was picked up by several newspapers. The *Belfast News-Letter* noted that the policies were advertised as 'this valuable property' and added 'it will be interesting to know the public estimate of the prospective life of the fraudulent speculator. Jabez's age is now fifty-four, and the fact is he is greatly reduced in weight since he appeared at the Old Bailey, for the hard work he has had to perform at Portland has much improved his physical condition'.[91] Or as the *County Gentleman* put it, 'what the buyers had to guess was the probable length of life still to be enjoyed by Mr. Balfour; whether, for instance, his present diet and exercise will prolong his years, or otherwise'.[92] The *Daily Mail* described the auction as 'Speculation on Jabez'. Sizing Jabez up as if this was a livestock auction, this reporting presented him as a speculative investment. The policies were sold for £630, reportedly 35 per cent over their surrender value.[93]

Once separated from the lives that they were intended to secure through their sale to another party, life assurance policies could become valuable properties, but in doing so they turned lives into commodities to be evaluated with an eye to their future value. It was illegal to assure a life where there was no insurable interest. In 1892 a Blackburn insurance agent had been promised 'third-party lives' to assure without their knowledge, and this had been reported as 'speculation in lives', for example, as we will see in Chapter 5. Once sold on or inherited, however, the policies travelled on into very different contexts.

Conclusions: Temperance life assurance's 'investment in form'

The movement of paper documents proved to be a surprisingly effective way of governing at a distance; like empire, life assurance depended on the production and circulation of paperwork and on effective bureaucratic practice.[94] As Dan Bouk puts it in the US context, 'by the turn of the twentieth century most applicants never set foot in a life insurers' home office – instead they arrived as pieces of paper, via the mail'.[95] The form stood in for a life, serving as a witness: it recorded that a named person underwent a medical examination in this place, on this day, and it specified the outcome. It travelled much more easily than the applicant could, and it had legal weight under the principle of *uberrima fides*. Like other written documents, the form 'allowed speech to inhabit any number of surfaces all at once, to replace one context for another, and to travel diverse trajectories'.[96] However, paper does not simply *extend* action; forms, letters and other documents were designed to *structure* the relations between different elements of this network. Life assurance forms recorded information about the policyholder, translating lives into numbers so they could be manipulated through calculation and circulated as references.[97]

At the same time forms governed the people who had to complete them. The applicant, medical referee, or agent who filled in a form or report incorrectly, or the clerk who misinterpreted or mislaid it, might lose their connection with the firm. The insurance form resembles the humble checklist 'that citizens … are to use to govern not only the spaces and subjects that are under their control, but also themselves', as Mariana Valverde points out in the context of alcohol licensing; 'one uses a checklist partly to govern one's own governing'.[98] These are textual 'social control agents' designed to discipline human actors, but rather than this becoming a problematic 'inflationary spiral', as Susan Shapiro feared (Chapter 3), these forms achieved what they were intended to – most of the time. As we will see in Chapter 5, standardizing a referee's responses by directing the way they completed their forms allowed firms to iron out local variations in practice and belief in favour of a single consistent approach. The chief medical officers of these companies effectively converted doctors' examination rooms into copies of their consulting rooms at the head office; highly trained doctors became simple recording devices plugged into wider networks. As Latour puts it, 'truth-value circulates here like electricity through a wire, so long as this circuit is not interrupted'.[99] The mobility of these forms and bundles, transmitting information back to a centre of calculation, was intended to stabilize the network and ensure the security of the firm.

This brings us back to statistics, considered as a form of *practice* rather than representations. As Libby Schweber points out, Laurent Thévenot's argument about the 'investment in form' required to make statistics useful 'draws attention not only to the technical tools used to stabilize statistical objects but to the importance of social, political, and commercial arrangements as well'.[100] In the context of life assurance, these forms *were* actually forms, as we have seen, and their development allowed the creation, recording, display and communication of information about applicants in a way that was stable and could be transmitted over space. Bruce Curtis has explored Thévenot's argument with reference to responses to the threat of cholera that gripped Canada in 1866, which provided Toronto's public health officials with the chance to develop administrative procedures for controlling the spread of infection. Curtis notes that investing in forms 'means investment in the economic sense of the expenditure of resources, especially expenditure directed towards those elementary forms that subtend human practice, such as the creation and maintenance of systems of time discipline, weights and measures, quality standards, or professional codes of conduct'. Investment also means to take by force, and these officials took the opportunity to take control of cholera, defining it as a problem only they could solve – though that would require knowledge of and control over citizens' movements and conduct. Investments like these are an attempt 'to render human conduct stable, predictable, and open to scrutiny … objects real or imagined are identified and defined in ways that render them susceptible to practical intervention'.[101]

Life assurance invested – laid claim to – health and mortality through its forms, and its temperance variants extended this to the consequences of drinking. This investment could be costly, though. We will see in Chapter 5 that the UKT's physician, Dr Joseph T. Mitchell, tried in 1856 to assess the effectiveness of the firm's referees, examining every claim made since 1840 to see if examiners had missed pre-existing medical conditions. His conclusions are discussed in Chapter 5, but here it is worth noting that Mitchell complained to his fellow directors about 'the enormous labour which has now been necessitated in searching each bundle of documents connected with each case reported upon'. Mitchell's review was meant to save the firm money, but he did not think it was worth repeating. 'The extended search through the papers of these cases', he decided, 'would involve so great an amount of labour that, the small benefit resulting therefrom, would not be a compensation'.[102] Making these arrangements required an investment of time and effort, an expenditure of resources.

These forms remained essential, though, materializing the networks through which temperance life assurance came into being. The making of these networks is the focus of Chapter 5.

Notes

1. James Dawson Burns, 'Some Remarks on Temperance Statistics', in *Proceedings of the International Temperance and Prohibition Convention, 1862*, edited by J. C. Street, F. R. Lees and D. Burns (London: Job Caudwell; Manchester: United Kingdom Alliance, 1862), 281.
2. Michael Zakim, 'Paperwork', *Raritan* 33, 4 (2014), 35, 37.
3. *Morning Chronicle*, 18 January 1850, 1.
4. Burns, company history, 6–7.
5. Alborn, *Regulated Lives*. See, for example, advert for R. Hellard, *Sherborne Mercury*, 6 June 1856, 1; UKT meeting, *Leicestershire Mercury*, 26 July 1856, 1.
6. Annual meeting, *Morning Chronicle*, 24 May 1859, 6.
7. 'Lecture on "life Assuances"' [*sic*], *Derbyshire Times and Chesterfield Herald*, 19 November 1859, 3.
8. *Western Daily Press*, 6 November 1858, 3.
9. Burns, company history.
10. James Alexander Mowatt, 'Life Insurance and Moderate Drinking – Facts!', *Phrenological Journal and Life Illustrated* 57, 5 (1 November 1873), 305.
11. M. A. Quetelet, *A Treatise on Man and the Development of his Faculties*, trans. Robert Knox (Edinburgh: William and Robert Chambers, 1842).
12. Ibid., 78.
13. Ibid.
14. Michael John Cullen, *The Statistical Movement in Early Victorian Britain* (Hassocks: Harvester Press; New York: Barnes and Noble, 1975), 65.
15. 1834 (559) *Report from the Select Committee on Inquiry into Drunkenness, with Minutes of Evidence, and Appendix*, 341, 62, 151. For John Clay, see, for example, 'Observations on the Annual Statistical Reports of the Gaol at Preston, in Lancashire, for the Last Four Years', *Proceedings of the Statistical Society of London* 1, 9 (1836–7).
16. William Hoyle, *Our National Resources; and How They Are Wasted. An Omitted Chapter in Political Economy* (London: Simpkin, Marshall; Manchester: John Heywood, 1871), 72.

17. Felix Driver, 'Moral Geographies: Social Science and the Urban Environment in Mid-Nineteenth Century England', *Transactions of the Institute of British Geographers* 13, 3 (1988), 278.
18. James Kneale and Shaun French, 'Mapping Alcohol: Health, Policy and the Geographies of Problem Drinking in Britain', *Drugs: Education, Prevention, and Policy* 15, 3 (2008), 233–49.
19. Suman Seth, 'Race, Specificity, and Statistics in Victorian Medicine', *Journal of Victorian Culture* 27, 2 (2022), 370–83; Heather Winlow, 'Mapping Moral Geographies: W. Z. Ripley's Races of Europe and the United States', *Annals of the Association of American Geographers* 96, 1 (2006), 119–41.
20. Kneale and Randalls, 'Making Climate Risks Work', 833–48; James Kneale and Samuel Randalls, 'Imagined Geographies of Climate and Race in Anglophone Life Assurance, c.1840–1930', in *Weather, Climate and the Geographical Imagination: Placing Atmospheric Knowledges*, edited by Martin Mahony and Samuel Randalls (Pittsburgh, PA: University of Pittsburgh Press, 2020), 115–31.
21. W. Felkin, 'Moral Statistics of a Section of the City of Norwich', 540–1, and 'Moral Statistics of a District Near Gray's Inn, London, in 1836', *Journal of the Statistical Society of London* 1 (1839), 541–2.
22. S. D. Chapman, 'Felkin, William (1795–1874)', *Oxford Dictionary of National Biography* (Oxford University Press, 2004), www.oxforddnb.com/view/article/53532, accessed 2 August 2016.
23. James Kneale, '"A Problem of Supervision": Moral Geographies of the Mineteenth Century British Public House', *Journal of Historical Geography* 25, 3 (1999), 333–48; Kneale, 'The Place of Drink'; Laura Vaughan, *Mapping Society: The Spatial Dimensions of Social Cartography* (London: UCL Press, 2015).
24. Cullen, *Statistical Movement*, 21, 109.
25. For the fate of this measure see James Kneale, 'Numbering Babylon? Failed Attempts to Map British Drinking, 1817–1914', in *Narcotic Cities. Counter-Cartographies of Drugs and Spaces*, edited by M. Germes, L. Klaus and S. Höhne (Berlin: Jovis, 2023), 42–53.
26. Tom Crook, 'Suspect Figures: Statistics and Public Trust in Victorian England', in *Statistics and the Public Sphere: Numbers and the People in Modern Britain, c. 1800–2000*, edited by Tom Crook and Glen O'Hara (London: Routledge, 2011), 179–98.
27. Cited in Libby Schweber, *Disciplining Statistics: Demography and Vital Statistics in France and England, 1830–1885* (Durham, NC: Duke University Press, 2006), 111.
28. Board meeting, 30 November 1840, UKT Minute Book 1, Aviva Archive.
29. Anna F. Fox, ed., *Memoir of Robert Charleton: Compiled Chiefly from His Letters* (London: S. Harris, 1876), 6; Thomas Hudson, *Temperance Pioneers of the West* (London: National Temperance Publication Depot, 1888), 99–100; G. C. Boase, 'Charleton, Robert (1809–1872)', rev. K. D. Reynolds, *Oxford Dictionary of National Biography* (Oxford University Press, 2004), www.oxforddnb.com/view/article/5156, accessed 9 January 2013.
30. Parliament, House of Lords (1842), *Children's Employment Commission: Appendix to the Second Report of the Commissioners Appointed for Inquiring into the Employment and Condition of Children in Mines and Manufactories: Trades and Manufactures, Part II. Reports and Evidence from Sub-Commissioners* (HL 1843 (30)), 537–43, 539.
31. Fox, *Memoir*; Hudson, *Temperance Pioneers*; Mason, *Sleigh Ride to Russia*, 9.
32. Fox, *Memoir*, 21, 33.
33. 1861 Census (Class: RG09; Piece: 1730; Folio: 17; Page: 29; GSU roll: 123).

34. Winskill, *Temperance Movement*, vol. 1, 221–2, 237; vol. 2, 147.
35. Hudson, *Temperance Pioneers*, 58–9.
36. Fox, *Memoir*, 28; Anon., *The Anti-Slavery Reporter* 18, no. 4 (1 January 1873), 115.
37. *Annual Monitor for 1874, or Obituary of the Members of the Society of Friends in Great Britain and Ireland, for the Year 1873*, 22, 24–5.
38. Hudson, *Temperance Pioneers*, 27; Fox, *Memoir*, 59, 20.
39. Hudson, *Temperance Pioneers*, 26.
40. Fox, *Memoir*, 10–11, 13, 11–12.
41. *Anti-Slavery Reporter* 18, 4 (1 January 1873), 116.
42. Probate 21 December 1872, England & Wales Government Probate Death Index 1858–2019; Winskill, *Temperance Movement*, vol. 1, 222.
43. 'Proceedings of the Statistical Society of London', *Journal of the Statistical Society of London* 5, 2 (1842), 230.
44. 'Theodore Compton', *Annual Monitor for 1910*; Withers, *Pioneers of British Life Assurance*, 84–5.
45. Timothy Alborn, 'Quill-Driving: British Life-Insurance Clerks and Occupational Mobility, 1800–1914', *Business History Review* 82 (2008), 33.
46. *Annual Monitor*, 47.
47. Report of Sixth Annual Meeting, January 1847, 2, Meeting, 15 May 1846, Standing Committee 2, Aviva Archives; *The Proceedings of the World's Temperance Convention, Held in London, August 4th, and Four Following Days* (London: World's Temperance Convention, 1846), 132.
48. Reproduced in 'Temperance Assurance Society', *British and Foreign Temperance Intelligencer* 6 (2 July 1842), 213.
49. *Morning Post*, 2 July 1860, 3; *The Times*, 31 August 1875, 8; *The Standard*, 24 September 1883, 3.
50. 'Temperance and Longevity', *Scientific American* 49, 23 (8 December 1883), 354.
51. *Manchester Times*, 1 July 1892, 8.
52. *Leeds Mercury*, 7 June 1876, 8.
53. 'Anniversary of the Rechabite and Temperance Society', *Wrexham Advertiser, Denbighshire, Flintshire, Shropshire, Cheshire & North Wales Register*, 19 June 1869, 6; *Glasgow Herald*, 9 May 1876, 4.
54. 'Does the Working Man Need Plenty of Beer?', *Sheffield & Rotherham Independent*, 31 August 1872, 8.
55. *Preston Chronicle and Lancaster Advertiser*, 9 October 1875, 6.
56. See, for example, Stanyon, *Leicester Chronicle and the Leicestershire Mercury*, 14 June 1879, 7; Whyte, *Manchester Guardian*, 21 March 1888, 7.
57. Charles R. Drysdale, *Morning Post*, 25 December 1886, 8; Charles R. Drysdale, *The Length of Life of Total Abstainers and Moderate Drinkers Compared: As Taken from the Records of Insurance Companies and Benefit Societies* (London: National Temperance Publication Depot, 1884).
58. Responding to Samuel Wilkes, 'Introduction to a Discussion on the Effects of Alcohol', *British Medical Journal* 2, 1600 (29 August 1891).
59. 'Temperance and Life Insurance', *Auckland Star*, 13 March 1882, 2.
60. Michel Callon, 'The Sociology of an Actor-Network: The Case of the Electric Vehicle', in *Mapping the Dynamics of Science and Technology*, edited by Michel Callon, John Law and Arie Rip (London: Palgrave Macmillan, 1986), 27.

61. Miranda Clow, 'The Design of Trust, Past and Present: A Dialogue between "Design for Trust" in Contemporary Design Practice and the Fire Insurance Industry in England 1680–1914', PhD thesis, Royal College of Art, 2020, 193–4.
62. Callon, 'Sociology of an Actor-Network', 28.
63. Advertisement, *British Women's Temperance Journal*, 1 January 1891, 12.
64. *Stirling Observer*, 24 January 1856, 3.
65. 'The Danger of Regular Habits', *Shields Daily Gazette*, 10 November 1887, 4.
66. Slide 2846, Friends Temperance Union lantern slides relating to medical aspects of temperance, MS 85L/2801–2808, Library of the Society of Friends.
67. Proposals in support of policy applications, 1885, Whittington MS 34430, London Archives.
68. Prospectuses in French, Dutch and in German, undated, Whittington Life Assurance Company Prospectuses 1867–91, MS 34427/001 and 34427/002, Summaries of the Whittington's accounts, policies, shares, investments etc., London Archives.
69. Alistair Macmillan, ed., *Mauritius Illustrated: Historical and Descriptive, Commercial and Industrial Facts, Figures, & Resources* (London: W. H. and L. Collingridge, 1914), 300.
70. French Whittington prospectus, undated but before 1889, London Archives.
71. Reference letters 1–249, Norwich Union Life 1809, MS NU5191, Aviva Archives.
72. Board meetings, 29 November 1842, 24 January 1843, 31 January 1843, 10 May 1842, Royal Farmers Minute Book 3, MS 14.989 3, London Archives.
73. Allen, *Medical Examinations*, first edition, 9, 10; Jonathan Adams Allen, *Medical Examinations for Life Insurance*, sixth edition (New York: J H and C M Goodsell, 1870), 162.
74. William Brinton, *On the Medical Selection of Lives for Assurance*, first edition (New York: John Hopper, 1863), 25.
75. Thomas David Lister, *Medical Examination for Life Insurance* (London: Edward Arnold, 1921), 34.
76. See James Kneale, '"These Are the Cases Who Call Themselves 'Moderate Drinkers', Because They Are Never Seen Embracing a Lamp-Post." The Problem of Moderate Drinking in Nineteenth- and Early Twentieth-Century Britain', in *Just Enough: The History, Culture and Politics of Sufficiency*, edited by Matthew Ingleby and Samuel Randalls (London: Palgrave Macmillan, 2019), 77–94.
77. Francis W. Moinet, *Guide to Medical Examination for Life Insurance* (Edinburgh: Maclachlan and Stewart; London: Simpkin, Marshall, 1876), 54; De Havilland Hall, *Medical Examination*, 78–9.
78. Alborn, *Regulated Lives*, 244, original emphasis.
79. Jureidini and White, 'Life Insurance', 191.
80. Theodore Porter, 'Life Insurance, Medical Testing, and the Management of Mortality', in *Biographies of Scientific Objects*, edited by Lorraine Daston (Chicago, IL: University of Chicago Press, 2000), 242.
81. Porter, 'Life Insurance', 227.
82. Christopher Lawrence, 'Incommunicable Knowledge: Science, Technology and the Clinical Art in Britain 1850–1914', *Journal of Contemporary History* 20, 4 (1985), 503–20.
83. Porter, 'Life Insurance', 237.
84. Alborn, *Regulated Lives*, 261.
85. Board Meeting, 5 July 1900, Minute Book 4, Sceptre Life Association, London Archives.

86. 39th Annual Report, 1904, Reports of Directors to Annual Meetings of Shareholders, 1872, 1886–90, 1903–4, 1914–17, SC 1/8/1/1 LMA.
87. McAllister, *Writing for Social Change*, 20–40.
88. George Robb, *White-Collar Crime in Modern England: Financial Fraud and Business Morality, 1845–1929* (Cambridge: Cambridge University Press, 1992), 138–42; McKie, *Jabez*.
89. Board meeting, 7 July 1893, UKT Minute Book 12, Aviva Archives; Harrison, *Dictionary of British Temperance Biography*, 18.
90. *The Standard*, 6 October 1897, 10 and 13 October 1897, 12.
91. *Belfast News-Letter*, 14 October 1897, 5.
92. *County Gentleman: Sporting Gazette, Agricultural Journal, and 'The Man about Town'*, 6 November 1897, 6.
93. 'Speculation on Jabez', *Daily Mail*, 22 October 1897, 3; *Financial Times*, 22 October 1897, 7.
94. Patrick Joyce and Chandra Mukerji, 'The State of Things: State History and Theory Reconfigured', *Theory & Society* 46 (2017), 1–19; Miles Ogborn, *Indian Ink: Script and Print in the Making of the English East India Company* (Chicago, IL: The University of Chicago Press, 2007).
95. Bouk, *How Our Days Became Numbered*, 57.
96. Zakim, 'Paperwork', 38.
97. Latour, *Pandora's Hope*.
98. Mariana Valverde, *Law's Dream of a Common Knowledge* (Princeton, NJ: Princeton University Press, 2003), 174.
99. Latour, *Pandora's Hope*, 69.
100. Schweber, *Disciplining Statistics*, 27; see Laurent Thévenot, 'Rules and Implements: Investment in Forms', *Social Science Information* 23, 1 (1984), 1–45.
101. Bruce Curtis, 'Social Investment in Medical Forms: The 1866 Cholera Scare and Beyond', *Canadian Historical Review* 81, 3 (2000), 362.
102. Joseph T. Mitchell, *Report of the Medical Director to the Directors of the Temperance and General Provident Institution* (16 September 1856), 17, 18, MS FL293, Aviva Archives.

5

Networks: Proselytizing fervour, minute inquisitorial inquiry

Introduction: Temperance societies and life assurance networks

When Theodore Compton, the UKT's first secretary, looked back at the problems the UKT had experienced in its first decade, he also acknowledged that 'the teetotal body was not prepared for such an institution. It took years of lecturing and writing, and tens of thousands of tracts, to educate the teetotalers of that age to an appreciation of the benefits of life insurance'.[1] The UKT did not simply take up a temperance network; it had to persuade that network of the value of life assurance. Robert Warner also noted that Dawson Burns's draft of the company's history did not include 'sufficient mention of the difficulties I had to keep it going, I being the pivot on which all things turned. No one but I could have got all those Friends as Country Directors'.[2] Those Friends – the Alexanders, Bowlys, Eatons and others – were useful intermediaries between the London board and local teetotalers and were brought into the firm's network through Warner's Quaker, business and temperance connections. He may not have been 'the pivot on which all things turned', but his role in building this network was clearly significant.

The UKT was created through temperance networks. Some of its founders had positions in the New British and Foreign Temperance Society, and this was their main source for contacts and employees. Warner sought the aid of William Baker, for example, who was not 'slow in using his position as Secretary of the New British and Foreign Temperance Society to advance the interests of the new Institution'.[3] Similarly, when the UKT sought salesmen and medical referees, they contacted members of local temperance societies around the country. This chapter examines their work, broadening our attention to include other firms alongside the UKT and extending it beyond the 1840s. In building effective networks these firms made a successful market for temperance life assurance.

The chapter considers two key actors: agents and medical referees. The work of these individuals ensured that the temperance principles and medical knowledge of the London board was put into practice in distant situations. Insurance agents needed intelligence, charisma and zeal in order to enrol members of their social networks while early medical referees were often outsiders within their profession; both had to navigate conflicting loyalties to employers, friends and clients. A good deal of 'tinkering' was needed to make sure this network operated smoothly. The chapter concludes with the UKT's review of its first fifteen years of business, which concluded that the firm might have been more prudent, because it had also sought to help 'reclaimed drunkards' who had been active in temperance. This reminds us that the UKT was not simply driven by the quest for actuarial and medical truths but was concerned with a broader sense of the values of temperance: socialized risks, the promotion of individual responsibility and careful investment.

The lives presented in this chapter include the Manx temperance agent, James Teare; the Harrap family of Leicester; and two early medical referees, Dr Ralph Barnes Grindrod and Dr Henry Mudge. We begin with James Teare, one of the best-known early teetotalers.

Temperance lives: James Teare (1804–1868)

James Teare was born on a farm on the Isle of Man, with six older brothers and two sisters. He was apprenticed to a boot and shoemaker, received 'the rudiments of a plain education' and joined the Wesleyan chapel. When his master decided to emigrate to America in 1823, Teare accompanied him as far as Liverpool before changing his mind and finding a new master in Preston. There he was one of the first to adopt temperance and then total abstinence, joining Joseph Livesey and the other 'men of Preston'.[4]

Teare was an influential temperance missionary. On their first missionary tour, in Lancashire in 1833, the Preston reformers drove through the streets waving a flag and ringing a bell, with 'James Teare, having a powerful voice, acting as crier'.[5] In 1835 he toured the Isle of Man, and in 1836, he set out on a 'self-imposed mission' to spread the word about teetotalism, using his own savings.[6] He visited twenty counties in England and Wales that year, concentrating on Wales, the West Country, and London and the home counties, covering around 8,000 miles by foot and stagecoach and attending over 400 meetings. The *Preston Temperance Advocate* mentions Teare's travels and meetings 108 times in 1836, publicizing his work even further.[7] In 1837 he told the Bristol Tee-Total Temperance Society that 'he had on the average attended six temperance meetings per week; had addressed Sunday Schools on the Sabbath; and regularly preached in the evening of that holy day'.[8]

Janette Martin suggests that historians have neglected the importance of 'oratory, the role of missionaries and the geographical organization of temperance'.[9] The first temperance agents certainly travelled impressive distances on foot – Arthur G. Barker noted that 'the story of the struggles and achievements of temperance agents in the West [of England] reads like a nineteenth-century addendum to the Acts of the Apostles'.[10] In the early days of the UKT, its agents' speeches were just as effective as the printed word. By 1859 Teare was thought to have travelled 20,000 miles and attended 8,000 meetings in twenty-four years' work as a temperance missionary.[11] His friend Thomas Hudson noted Teare's qualifications for this work. He was eloquent and 'could preach a powerful sermon [with] a very strong voice; and a speaker who can make a great noise in a popular assembly has obvious advantages, in that respect, over

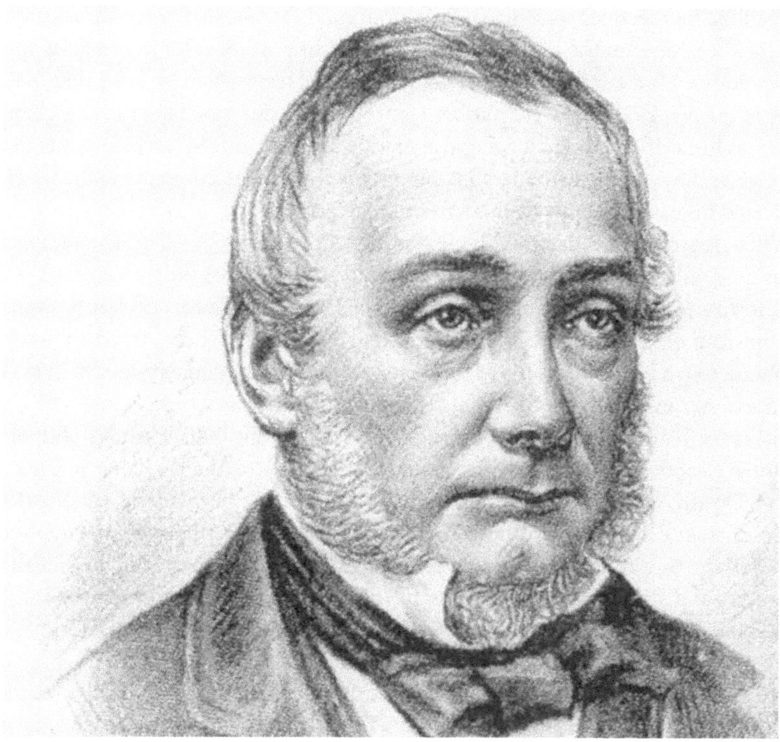

Figure 5.1 James Teare.

Source: P. T. Winskill, *The Temperance Movement and Its Workers*, volume I, 1891, 96. Courtesy of the Livesey Collection, UCLan.

other men'.[12] Winskill noted that as 'a strong-built, healthy, vigorous man', Teare was proof of the healthiness of abstinence, and he was brave, 'uncompromising, fearless'.[13]

That fearlessness was tested in the 1830s. Penryn's Wesleyans refused to let him use their chapel for a meeting, but his fiercest opponents were the licensed victuallers and brewers, for whom the arrival of Teare, 'that Stormy Petrel from the north', was 'the harbinger of a coming storm', as Hudson humorously suggested.[14] In Liskeard, clerks broke up Teare's meeting, and in Bridgwater local 'roughs' encouraged by the trade smashed up the Friends' meeting house where Teare was speaking.[15] At Taunton's Wesleyan chapel, the pews were broken and iron hat pegs were hurled at the speakers; at Street teetotalers who had turned out to hear him were attacked.[16] Still, this opposition served to demonstrate how seriously Teare was taken by supporters and enemies alike; it was reported that 'James Teare has set the west on fire with cold water!'[17]

Teare was a remarkably successful advocate of total abstinence, particularly in Cornwall, where audiences shared his Methodism and respected his working-class origins. Thomas Hudson went so far as to suggest that 'there were two portraits to be seen hanging side by side on the walls of hundreds of the houses of the Cornish people, namely, those of John Wesley and James Teare'.[18] Teare's visits to Devon also inspired the first teetotal societies in Devonport and Plymouth, Exeter, Ilfracombe and Tavistock.[19] Several of the individuals who played important roles in the development of temperance life assurance were persuaded to adopt teetotalism by Teare, like William Baker of the NB&FTS and UKT and Dr Henry Mudge, described later in this chapter.[20] Teare was himself appointed a general agent for the UKT in 1841, which made perfect sense, given how many teetotalers he met on his travels; the company enthusiastically publicized his association with them in their advertising.[21]

When Teare's health declined he feared he would die in poverty. The temperance writer Dr Frederic Richard Lees criticized Teare's 'passion for little economies, which is apt to run into meanness', but this might have reflected Teare's modest background and the fear of a pauper's burial, which the middle-class Lees, freed to work for temperance by a legacy from his grandfather, would not have understood.[22] Teare died in Manchester in March 1868, probate establishing him to be comfortably off.[23]

In James Teare, 'intensely earnest and impressive', the UKT found a temperance missionary who could also sell life assurance.[24] Many of their agents, referees and lives in Devon, Cornwall and other counties would have been members of societies whose existence had been prompted by Teare's visits in the 1830s. Teare's qualities as a missionary would also have made him an excellent salesman, and his meanness, plain dress and simple habits might also have been read as signs of prudence. It is hard to assess his effectiveness in bringing lives to the UKT, but also difficult to imagine a better sign of the firm's commitment to abstinence.

Before we turn to other temperance life assurance agents it is worth briefly comparing Teare to James McKenna, another of the UKT's early travelling agents. McKenna must have seemed like another good choice: active in temperance since 1837, he toured Britain and Ireland as the secretary of the wildly popular Irish temperance advocate Father Mathew, meeting thousands of teetotalers in the process. However McKenna was not an effective travelling agent for the UKT, and the board let him go after it found that he had produced only £230 worth of premiums for £400 of expenses.[25] He became the firm's Glasgow agent instead, where he remained until 1853.[26] Thomas Hudson suggested that McKenna's unsuitable wardrobe, limp and quick temper meant that 'he did not appear to advantage in the presence of ladies', dwelling also on McKenna's divorce, Irishness and Catholicism.[27] Teare might have had his foibles, but he had charisma, and his working-class Methodism endeared him to temperance audiences; McKenna, an Irish Catholic ex-soldier, would often have seemed like an outsider.

Agency: Intelligence, urbanity and zeal

In his draft manuscript of the history of the UKT Dawson Burns noted that the firm's success 'has been due in a large degree to the intelligence urbanity and zeal of the District Superintendents, and local Agents. They have shown the excellence of their case, and have known also how to make this excellence clear to those willing to listen and understand'.[28] Burns knew that Warner's 'bright idea' had to be actively marketed.

Liz McFall's account of industrial assurance rightly devotes a good deal of attention to 'the Man from the Pru', who sold industrial life assurance policies to working-class families, collected payments on their doorsteps, and provided the firm with detailed knowledge of, and a flexible relationship with, precarious household economies.[29] McFall reminds us that insurance is more than just cold governmentality; the men who sold industrial assurance needed charisma and zeal as well as intelligence. Other researchers have emphasized the importance of emotion and intuition in the buying and selling of everyday finance.[30] Selling temperance life assurance brought ideas of uncertainty, risk and security to life in affecting ways.

Zeal was also a quality commonly associated with temperance activists. The UKT insisted that agents must also be policyholders and thus members of the institution, and 'so communicate the advantages of life assurance not only by argument but by example'.[31] The report of the firm's third annual meeting reminded readers 'that every agent of this Society lectures on the general subject of Temperance, and that every paper issued by the Society enforces the same principle'. Agents who volunteered to address local temperance societies would have some of their expenses paid by the firm. As a result 'this Institution is not only a standing proof of the benefits of Total Abstinence, but a most powerful engine in promoting the cause throughout the kingdom'.[32] Peter Winskill also noted that 'most of the agents, and more particularly the district or superintendent agents, of the United Kingdom Temperance and General Provident Institution were and are earnest temperance advocates, many of whom did great service to the cause'.[33] Similarly, the firm's twentieth-century historian, Hartley Withers, suggested that 'for a long time the Bands of Hope and similar bodies acted in effect as its enthusiastic agents; life assurance acquired a streak of the proselytizing fervour which meant much in Victorian days'.[34] In general, though, agents became increasingly professional as the century went on; early agents tended to be active members of temperance societies with business connections beyond insurance, becoming increasingly specialized life assurance salesmen as the market grew. After the General section opened, moderate drinkers could also be appointed as agents, as A. H. Kidson of Warrington was in 1849 for example.[35]

This section begins by setting out the ways in which these offices established their networks of agents beyond the metropolis. We will then look at these agents, comparing them to the salesmen (and occasional saleswoman) included in Timothy Alborn's study of British life assurance firms, before turning to see what their work involved.

'A few active temperance men wanted': Establishing networks of agents

While it would eventually develop a system of district superintendents to supervise its local agents, with 'chief offices' in Edinburgh, Glasgow, Aberdeen, Dundee, Manchester, Liverpool, London, Dublin and Belfast, in its early years the UKT had a simpler, flatter structure: the London board and its staff on the one hand, and its agents scattered across England, Scotland, Wales and Ireland on the other. In its first meetings the UKT promised to appoint agents in 'the different districts where the cause of Temperance has taken root'.[36] It agreed that the travelling agents of three temperance societies – the New British & Foreign Temperance Society, the Society for the Suppression of Intemperance, and the British Temperance Association – could also be UKT agents.[37] In 1848 the board stated that it wanted to have an agent in all 5,365 of the English and Welsh parishes with more than 500 inhabitants listed in the 1841 Census. At that point the firm had only 277 agents, which certainly left room for growth.[38] Advertisements were placed for particular areas, for example in Essex in 1848 and again in 1866, when there were already fourteen agents in thirteen places in the county. In 1869 'a few active Temperance Men' were sought in Liverpool, and the firm advertised for a chief agent for each county in North Wales in 1879.[39] By 1856, following a very prosperous year's business, the report of the UKT's annual meeting stated: 'Experience has fully proved that the most efficient mode of extending life assurance business is by means of active agents, and during the past year your directors have appointed no less than 171, many of whom already give promise of being very successful.'[40]

Sceptre's minute books show similar efforts to recruit and manage the firm's first agents, appointing men in Yorkshire, London, Lincolnshire, Durham and Nottinghamshire in the first meetings.[41] The board enquired about buying 'a good office map of England and Wales', perhaps to locate existing agents and identify places where they still needed them – the Prudential provided its superintendents with maps, and advised them to become 'thoroughly conversant with the various places under your supervision, and of the boundaries of your district'.[42] Closely associated with the Methodist churches that had separated from the Wesleyans, Sceptre knew what kind of agents they wanted; in 1865 a newspaper advertisement sought 'an active pushing Man (a liberal Methodist preferred), as AGENT for Leeds'.[43] The firm made good use of its travelling agents and district superintendents were appointed. In 1865, the first full year of the Sceptre's business, James Perry Distin, the firm's superintendent in Bristol, managed forty-eight agents in the district.[44]

James Mills, the Sceptre's general agency superintendent, paid tribute to the qualities of his agents when he noted that Sceptre's success owed a good deal to 'the employment of energetic and trustworthy men as agents', who worked with 'steady perseverance and tact'.[45] It's not always clear that temperance was an important motivation for these Sceptre agents, but it was clearly significant for some. At the office's twenty-second annual meeting in 1887, the two superintendents – William Bingham, who had replaced Mills in 1885 after previously working for the UK Alliance, and William Jepson – were singled out for praise:

> Mr Bingham was doing them good service. He had been long and honourably connected with the temperance world. The fact that he and Mr Jepson were largely interested in that matter would account for the large proportion of temperance lives they secured. According to the character of these gentlemen, so would be the character of the Agents they appointed.[46]

A year later it was noted that 59 per cent of the year's new business came from assuring total abstainers, which 'indicated the strata in which [the agents] were accustomed to work'. However Jepson warned it was possible for agents to exhaust their social circle: 'In the congregation of which he was a member, at Leeds, they had no less than eight agency superintendents or district managers, all representing capital insurance companies.' Local competition could become a problem, especially when firms sought the same thrifty nonconformist lives. At the same time, Bingham acknowledged that more agents were needed, as 'many parts of the kingdom were imperfectly represented'.[47]

We now look to see who some of these agents were and what they did. In the process we will see that early temperance activism may have given way to professionalism as the century progressed.

Activists and professionals: Agents for temperance life assurance

Timothy Alborn notes that early British life assurance offices, targeting upper- or middle-class markets, preferred to appoint lawyers, bankers, merchants, or shopkeepers as agents, while newer firms sought 'estate agents, grocers, drapers, and chemists' who might find more modest customers; he suggests shopkeepers would have been the first choice for the UKT.[48] The professions of these early agents were important because they were expected to sell policies to their social networks; when these were exhausted firms needed to find new agents. Women agents were very rare until after 1918 at least in part because of this emphasis on utilizing existing business networks, though women were of course potential customers.

There are no lawyers or bankers amongst the UKT agents named in the 1840 prospectus who can be traced in other sources, but there was a gentleman, three schoolmasters and a minister, alongside men used to handling money – a surveyor, accountant and house agent, a solicitor's clerk and an auctioneer – as well as two builders. There were also many shopkeepers, particularly grocers, drapers and ironmongers, as well as men of more modest positions. In 1841, for example, William Norris resigned his Coalbrook Dale [*sic*] agency, recommending John Child as his replacement. The board agreed to this, resolving though 'that his name be omitted from the list of Agents, his station being that of a mechanic'.[49] This John Child may have been the twenty-five-year-old mechanic living at Coalbrook Dale, Madeley, with his wife Elizabeth and their new baby in 1841.[50] The only William Norris listed locally in the census for this area was a forty-five-year-old accountant in Madeley, much more the kind of man the firm was looking for as an agent. It seems likely that the board could see the advantage of employing someone like Child, who could sell policies in his working-class workplace and neighbourhood, but did not wish to advertise his employment.

Some of the first agents recruited by the UKT were, like James Teare and James McKenna, early teetotal activists, including a turner and chairmaker (and future travel agent) named Thomas Cook, who became the agent for Market Harborough at the end of 1840.[51] Moving to Leicester in 1841, Cook became the agent there, alongside his printing and bookselling business; he began his temperance excursions in the same year.[52] In 1843 Cook reported that members of Leicester's Temperance Society had already established about £1,000 worth of policies with the UKT.[53] Cook was a natural choice for an agent, but when his first business failed in 1846 he stopped advertising his UKT agency.

Other agents were also prominent businessmen and early teetotalers. The agent for Norwich listed in the prospectus seems likely to be the bookseller, publisher and printer John Jarrold II, who had originally been invited to be a director of the UKT.[54] By 1849 the firm of Jarrold & Sons were acting as agents for the UKT in Norwich.[55] John's son Samuel was one of the first to sign the pledge in Norwich and a founder of the city's Temperance Society; the Jarrolds also supported abolition, the Norwich City Mission and temperance publishing, giving John Cassell his start in this field.[56] In Belfast, Alexander Smith Mayne was another early agent for the UKT, a founder member of the city's Temperance Society and publisher of several temperance magazines.[57] The Quaker Francis J. Thompson was listed as the agent for Bridgwater, Somerset; inspired by James Teare and John Hockings, Thompson was the first to sign the pledge in Bridgwater, becoming secretary of the town's Total Abstinence Society, a founder and president of the Western Temperance League and a vice president of the National Temperance League. While serving as Mayor in 1883 Thompson abstained from licensing sessions, as he would have had felt honour-bound to refuse every application.[58]

In Sleaford, Lincolnshire, William Fawcett was the secretary of the first teetotal society established in the county and another natural choice as agent.[59] William was a baker, grocer and medicine vendor by 1851, and his wife Lydia was a temperance hotel keeper. Winskill reported that 'after placing the [Sleaford] temperance society on a good working basis, Mr. William Fawcett devoted much of his time to the larger villages in the neighbourhood, and after walking many a weary mile, delivering lectures and scattering temperance literature, he was enabled to form societies in most of these places'.[60] Lincoln itself seems to have been a lively Temperance city, returning Whig and Liberal MPs for much of the period covered by this book, with temperance stalwarts in key civic positions – several of them also UKT agents, like printer, bookbinder and stationer Charles Akrill, who was the firm's representative between 1856 and 1861 and Sherriff of Lincoln in 1868.[61]

The final UKT agent considered here was another important local Liberal, this time in Birmingham. A former Stourbridge engine fitter, Charles Lamsdale became one of the UKT's Birmingham agents by 1865; by 1861 he was comfortable enough to employ a domestic servant.[62] At his death in 1898 it was said that Lamsdale 'was almost the *doyen* of Life Assurance circles in the Midlands, and did, perhaps, more than anyone else to popularize that extraordinarily successful office, the United Kingdom Temperance and General Provident Institution. The Liberalism of Birmingham generally and of Handsworth in particular is the poorer by the regretted death of Charles Lamsdale'.[63]

The Sceptre office seems to have employed two kinds of agents: professional salesmen who operated for many years, and others who sold policies to a small number of friends and acquaintances. The sample lists 274 agents outside the London office, which sold seventy-five of the sample's 959 abstainers' policies between 1865 and 1881; another thirty-eight did not record an agent and may also have been sold through the office. Of the remainer, only sixteen agents, many of them district managers, sold ten or more, establishing nearly a third of the policies in the sample between them

Table 5.1 The most successful agents in the sceptre sample, 1865–81

Agent	Location	Policies sold in	Lives assured
John Trythall	Croydon	Kent, Surrey, East Sussex	40
Kennedy		Middlesex, Surrey	33
Thomas Nicholson	Southampton	Hampshire, Berkshire	29
Ashworth		Lancashire, Yorkshire	23
William Bartlett	Bristol	Gloucestershire, Somerset	23
Edward Hall	London	Middlesex, Essex	22
Bradbury	Manchester	Lancashire, Cheshire	20
Samuel Antliff	Newark	Yorkshire, Lincolnshire	19
James Ward Rhodes	Nottingham	Nottinghamshire, Derbyshire	17
William Jepson	Leeds	Yorkshire	16
Sutton	Long Eaton	Derbyshire	16
James Looney	Liverpool	Lancashire, Cheshire	15
Aaron Mobbs	Reading	Berkshire	12
Eatwell	Swindon	Wiltshire	11
James Moorhouse	Sabden	Lancashire	11
Henry Haynes	Cardiff	Glamorgan, Monmouthshire	10

Source: Sceptre sample.

(Table 5.1). One hundred and forty-two agents – more than half – sold only one policy each. That might reflect sampling and archiving issues but also suggests that insurance was not a significant concern for many of these men.

It is possible to discover a little about some of these men. John Trythall, a Croydon auctioneer active from the late 1870s, sold forty of the sample's policies in London, Kent and East Sussex; his son John Anthony Trythall continued the auction business, but probably not the agency, after his father died in 1891.[64] Edward Hall, the East London district manager in Bow, sold twenty-two of the sample policies in the area.[65] Another manager, James Ward Rhodes, was very successful in the short time that he was the Sceptre's superintendent of the Nottinghamshire district, from 1881. By 1891, though, he was the local superintendent for the Scottish Provident office, remaining with them until he took his own life, at work, in 1898. Scottish Provident had asked him to resign, though the firm was quick to protect James's reputation – and its own – by assuring the coroner that the office's finances were in order, and that the row had simply been 'differences of opinion … as to the management of the district'.[66] In 1886 Sceptre had agreed to honour claims resulting from suicide, so it would have covered the £250 policy James established when he first became their agent.[67]

Local factors could make Sceptre agencies distinctive: Ashworth and Moorhouse sold policies in the temperance towns of Lancashire (Chapter 2), and Thomas Nicholson's Hampshire agency assured eleven military personnel stationed at Aldershot. Nicholson was a Rochdale-born textile worker who became a Methodist local preacher in Southampton, and then an insurance and merchant shipping broker; his career path combines many of the things that made Sceptre distinctive.[68] Other moderately successful salesmen shared the liberal ethos of men like Jepson and Bingham. The Scarborough auctioneer John Dawber, who sold six of the policies in the sample, was also the proprietor of the Albert Hall, a 700-seat music theatre. The Hall's first advertised event was a public meeting for the repeal of the Contagious Diseases Act in 1880, and it hosted a meeting of the Women's Christian Temperance Union in the following year, as well as comedians, variety performances and at least one minstrel show.[69] While Dawber's role as a music hall proprietor was unusual, he was clearly part of the town's liberal and temperance culture – the Hall also provided a home for the Scarborough Liberal Association.[70]

The Whittington's agents are more anonymous, but an 1889 booklet of *Instructions to Agents* sets out how they were meant to act. Agents were told to assure themselves with the company, as 'every man who has assured his life is likely to be earnest in impressing the advantage of assurance upon another. To an Agent, this earnestness would be worth ten times the cost of a policy'.[71] As each life required friends' references, every sale brought the agent into contact with a widening pool of potential lives, who would 'follow by the force of attraction … this *personal canvass* amongst friends, neighbours, and even from house to house, will afford the best opportunities for explanation and persuasion'.[72] The guide told agents to take advantage of a death, whether the deceased had been assured or not, quoting one of W. E. Hillman's hints: 'Whenever a neighbour was unwell, I reminded him of the uncertainty of life. When prosperous, I urged him to devote some portion of his spare wealth to the purpose of Assurance; every situation of life more or less supplied me with arguments for attending to this duty'.[73]

Our next Life provides further detail of the character and business of these agents.

Temperance lives: The Harraps of Leicester (1853–1935)

The lives of Joseph Harrap and his sons Amos and Joseph, who were UKT agents for over eighty years between them, offer us useful glimpses not only into Leicester's temperance world, but also into the transformation of temperance life assurance as it shifted from radical, working-class roots into something more professional.

Joseph Harrap (1823–1883) was born in Ossett, near Wakefield, Yorkshire, and was raised by his grandfather after his father died. Working in a cotton factory by the time he was eight, Joseph led other child workers in an unsuccessful strike before being apprenticed to a shoemaker at fourteen.[74] Joining the Primitive Methodists at about this time, with the encouragement of the Reverend William Antliff (Chapter 3) he served as an itinerant preacher for some years, until he resigned due to ill health in 1844.[75] Joseph had been teetotal from 1839, joining the Rechabites by 1844.[76] It was later said that he had 'walked 2,346 miles, preached 443 times, besides delivering temperance lectures, and visited 4,357 families' in the twenty-two months of his ministry.[77] Joseph settled in Whitwick, near Leicester, where he was active in temperance circles. He married Harriett Briggs in 1847, and their son Amos Briggs Harrap was born in 1855.[78] In 1853 Joseph became an agent for the UKT, his success as a salesman leading the firm to persuade him to become a fulltime district manager from 1856. He moved to Leicester, 'where by patient, persevering effort, and by adding other businesses to

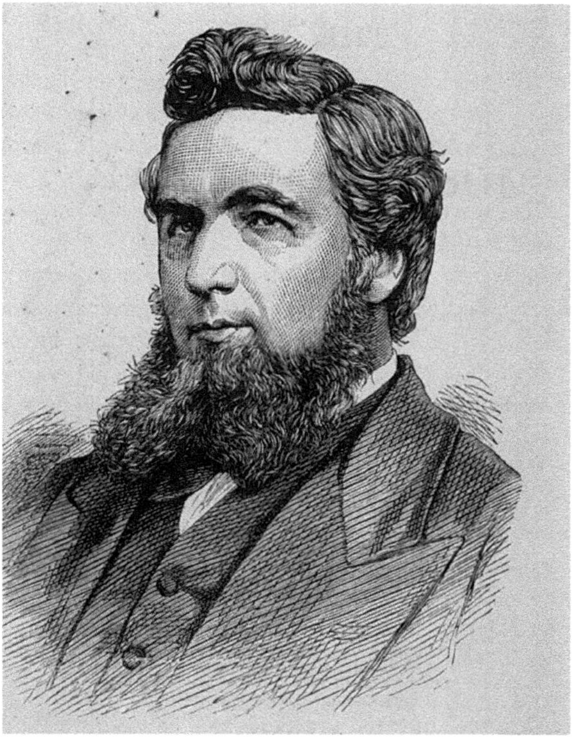

Figure 5.2 Joseph Harrap.

Source: John W. Kirton, *The Life of Joseph Harrap, of Leicester*, 1873.

that of insurance, he secured a respectable position in society', as Winskill put it.[79] It was later claimed that he gave a hundred lectures in a year, though his health suffered again.[80] By the 1860s Joseph was operating a 'Commercial Auction Mart' on Belvoir Street as well as selling insurance.[81]

Joseph supported Leicester's local Auxiliary of the UK Alliance, and in time became vice president of the town's Temperance Society and a founder and first manager of the Leicester Temperance Building Society.[82] He was elected to national and local positions in the International Order of Good Templars, having helped establish the first Lodge in Leicester, and to the British Temperance League executive. He was a frequent correspondent on temperance matters to Leicester's papers.[83] By 1871 Joseph and Harriett had five children, including Amos, now a sixteen-year-old clerk, and Joseph junior, who had been born in 1869, and their household included a general servant and a nurse.[84]

Poor health was again starting to interfere with Joseph's ability to work, however, and he gave up public speaking on the advice of Dr James Edmunds, the UKT's physician (Chapter 8).[85] Harriett died in 1878, after a long illness, and Joseph married Mary Ann Burton.[86] While Joseph was still listed as the UKT's branch superintendent for the Midlands District in their 1881 prospectus, it seems likely that management of the 'mart' had now fallen to Amos, with the firm listed as 'Joseph Harrap and Sons'.[87] Joseph died in March 1883, leaving the agency to Amos; his personal estate was worth just over £2,500.[88] The *Leicester Chronicle*'s obituary noted, 'Leicester has lost one of its old and esteemed townsmen; the temperance cause in Leicester has been deprived of one of its most popular local champions.'[89] The UKT acknowledged the loss of one of 'its most prominent representatives' at their its annual meeting.[90]

Amos Briggs Harrap (1855–1900) became the UKT's district manager after his father's death. Unsurprisingly, he had been an active Good Templar as a teenager, and his brother Ernest and sister Selina were also active temperance workers.[91] Amos married Emma Susan Jardine at the London Road Congregational chapel in 1879.[92] He continued to be an active Templar and supported the Alliance's work.[93] Amos died young, aged forty-five, and his funeral drew representatives of the Leicester Temperance Society, Rechabites, Band of Hope Union, British Women's Temperance Association, UKT and the Good Templars.[94] Amos left £3,536 to his wife, and his younger brother Joseph took over the UKT's district office.[95]

Joseph Harrap (1870–1935) was already an insurance agent at twenty-one, and by 1909 Harrap Brothers, insurance and shipping brokers, occupied the handsome Queen's Chambers building on Leicester's Horsefair Street.[96] Joseph does not seem to have been as active in Leicester temperance as his father and older brother. He died in April 1935, leaving just over £3,100; he left shares in the firm to his wife Sarah, his son Joseph Arnold Harrap and a friend. It's not clear what happened to Harrap Brothers after that date.[97]

Between them Joseph, Amos and Joseph junior were agents for the UKT for over eighty years. Joseph senior's itinerant preaching resembles James Teare's; as a labour organizer he also reminds us of the radical strands within teetotalism, though Samuel Smiles would have applauded his later social mobility. His temperance work was probably fostered within Primitive Methodism, though he seems to have ended his days as a Congregationalist. His sons inherited Joseph's well-established business but enjoyed a rather different upbringing – Joseph junior was educated at Wyggeston Boys Grammar School, for example.[98] While Amos was clearly brought up in his father's temperance world, Joseph junior does not seem to have been as active. The relative scarcity of twentieth-century temperance archives makes its members harder to research than Winskill's 'pioneers', but the contrast between the older and younger Joseph is striking.

The lives of the Harraps give us a strong sense of a life assurance business intertwined with the world of temperance. It is time to turn to the medical referees these firms employed, who would not always be so enthusiastic about total abstinence.

Minute inquisitorial inquiry: The medical referees

In 1870 the UKT's surgeon Joseph T. Mitchell wrote to the *British Medical Journal* to complain about an article that had suggested that the General section contained 'drunkards', insisting that 'no insurance company makes more minute inquisitorial inquiry into the habits of candidates than the United Kingdom Temperance Provident

Office'.[99] Life assurance depended upon medical referees and directors carefully examining applicants, but the UKT continued to attract additional attention and suspicion throughout its existence because not everyone was convinced by the statistical evidence presented by the firm's 'experience'. One otherwise positive 1890 newspaper report concluded, for example, that offices did not seem to be able to ascertain 'whether the so-called abstainers do abstain, and how far the moderate section are merely moderate'.[100] Given these persistent fears, the role of the medical referee was vital.

While Chapter 4 examined the attempts made by temperance life assurance companies to ensure this 'minute inquisitorial inquiry' was carried out, and Chapter 8 will consider the contribution of temperance life assurance to medical arguments about alcohol's effects on the human body, the next section of this chapter focuses on the medical referees employed by these firms. In general, the character of these referees changed as firms became more successful and 'medical temperance' became more acceptable. In the early years of the UKT, medical referees might be enthusiastic temperance supporters, but the men who came later, when abstinence was increasingly accepted as at least as safe as, and perhaps healthier than, moderate drinking, far exceeded the number of doctors who might publicly declare for 'medical temperance'. At the same time, they had to be proficient doctors; 'no gentleman should be appointed to the Office but one who is held in the very best repute by his professional brethren', as Mitchell warned in 1856.[101] We will look first at the UKT's efforts to recruit these early referees, before looking at two of them in more detail.

The UKT appointed thirty-two medical referees in December 1840, before the firm opened for business, and another 104 in 1841, though sixty-seven of those were appointed in the first three months of that year. These referees were unevenly distributed (see Table 5.2).

Table 5.2 Medical referees appointed by the UKT, December 1840–December 1841

County or territory	Referees
Cornwall	13
Yorkshire	11
Lancashire	8
Lincolnshire	7
Devon	6
Berkshire, Durham, Kent, Middlesex, Somerset	5 each
Bedfordshire, Buckinghamshire, Gloucestershire, Hampshire, Hertfordshire, Isle of Man, Norfolk, Wiltshire	4 each
Warwickshire	3
Essex, Glamorgan, Northamptonshire, Northumberland, Staffordshire, Suffolk, Worcestershire	2 each
Aberdeenshire, Antrim, Cambridgeshire, Cheshire, City of London, East Sussex, Jersey, Lanarkshire, Limerick, Midlothian, Montgomeryshire, Nottinghamshire, Offaly, Renfrewshire, Selkirkshire, Shropshire, West Sussex	1 each

Source: Sceptre sample.

Most of these referees were in England, with only three appointed in Ireland, five in Scotland, three in Wales, one in Jersey and four in the Isle of Man.[102] This distribution broadly reflected the spread of agents appointed by the firm in its first year, as well as the geography of temperance support. Lancashire, with a census population of 1,667,054, had only one more agent than Lincolnshire, with a population of 362,602; Cornwall, with more referees than any other county, had fewer inhabitants than Lincolnshire, though that may have reflected the influence of James Teare on the UKT's early success, as he was travelling in Cornwall in June 1841, when referees were appointed in Truro, Penryn, Helston, Hayle and St Austell.[103]

We will find out more about some of these men, and the relationship between medicine and life assurance, in Chapter 8, but one referee worth mentioning here is John Snow, investigator of the Broad Street cholera outbreak and later anaesthetist to Queen Victoria. John and his brother the Reverend Thomas Snow became teetotalers in 1836 through the York Temperance Society, and John remained abstinent except when told to take wine for medical reasons later in his life.[104] In 1841 Theodore Compton suggested that the UKT needed to appoint metropolitan medical referees to stand in for the firm's surgeon, Joseph Mitchell, and physician, R. Dundas Thomson, when they could not examine applicants. Snow, who was then living on Frith Street, Soho, where he had been in practice since 1838, was one of two doctors appointed.[105] In fact when Mitchell wrote his report on the firm's first fifteen years of mortality, he noted that Snow had examined one of the ten London cases where a serious condition had been missed; Mitchell and Thomson had examined the others.[106] Snow's adherence to teetotalism at a time when many doctors considered alcohol necessary for diet presents a parallel with his refusal to abandon his theory about cholera as a water-borne infection, despite opposition from William Farr, *The Lancet* and many authorities; it may also explain his experiments with ether as an anaesthetic, as an alternative to spirits.[107]

While it is hard to discover much about the UKT's referees from medical directories, some, like Snow, are mentioned in temperance records. We now turn to consider another two early teetotal referees, Ralph Barnes Grindrod and Henry Mudge.

Temperance lives: Dr Ralph Barnes Grindrod (1811–1883), Dr Henry Mudge (1806–1874)

Doctors Grindrod and Mudge were appointed as medical examiners for the UKT on the same day in December 1840.[108] They were alike in many ways, though Grindrod achieved national recognition while Mudge was most active in Cornwall and Devon.

P. T. Winskill divided the career of Ralph Barnes Grindrod into three distinct periods: his early work in Manchester (1830–44), his 'medical mission' (1844–50) and finally his hydropathic work in Malvern (1850–83).[109] Born in Cheshire, Grindrod was apprenticed to his older brother, a physician, becoming first a medical officer to working men's clubs in Runcorn, then the Chorlton Infirmary's surgeon and later a general practitioner at Ancoats, Manchester. He joined the moderationist Salford and Manchester Temperance Society but was teetotal by 1832. A rare Anglican early teetotaler, his juvenile teetotal society was supported by the established church.[110] Grindrod became famous for public lectures and debates; the 'Teetotal Discussion' with a local brewer in Stephenson Square was reported to have attracted 10,000–15,000 people in 1835.[111] Grindrod joined Francis Beardsall's Society, alongside Joseph Barker (Chapter 3), which helped establish a national body, the British Temperance Association (later the British Temperance League).[112] Grindrod was awarded a prize by the British and Foreign Temperance Society in 1838 for his essay on the benefits of total abstinence, which received widespread attention when it was published in 1839 as *Bacchus*.

Grindrod gave up his medical practice for a temperance tour of northern and Midlands counties between 1844 and 1850, with his wife Mary acting as his secretary. His lectures had a strongly medical and scientific character; he employed an artist to prepare coloured diagrams of organs showing the effects of alcoholic indulgence. He also employed other props including 'a number of models to illustrate the action of the heart and respiration, exhibiting the movements of these organs by mechanical contrivances'.[113] Winskill credited Grindrod with reaching 'the clergy, medical men, and others in the higher circles of society' with these lectures, but their audiences could be substantial; Thomas Cook reported an audience of 3,000 juveniles at Leicester in 1845 and Winskill would later claim that Grindrod converted nearly 200,000 people to teetotalism.[114] It might be significant that he established a sizeable UKT policy for £1,000 in 1844, at the start of his tour.[115] Grindrod was clearly very comfortably off – he owned property from at least 1832 and was paying rates for five properties in Ancoats in 1840 – but the life of a travelling lecturer probably seemed less certain than that of a general practitioner, and Ralph and Mary's only child was born in 1846. The prospect of unsettled family life may explain why he established the policy; his status as a gentleman explains its size.[116]

In 1850 Grindrod opened a hydropathic clinic and practice in Malvern, which was already strongly associated with the 'water cure' through its association with doctors James Wilson and James Gully since 1842; Grindrod was friends with Wilson, having first visited Malvern in 1846.[117] Busy with the scientific and liberal life of the town, Grindrod opened a geology museum and was the owner and editor of the *Malvern Advertiser* from 1855.[118] He continued to lecture on temperance and hosted meetings at Malvern. After suffering a long illness, Grindrod passed away in November 1883.[119]

Henry Mudge had been a medical examiner for the Eagle life assurance office since at least 1830, and this experience, together with his active teetotalism, probably made him an obvious choice for the UKT.[120] Mudge was educated at St Bartholomew's Hospital, London, but spent the rest of his life in Bodmin, Cornwall, becoming surgeon to Bodmin Hospital and Dispensary and the Union Medical Officer.[121] A Wesleyan, he was converted to teetotalism by James Teare, becoming the first member of Bodmin's Temperance Society to sign the pledge. Despite opposition, Mudge 'stood bravely by teetotalism, freely using his voice, pen, and purse to further the interests of the cause'.[122] As a temperance speaker in Cornwall and Devon, he encouraged the establishment of societies in St Austell and Liskeard.[123] He married Susan Lyon in 1831, and the couple moved in local temperance circles. Their daughter Susan married John Stanger Pethybridge, J.P., another Bodmin temperance worker, and Mudge's brother-in-law, William Pearce, was also a teetotal Cornish doctor and the agent for the Standard Life office.[124] A popular figure locally, Mudge was Mayor of Bodmin in 1862 and 1863.[125]

Thomas Hudson described Mudge as 'a person of spare habit of body and of pale countenance', 'highly-intelligent and benevolently disposed'.[126] Winskill thought Mudge was 'probably one of the first medical men in the country to carry out temperance principles in their regular medical practice', at a time, as Hudson noted, 'when teetotal doctors had often to suffer pecuniarily and otherwise for conscience sake', suffering 'loss of patronage and petty persecution'.[127] Thomas Whittaker agreed that Mudge and other figures in early medical temperance 'taught the truths to an unbelieving people, when teetotal doctors walked in an untrodden path and practised what they preached, and suffered, if not in person, very seriously in purse'.[128] Mudge promoted medical temperance at the World Temperance Convention in London in 1846, denounced friendly societies in the pamphlet *An Exposure of Odd Fellowship* (1845), edited temperance journals and published two books, *Physiology, Health, & Disease* (1859) and *A Guide to the Treatment of Disease without Alcoholic Liquors* (1863).[129] Though Mudge also gave magic lantern lectures on astronomy and microscopy, *Physiology* combined scientific observation with scripture and rather theatrical public experiments, which gives some sense of the character of mid-century medical temperance.[130] Mudge lectured on *Physiology* as far afield as Huddersfield and York.[131]

Henry Mudge died in June 1874, leaving under £4,000.[132] At an anniversary meeting of the Scottish Temperance League in 1854, the publisher and UKT director William Tweedie had described Mudge as 'a missionary among the medical profession, believing that the doctors needed enlightenment upon this subject ... as much as any other class of the community', a comment that greatly amused his audience.[133] Grindrod and Mudge, like James Teare, were pioneers.

Disciplining and tinkering: Arranging agents and referees

As has already been noted, the successful *agencement* of temperance life assurance required constant attention to the relations between its different elements: the London office, superintendents or district managers, agents, referees and lives, among others. Occasionally these actors were in conflict with one another, sometimes because this provided useful checks and balances for the firm, but not always. In 1860 Robert Hellard, an insurance agent, ironmonger and proprietor of a temperance hotel in Taunton, travelled to London to attend the UKT's annual meeting, complaining that his commission had been reduced after he had been temporarily removed from the office's employment after fifteen years working for them. Hellard moved an amendment demanding that agents should not be removed by the directors without the chance to defend themselves at the members' meeting. The directors replied that Hellard had acted for two other firms while representing the UKT, and his proposed amendment came to nothing.[134] Similar hints of the tensions between the centre and its distant agents can be seen in the calls for reform heard at the 1894 annual members' meeting, which would have given agents a share of the net profits and establish a tribunal to settle their disputes with the company. Nothing seems to have come of these requests, described by *The Times* as 'vexatious and needless proposals for reform'.[135]

In the main, though, agents caused trouble for offices by holding onto policyholders' premiums, delaying payments to referees, or – more seriously – defrauding the office. In 1894 John Wesley Willis, the UKT's Bristol district manager since 1856, was charged in court with appropriating a client's policy to pay off some of his own debts before declaring bankruptcy.[136] Sometimes agents threatened the reputation of this temperance firm. In May 1848, for example, the board reported 'a notice was received that S. Grocott the agent at Stoke had been seen drunk'; Grocott had established a £100 policy in 1845, so had taken the pledge and publicly professed teetotalism.[137] Grocott sent in a letter and a ten shilling fine for breaking the pledge, but his agency was cancelled.[138] An ordinary member would have simply been fined, but the company may have felt that a drunken agent was too much bad publicity.

Sometimes agents combined drinking with fraud. In 1892 Richard Ingram took James Abbott, a Blackburn insurance agent, to court, accusing him of obtaining £3 14s. 9d. on false pretences. Ingram found several men for Abbott to assure with Lancashire Fire and Life and the UKT, paid their premiums to Abbott and waited for the policies to come through. When Abbott kept putting him off, Ingram wrote to the companies, discovering that no policies had been received, and that Abbott was no longer in their employment. The case is hard to follow, but it was claimed that Ingram had promised Abbott that he could find him third-party lives as 'good spec'. (speculation); Ingram admitted that he had no insurable interest in these other lives, which would invalidate those policies, and was asked if he knew that these men were likely to die soon, implying that Ingram was planning to claim their policies. The detail that the UKT's proposal had been signed in the Paganini Inn on Northgate presented an additional irony; Ingram denied that they had all been drunk. It is not clear how this case concluded, and any fraud would appear to have been Ingram's fault, not the UKT's, but the story does at least demonstrate what agents might get up to.[139]

On the other hand, agents sometimes went too far as a result of temperance zeal. David Long, a Sceptre salesman, joined Albert T. Bartlett, a detective employed by the Public Morals Council, in investigating Henry Warsnop's respectable Clarendon Hotel, Nottingham, and taking him to court for allowing alcohol to be served after hours. Warsnop was fined twenty shillings, though his licence was not endorsed, and it was pointed out that Long and Bartlett had overstepped their authority as citizens.[140] The Sceptre does not seem to have been dragged into this case, but they did go to court where necessary, suing both Thomas Nicholson and William Bartlett, their district managers for Southampton and Bristol.[141]

Medical examiners were warned about agents for precisely these reasons. The American doctor Charles Lyman Greene noted that agents could be trouble, talking up the quality of a life they had found or bringing a ringer – someone who wasn't the applicant – in for the medical examination, as Isaac Franklin had done in Ipswich. He advised referees to write in confidence to the chief medical examiner if they had doubts.[142] However other insurance medicine authorities, like Pollock and Chisholm, acknowledged that agents could be very useful to referees; 'the agent is often most useful in obtaining information as to the habits of a proposer and his moral character'. Dr Robert Bentham, the Sceptre's medical director, acknowledged that much of the work of investigating applicants had already been done before the forms arrived on his desk, much of it by the firm's agents, 'who were most scrupulous and conscientious'.[143]

Agents monitored assured lives after assurance, too. In the ledger recording the details for John Samuel Horsham's £200 Sceptre policy, for example, are two pencil notes, underlined, reading 'Hall says he drinks' and 'Do not restore – drinks'. Horsham's policy was established in 1870, through Edward Hall in Bow. Horsham was a twenty-three-year-old engineer, living in Poplar, who married around the time he established the policy.[144] We do not know when the note was added, but it seems likely it would have been the reason for Horsham's surrender of the policy between 1888 and 1893.

Theodore Porter's discussion of the views of agents and referees shared by US medical directors suggests that firms were prepared to expect the worst of their employees. Referees were encouraged to be suspicious of agents and vice versa; Pollock and Chisholm noted that agents could assist the board by establishing 'the repute in which the Medical Examiner is held in his own neighbourhood'.[145] Not even the staff in the office could be trusted; in 1866 Sceptre fired their manager, William J. Moore, after discovering he had misappropriated the Association's funds.[146] For the *agencement* of temperance life assurance to work, everyone had to do what was expected of them. Lyman Greene sympathetically identified the challenges facing medical referees: 'Having received his appointment, the examiner is … at once brought face to face with a most interesting and difficult problem – namely, how to suit the agent, the applicant, and the company at the same time.'[147]

Though it could be difficult to ensure that the *agencement* worked smoothly, this kind of mutual surveillance helped identify drinkers as risks before or after they applied for a policy, while monitoring agents and referees. As we will see in the next section, though, at least in the early years of the UKT this was not always enough to protect the firm, and those it assured, from the risks associated with the 'reformed drunkard'.

Conclusion: 'Doing moral good' and actuarial prudence

In 1856 Joseph T. Mitchell, the UKT's medical director, prepared an internal report on the firm's mortality experience over its first fifteen years of business. While there had been fewer than 400 deaths from nearly 11,000 lives assured in that time, Mitchell concluded that some of those policies should have been refused by their medical examiners. Nine were 'reformed drunkards', and another who had died of apoplexy was a regular drinker; Mitchell suspected that the 'epilepsy' which claimed a thirty-eight-year-old surgeon who had become intemperate after he was insured was really *delirium tremens*.[148] He reiterated the care that needed to be taken with ex-drinkers, noting that 'where a proposer had ever lived an intemperate life, there should be special caution observed in considering the case, for it often happens that chronic hidden mischief exists in the head, liver and other viscera, under these circumstances, which evades the most searching medical examination'.[149]

More worrying than this, though, was Mitchell's realization that over the first nine years of the firm's business, the mortality rate had been 23.3 deaths in a thousand in the Abstainers' section, while that figure in the General section had been slightly *lower* at 22.7 per thousand over its first nine years.[150] Different outcomes could be found, depending on the years chosen for the calculation, but Mitchell reminded the board that 'the insurances of the first seven years were made entirely on the lives of total abstainers and they chiefly of the labouring and humble class, who in many instances had been converted from the extremely opposite habit of life; from which cause their lives had been rendered less valuable than others'.[151]

Perhaps the UKT had been 'too confident that total abstinence from the use of intoxicating drinks was in itself a sufficient remedy for any damaging effect', granting policies to reclaimed drunkards who turned out to be 'bad lives'. Henry Rickman might have been right, in other words (Chapter 3). On the other hand, Mitchell wondered if he and his colleagues, 'being anxious to do as much moral good to that class as possible' had perhaps 'admitted some as members whom now on that account they would certainly reject'.

Later teetotalers did feel the need to support the first abstainers when they fell on hard times. In 1873 S. Norbury Williams collected £230 for John King, the first British man to take the teetotal pledge; King was seventy-eight in 1873 and losing his sight. Williams's collection was converted into a UKT annuity paying King £40 annually for twelve years until his death in 1885. Williams then started another collection to support King's widow Mary Ann and to have a stone laid on John's grave, saying 'it is not fitting that such a man should depart and that no stone should mark his place of rest. It is eminently fitting that the Temperance community should relieve his widow, and mark the place where lies a general who has, for 53 years, helped to lead a victorious army'.[152] King lived to be ninety, but he and his wife had little to show for it, and Williams and others had felt bound to assist them. Perhaps Mitchell felt a similar sense of obligation to abstainers who had been part of the movement from the beginning.

In 1870 Mitchell would publicly defend the UKT's 'minute inquisitorial inquiry', but in his private report to the board fourteen years earlier he had suggested that the UKT had set out to help working-class teetotalers, including reformed drunkards, by granting them policies that would bring them material benefit. Life assurance could 'do moral good', at least as long as the company broke its own rules and assured friends, family, or allies in the struggle against alcohol when it should perhaps have turned them away. The company had not completely relaxed its scrutiny, of course; there were only 218 claims in the Abstainers' section between 1841 and 1855, and Mitchell thought only nine of those were reformed drunkards.[153] It is hard, too, to discern much about the teetotal lives who died earlier than expected in those years, precisely because many of them were members of the 'labouring and humble class', so it's impossible to tell how many had been 'bad lives'. Still, Mitchell's admission that life assurance involved motivations and outcomes beyond prudence and self-improvement reminds us that temperance life assurance could be different things to different people – in fact, that it could be several different things at once. We will explore this further in Chapter 6.

Notes

1. Compton, 'Early Days'.
2. Warner, letter to Cash, 1896.
3. Burns, company history, 38.
4. Winskill, *Temperance Movement*, vol. I, 87, 89.
5. Ibid., 105.
6. Winskill, *Temperance Movement*, vol. 2, 14, vol. 1, 216.
7. *Livesey's Preston Temperance Advocate*, 1836.
8. *Bristol Temperance Herald* 1, 7, May 1837, 29, 32–3, 35, MS 41001/WTL/J/1/1, Bristol Record Office.
9. Janette L. Martin, 'Popular Political Oratory and Itinerant Lecturing in Yorkshire and the North East in the Age of Chartism', PhD thesis, University of York, 2010, 118.
10. Barker, *Temperance Century*, 15.
11. Winskill, *Temperance Movement*, vol. 3, 165.
12. Hudson, *Temperance Pioneers*, 34, 272.
13. Winskill, *Temperance Movement*, vol. I, 87; Winskill, *Standard Bearers of Temperance*, 485.
14. Hudson, *Temperance Pioneers*, 268, 124.
15. Ibid., 254, 125.
16. Winskill, *Temperance Movement*, vol. I, 223–4.
17. Cited in Winskill, *Temperance Movement*, vol. I, 223.
18. Hudson, *Temperance Pioneers*, 273.
19. Anon., *History of Teetotalism in Devonshire*.
20. Hudson, *Temperance Pioneers*, 141; Winskill, *Standard Bearers*, vol. 2, 267.
21. Meeting, 31 May 1841, Minutes of the Standing Committee 1, Board meeting, 2 June 1841, UKT Minute Book 1, Aviva Archives.
22. Winskill, *Temperance Movement*, vol. 3, 165; Harrison, *Dictionary of British Temperance Biography*, 77–8.
23. Probate 7 April 1868, England & Wales Government Probate Death Index 1858–2019, Civil Deaths & Burials.
24. Burns, *Temperance History*, 62.
25. Meetings, 28 March 1842, Minutes of the Standing Committee 1; 27 June 1842, Minutes of the Standing Committee 2; Report of AGM, 2 January 1844, Board Meeting, 1 March 1844, 3 May 1844, UKT Minute Book 1, Aviva Archives.
26. Report of Sixth Annual Meeting, 1 January 1847, 2, United Kingdom Temperance and General provident Institution, Annual Reports and Balance Sheets 1840–1910, Aviva Archives; *Abstainer's Journal* (1853), 70.
27. Hudson, *Temperance Pioneers*, 289.
28. Burns, company history, 9.
29. McFall, *Devising Consumption*.
30. Shaun French and James Kneale, 'Speculating on Careless Lives: Annuitising the Biofinancial Subject', *Journal of Cultural Economy* 5, 4 (2012), 391–406; Louise Amoore, 'Security and the Incalculable', *Security Dialogue* 45 (2014), 423–9; Turo-Kimmo Lehtonen, 'Picturing How Life Insurance Matters', *Journal of Cultural Economy* 7, 3 (2014), 308–33; John Hogan Morris, 'Decentring Ingenuity: Calculation, Intuition and Atmospheres in the Bank of England's Financial Literacy Assemblages', *Geoforum* 90 (2018), 45–54.

31. Board meeting, 6 May 1841, UKT Minute Book 1, Aviva Archives.
32. Third Annual Report, 3, United Kingdom Temperance and General Provident Institution, Annual Reports and Balance Sheets 1840–1910, Aviva Archives.
33. Winskill, *The Temperance Movement*, vol. 2, 121.
34. Withers, *Pioneers of British Life Assurance*, 92.
35. Board meetings, 19 and 26 January 1849, UKT Minute Book 1, Aviva Archives.
36. Meeting, 21 December 1840, Minutes of the Standing Committee 1, Board meetings, 14 January 1841, 1 April and 6 May 1841, UKT Minute Book 1, Aviva Archives; Advertisement, *British & Foreign Temperance Intelligencer* 4, 26 December 1840, 409–10.
37. Meeting 21 December 1840, Minutes of the Standing Committee 1, Aviva Archives.
38. Board meeting, 1 December 1848, UKT Minute Book 1, Aviva Archives.
39. Advertisement, *Chelmsford Chronicle*, 15 December 1848, 1 and 23 March 1866, 1; *Liverpool Mercury*, 4 December 1869, 4; *Y Genedl Cymreig*, 27 March 1879, 3.
40. *The Times*, 30 May 1856, 5.
41. Board meetings, 2 September 1864, 2 December 1864, Sceptre Minute book 1, London Archives.
42. Board meeting, 17 February 1865, Sceptre Minute book 1, London Archives; Special Directions to Superintendents, Prudential Assurance Company, Industrial Branch, May 1881, Prudential Archives.
43. Advertisement, *Leeds Mercury*, 6 May 1865, 6.
44. Advertisement, *Western Mail*, 15 December 1870, 3.
45. Advertisement, *Western Mail*.
46. Sceptre Life Association Ltd., Report of Proceedings at the Twenty-Second Annual Meeting, 17 February 1887, Reports of Proceedings at AGMs, 1887–91, MS SC1/7/2/1, London Archives.
47. Sceptre Life Association Ltd., Report of Proceedings at the Twenty-Third Annual Meeting, 23 February 1888, Reports of Proceedings at AGMs, 1887–91. London Archives.
48. Alborn, *Regulated Lives*, 88, 96.
49. Meeting, Minutes of the Standing Committee 1, Aviva Archives.
50. 1841 Census (Class: HO107; Piece: 928; Folio: 39; Page: 7; GSU roll: 1715).
51. *Pigot and Co.'s Royal National and Commercial Directory, 1841* (London, 1841), 480; Meeting, 23 December 1840, Minutes of the Standing Committee 1, Aviva Archives.
52. Piers Brendon, 'Cook, Thomas (1808–1892), Travel Agent', *Oxford Dictionary of National Biography* (Oxford University Press, 2008), www.oxforddnb.com/view/10.1093/ref:odnb/9780198614128.001.0001/odnb-9780198614128-e-6152, accessed 7 April 2020.
53. Cook, *Guide to Leicester, 1843* (Leicester: Cook, 1843), 115; *Leicestershire Mercury and General Advertiser for the Midland Counties*, 9 September 1843, 3.
54. Meeting, 20 November 1840, Minutes of the Standing Committee 1, Aviva Archives.
55. Board meeting, 16 March 1849, UKT Minute Book 1.
56. Anon., *The House of Jarrolds 1823–1923: A Brief History of One Hundred Years* (Norwich: Jarrolds, 1924), 12–13, 18–21.
57. Winskill, *Comprehensive History*, 14, 524, 538; Winskill, *Temperance Movement*, vol. 1, 52–3.
58. Winskill, *Temperance Movement*, vol. 1, 225; Hudson, *Temperance Pioneers*, 123, 113; Harrison, *Drink*, 448.
59. Winskill, *Temperance Movement*, vol. 1, 251.

60. Winskill, *Temperance Movement*, vol. 4, 207.
61. See Vieira Paisana, 'Tipplers, Drunkards and Backsliders'.
62. 1861 Census (Class: RG09; Piece: 2064; Folio: 6; Page: 7; GSU roll: 40); Caverly and Bankes, *Leading Insurance Men*, 364; 1871 Census (Class: RG10; Piece: 3154; Folio: 109; Page: 3; GSU roll: 11).
63. *The Owl*, 25 February 1898, 11.
64. Sceptre sample; Advertisement, *The Times*, 16 August 1877, 14; 1881 Census (Class: RG11; Piece: 825; Folio: 26; Page: 48; GSU roll: 257); England & Wales Deaths 1837–2007, Civil Deaths & Burials.
65. Board meeting, 27 July 1866, Sceptre Minute book 1, London Archives.
66. Sceptre Life Association Limited Policy Ledger No. 4, London Archives; *Kelly's Directory of Derbyshire, Leicestershire & Rutland, and Nottinghamshire. 1891. Part 3: Nottinghamshire* (London: Kelly, 1891), 1283; 'Suicide of a Nottingham Insurance Agent', *Nottinghamshire Guardian*, 12 March 1898, 5.
67. Special Board Meeting, 19 May 1886, Minute Book 3, Sceptre Life Association, MS SC 01/05/01/003, London Archives.
68. 1871 Census (Class: RG10; Piece: 1188; Folio: 8; Page: 10; GSU roll: 61); 1881 Census (Class: RG11; Piece: 1221; Folio: 33; Page: 9; GSU roll: 257).
69. Advertisement, *York Herald*, 29 July 1880, 1; 'District News', *Hull Packet and East Riding Times*, 18 November 1881, 3; Advertisement, *Era*, 9 October 1886, 23.
70. 'Local Intelligence', *Sheffield Independent*, 21 October 1878, 3.
71. Instructions to agents of the Whittington Life Assurance Company 1889, 15, Whittington Life Assurance Company Prospectuses 1867–91, London Archives.
72. Ibid., 16; 17, original emphasis.
73. Ibid., 5.
74. Winskill, *Temperance Movement*, vol. 2, 121; Winskill, *Comprehensive History*, 369–71.
75. John W. Kirton, *The Life of Joseph Harrap of Leicester* (Leicester: Richard Lawrence, 1873), 9.
76. Ibid., 13.
77. 'Death of Mr. Joseph Harrap', *Leicester Chronicle*, 24 March 1883, 2.
78. Kirton, *Life*, 24.
79. Winskill, *Comprehensive History*, 370; Winskill, *Temperance Movement*, vol. 2, 122.
80. Kirton, *Life*, 22, 24.
81. *Leicester Chronicle and the Leicestershire Mercury*, 1 October 1864, 1.
82. 'The Permissive Bill', *Leicestershire Mercury*, 4 June 1864, 8.
83. *Leicester Chronicle*, 13 June 1868, 3; *Leicester Mercury*, 31 October 1868, 8; *Leicester Chronicle and Mercury*, 24 July 1869, 6; *Leicester Chronicle*, 20 November 1869, 6.
84. 1871 Census (Class: RG10; Piece: 3269; Folio: 84; Page: 13; GSU roll: 69).
85. Winskill, *Temperance Movement*, vol. 2, 122; *Bradford Observer*, 17 July 1873, 5.
86. *Leicester Journal*, 15 March 1878, 8 and 20 June 1879, 8.
87. UKT 1881 Prospectus; *Leicester Chronicle and Leicestershire Mercury*, 5 February 1881, 2.
88. Leicester Probate Registry Will Register 1883, DE462/26 Record Office for Leicestershire, Leicester & Rutland, Leicestershire Wills and Probate Records, 1500–1939, 303–6.
89. *Leicester Journal*, 23 March 1883, 8; *Leicester Chronicle*, 24 March 1883, 2.
90. *Leicester Chronicle*, 2 June 1883, 10.
91. Winskill, *Temperance Standard Bearers*, vol. 2, 458.
92. *Leicester Daily Mercury*, 10 May 1879, 6.

93. *Leicester Chronicle*, 5 July 1890, 2 and 15 April 1893, 7.
94. *Leicester Chronicle and the Leicestershire Mercury*, 24 February 1900, 8.
95. Probate 31 March 1900, Leicester, England & Wales Government Probate Death Index 1858–2019.
96. *Wright's Directory of Leicester* (London: Kelly's Directories, 1909), 99.
97. *Nottingham Evening Post*, 3 August 1935, 7; England & Wales Government Probate Death Index 1858–2019, Leicester Probate Registry Administration Registers, Archive reference DE 462/76, Record Office for Leicestershire, Leicester & Rutland, Leicestershire Wills and Probate Records, 1500–1939.
98. The Record Office for Leicestershire, Leicester & Rutland, Archive reference DE7146/8, National School Admission Registers & Log-Books 1870–1914.
99. 'Doctors and Water-Drinkers', Correspondence, *British Medical Journal* 2, July 2, 1870.
100. *Bristol Mercury and Daily Post*, 13 October 1890, 6.
101. Mitchell, *Report of the Medical Director*, 9.
102. Minutes of the Standing Committee 1, Aviva Archives.
103. 1841 Census; Board meeting, 2 June 1841, UKT Minute Book 1, Aviva Archives.
104. Stephanie J. Snow, 'John Snow MD, (1813–1858). Part II. Becoming a Doctor – His Medical Training and Early Years of Practice', *Journal of Medical Biography* 8 (2000), 71–7.
105. Meeting, 15 March 1841, Minutes of the Standing Committee 2, Aviva Archives.
106. Mitchell, *Report of the Medical Director*, 10.
107. Kari S. McLeod, 'Our Sense of Snow: The Myth of John Snow in Medical Geography', *Social Science & Medicine* 50 (2000), 924.
108. Meeting, 7 December 1840, Minutes of the Standing Committee 1, Aviva Archives.
109. Winskill, *Temperance Movement*, vol. 2, 171.
110. Winskill, *Temperance Movement*, vol. 1, 118.
111. Ibid., 117.
112. Ibid., 142.
113. Winskill, *Temperance Movement*, vol. 2, 166.
114. Ibid., 168, 167; Winskill, *Comprehensive History*, 505, cited 70.
115. Meeting, 24 May 1844, Minutes of the Standing Committee 2, Aviva Archives.
116. Greater Manchester Electoral Registers 1820–1940, Greater Manchester County Record Office, Poor Rate Assessments, Greater Manchester Rate Books, M 9/40/2/128, Greater Manchester County Record Office.
117. See Robin Price, 'Hydropathy in England 1840–70', *Medical History* 25, 3 (1981), 269–80; Gregory, *Vegetarians and Victorians*, 70–3.
118. Janet Grierson, *Temperance, Therapy and Trilobites: Dr Ralph Grindrod, Victorian Pioneer* (Cora Weaver: Malvern, 2001), 64.
119. Winskill, *Temperance Movement*, vol. 2, 173.
120. *Royal Cornwall Gazette*, 27 February 1830, 3.
121. Mark Clement, 'Mudge, Henry (1806–1874)', *Oxford Dictionary of National Biography* (Oxford University Press, 2004), www.oxforddnb.com/view/article/19483, accessed 9 January 2013; *London & Provincial Medical Directory 1849* (London: John Churchill, 1849), 379.
122. Winskill, *Temperance Standard Bearers*, vol. 2, 267.
123. Hudson, *Temperance Pioneers*, 254; Burns, *Temperance History*, vol. 1, 111.
124. *Royal Cornwall Gazette*, 10 December 1831, 3; Winskill, *Temperance Standard Bearers*, vol. 2, 318–19; *Royal Cornwall Gazette*, 19 June 1840, 1.
125. Winskill, *Comprehensive History*, 147.

126. Hudson, *Temperance Pioneers*, 219, 222.
127. Winskill, *Comprehensive History*, 510; Hudson, *Temperance Pioneers*, 221, 224.
128. Whittaker, *Life's Battles*, 330.
129. Advertisement, *National Temperance Chronicle and Temperance Recorder* 1 (1846), 1; Winskill, *Comprehensive History*, 133; *Temperance Movement*, vol. 2, 152; Clement, 'Mudge'.
130. For example, *Royal Cornwall Gazette*, 29 October 1858, 5; Henry Mudge, *Physiology, Health, & Disease, Demanding Abstinence from Alcoholic Drinks, and Prohibition of Their Common Sale: Being a Course of Five Lectures* (London: William Tweedie, 1859), 4, iii.
131. *Huddersfield Chronicle*, 3 November 1860, 8; *York Herald*, 17 November 1860, 10.
132. 8 October 1874, England & Wales Government Probate Death Index 1858–2019, Civil Deaths & Burials.
133. 'Breakfast Party in the Music Hall', *Abstainer's Journal*, June 1854, 142.
134. Slater's Royal National and Commercial Directory 1852–3 (London: Slater, 1852–3), 802; *The Standard*, 29 May 29, 1860, 6.
135. *The Standard*, 7 April 1894, 7; *The Times*, 23 May 1894, 11.
136. *Bristol Mercury and Daily Post*, 3 February 1894, 1.
137. Board meetings, 5 May 1848, 3 October 1845, UKT Minute Book 1, Aviva Archives.
138. Meetings, 20 May 1848, Minutes of the Standing Committee 1, Aviva Archives.
139. 'Speculations in Lives at Blackburn', *Manchester Courier and Lancashire General Advertiser*, 19 May 1892, 8 and 21 May 1892, 6; 'Speculation in Lives at Blackburn', *Lancaster Gazette and General Advertiser for Lancashire, Westmorland, and Yorkshire*, 21 May 1892, 3.
140. *Nottingham Evening Post*, 29 July 1891, 2.
141. *Morning Post*, 8 April 1886, 6; Board Meeting, 9 October 1890, Sceptre Minute Book 3, London Archives.
142. Charles Lyman Greene, *The Medical Examination for Life Insurance and Its Associated Clinical Methods, with Chapters on the Insurance of Substandard Lives and Accident Insurance*, second edition (London: Rebman, 1905), 41, 47.
143. Report of Proceedings at the Twenty-Third Annual Meeting, 23 February 1888, Reports of Proceedings at AGMs, London Archives.
144. Policy Ledger 2, Marriage, 3rd quarter 1870, Poplar, vol. 1C, p. 1021, Birth, Marriage, Death & Parish Records.
145. Pollock and Chisholm, *Medical Handbook*, 21.
146. Board Meeting, 1 June 1866, Sceptre Minute book 1, London Archives.
147. Greene, *Medical Examination*, 40.
148. Mitchell, *Report of the Medical Director*, 9.
149. Ibid., 9–10, 11.
150. Ibid., 14–15.
151. Ibid., 13.
152. S. Norbury Williams, 'The Late John King, the First Pledged Total Abstainer. An Appeal on Behalf of His Widow. To the Editor of "The Good Templars' Watchword"', *Good Templars' Watchword* 12, 586 (13 April 1885), 236.
153. Mitchell, *Report of the Medical Director*, 13–14.

Part 3

Improving Temperance Lives, 1850–1918

6

Improvement: A very business-like argument

Introduction: Varieties of temperance

Having reviewed the early years of the UKT in Parts 1 and 2, it is now possible to start to explore what temperance life assurance might have meant to those involved with it, concentrating on ideas of improvement. This chapter considers this idea in its widest sense, while the next two chapters examine the lives of ordinary teetotalers – to see if their policies might have made a difference to their lives – and the growing medical acceptance of abstinence as a way of improving health. As Chapter 1 demonstrated, life assurance made temperance more than a political movement seeking parliamentary reform or a religious 'crusade' designed to impose order on an unruly working class. This chapter shows that temperance could in fact be several different things, sometimes all at once, and considers four key ideas of 'improvement', before demonstrating that they could be complicated by the messy realities of business, and particularly property ownership and investment.

We look first at temperance life assurance as moral reform, illustrated by the life of Robert Dundas Thomson, the UKT's first physician, before turning to assurance as an 'affective technology', producing security, hope and more; a Sceptre life then suggests how assurance might have offered new possibilities. The third way in which temperance life assurance might have been understood was as part of a virtuous circle of investment, where prudent individuals created capital that might fund progressive improvement schemes improving the lives of others. The final idea concerns temperance life assurance as an improving *business*, one that appeared not to have a distinctive morality because it simply took advantage of the natural laws of both the market and human mortality. From this final perspective, temperance was ordinary and unremarkable, and its benefits were thought to be obvious and uncontroversial.

The chapter concludes by bringing these four ideas together, because temperance life assurance was many things at once: it was a moralizing technology that could also be a source of social and geographical mobility, and an unremarkable business 'product' that simultaneously created funds for social and individual improvement. It dd not always work this smoothly, though. The final temperance 'life' considered in the chapter considers the UKT's first three offices in London as signs of these multiple meanings. Finally, we consider some of the more unexpected outcomes of temperance life assurance, as the UKT became the owner of several public houses. This is read not as a sign of hypocrisy on the part of the company's directors – a charge levelled at them by critics – but as a sign of the complexity of the assemblages in which they were working, where something as ubiquitous as alcohol was likely to get caught up in the socio-material networks this temperance firm was building.

Teaching a practical lesson: Temperance life assurance as moral reform

As noted in the introduction, some historians of temperance have seen it as a moralizing middle-class campaign designed to improve the character of the working class. If those historians had considered temperance life assurance, they would probably have seen it as another form of discipline that could be placed alongside the policing of everyday life and the provision of 'improved' forms of leisure and 'rational recreation'. From this perspective the marketing of temperance life assurance looks like an attempt to shame audiences into good conduct. A few months into the UKT's first year of business, for example, Robert Dundas Thomson gave a lecture at the Aldersgate Literary and Scientific Institution on the deleterious effects of alcohol on digestion, before discussing the role of life assurance in offering the prospect of independence and an alternative to the workhouse. He acknowledged, however:

> It is not to be supposed, that the majority of labouring men can appreciate without instruction the bearing of such a proposition. I therefore suggest, that the heads of families may essentially contribute to the desirable end of dispensing in a great measure with the present obnoxious poor rates, by teaching a practical lesson to their servants. I propose that servants should be advised to forego the purchase of beer with their daily beer money, and to invest it in a Policy of Insurance, or in a deferred annuity.[1]

By urging their servants to buy life assurance, employers would be 'teaching a practical lesson', imparting bourgeois habits to their employees.

Others promoted life assurance by presenting the refusal to establish a policy as a moral failure. In 1854, for example, William Gawthorpe, the secretary of the Manchester and Salford Temperance Society and the UKT's agent in Manchester, addressed a meeting promoting the firm in Bradford.[2] 'He knew there were some persons who did not approve of life assurance', he said; 'perhaps they were not provident; *they perhaps did not love their wives and families* to such a degree as to feel an inducement to save 3d. or 6d. or 1s. a week to make provision for them in the future'.[3] Samuel Smiles would make a similar point about the refusal to save, which might generate costs that would have to be paid for by others: 'To leave the family to the workhouse, the prison, or the street … is nothing short of a crime done against society, as well as against the unfortunate individuals who are the immediate sufferers.'[4]

Perhaps more importantly, saving might change the character of the assurer in productive ways. As we have noted, Jeremy Bentham was keen to find ways to 'accustom men to submit to the yoke of foresight'; planning for the future became a key technique of the self, shaping new liberal subjects prepared to turn uncertainty into risk through thrift and prudence.[5] Teetotalers were already accustomed to looking forward through taking the pledge, and temperance assurance firms used similar terms to those employed by Bentham. Speaking in Cardiff in 1870, for example, the Sceptre's James Mills told his audience that 'men must be taught habits of economy, forethought, and self-reliance'. Furthermore,

> Men must be taught to save before we can assure their lives. There were a large number of working men who wasted more than 2s a week, and for half that they could assure their lives for £100. Temperance was the handmaid of assurance, as it was always the temperate, saving class who assured their lives, and they were the best lives.[6]

A similar tone could still be detected in the 1915 Eagle Star prospectus, the firm that absorbed Sceptre, which quoted the Reverend Dr Norman McLeod's description of life assurance as 'an excellent means of educating men out of selfishness, and training them to have due consideration for others'.[7] Life assurance could encourage this 'due consideration', and policies that grew in value might have a special attraction, as Thomas David Lister explained in his handbook for medical examiners: 'They have the advantage of tending to produce that *desire for longevity* which may come from the certainty that the longer the proposer lives the more his dependents will derive from his insurance.' 'The chief advantage of this method', he concluded, 'seems to me to be the *introduction of the force which tends to keep proposers alive*'.[8] Teetotalers were thought to possess this 'force' – foresight, prudence, an aversion to risk – in abundance. In establishing 'habits of forethought', temperance life assurance encouraged them to become even more risk-averse in their 'desire for longevity'.

There is little mention, though, of temperance life assurance as a political or religious mission. Links between these firms and campaigning groups like the UK Alliance were of course strong; William Bingham of the Sceptre resigned from the Alliance when his health failed in 1885, for example, and many UKT directors were associated with it in some capacity.[9] However these firms had little to do with parliamentary politics, except when it threatened their business. Religious motivations are also largely absent, though the Reverend Baker described his work with the UKT as an extension of Christian commitments, explaining that 'he believed that it was really and truly a religious work for a man to provide for himself in his old age, or for those whom his death might deprive of the means of livelihood'.[10] These firms may have been reluctant to get dragged into divisive and distracting theological arguments, as the UKT had been with Joseph Barker. Many of the men who ran these companies were committed Christians, and some of the UKT's Friends, like Bowly, Charleton and Compton, worried about the worldliness of temperance business. The Sceptre lent money to dozens of Methodist chapels and remained closely identified with the denominations that had left the Wesleyans; Thomas Snape, a Sceptre director, was a lay member of the Connexional Committee of the United Methodist Free Churches.[11] Alfred T. Bowser, the Whittington's secretary and manager for twenty-five years, was a deacon at the Baptist Chapel on Mare Street, Hackney, London.[12] This was characteristic of other business leaders into the twentieth century, though, as David Jeremy shows, and it is rare that religious arguments were made in the business records that survive, or in newspaper reports.

So while representatives of these firms clearly spoke of foresight and discipline in a way that chimes with O'Malley's reading of Bentham, the paternalistic or coercive attitude encouraged by Thomson seems to have been relatively rare. Perhaps this reflects Thomson's other interests, which are explored in the next life.

Temperance lives: Robert Dundas Thomson (1810–1864)

Robert Dundas Thomson was born to James, a minister, and Elizabeth, in Eccles, Scotland. Robert studied medicine in Edinburgh and Glasgow and was taught chemistry by his uncle Thomas Thomson, Regius Professor at Glasgow, whose daughter, Margaret, Robert later married. Robert then studied in Gliessen under Justus von Liebig, whose work on alcohol would be very influential in Britain (Chapter 8) before working for the East India Company as a surgeon in China and India. Thomson returned to London in 1837.[13]

Thomson became the UKT's first physician, though the Reverend Baker had to persuade him to take the teetotal pledge before he could be offered the job. It seems likely that he was the R. D. Thomson who signed the Medical Declaration against the use of spirits in medicine in 1837, so he was already a moderationist.[14] Thomson served the UKT for only a year, however, before returning to Glasgow University to assist his uncle. Robert took an active role in efforts to improve the quality of vital statistics collected by the Philosophical Society of Glasgow, of which his uncle was president. When Thomas Thomson died in 1852, Robert failed to secure his uncle's chair, and he rejoined the UKT in 1853; he helped found the Blenheim Dispensary and was appointed professor of chemistry at St Thomas's Hospital.

In 1855 Thomson contributed to the Medical Council's General Board of Health's report on the Soho cholera outbreak, supporting William Farr's miasmatic theory over that of his UKT colleague John Snow.[15] Thomson had already published on the relationship between climate and mortality while working in Glasgow, extending this to cholera and atmospheric processes in 1855; he was a member of the British Meteorological Society for ten years and was eventually elected its first president, though '[his] academic input … appears to have been limited', compared to the efforts he made to improve the quality of the data collected by the Society.[16] He was appointed one of the new Metropolitan Medical Officers of Health, and then the first president of their association. He was an effective administrator, collaborating with Francis Galton to establish the importance of regular and accurate returns of meteorological conditions, water quality, disease and mortality. His monthly analyses of organic matter in the water supplied by London's Water Companies were published in *The Times* and in many Reports of Medical Officers of Health.[17]

In many ways Thomson was a Chadwickian figure, a keen student of London's water supply and the relationship between meteorology and disease; his attitude to poverty was also close to that of the architect of the New Poor Law. While at Glasgow Thomson published the influential study *Experimental Researches on the Food of Animals and*

Fattening of Cattle. With Remarks on the Food of Man (1846), as well as five papers on the nutritive powers of bread and flour in the *Proceedings* of the Philosophical Society, while trying to improve the diet of Glasgow's Night Asylum for the Houseless. M. Norton Wise and Crosbie Smith see this project as a Gradgrindian attempt to find the most efficient – or cheapest – workhouse diet possible.[18] It is worth remembering that Thomson exhorted employers to impress teetotalism on their domestic servants as a way of 'dispensing in a great measure with the present obnoxious poor rates', because a sober working class would require less support from the ratepayer. Thomson concluded his 1840 lecture by suggesting that life assurance policies should be established to provide annuities when workers were too old to be able to support themselves, again to keep them from the workhouse – and to ease the burden on the payer of the Poor Rate.[19] For Thomson life assurance and workhouse diets were matters of efficiency, measured by cost.

Robert Dundas Thomson died in 1864, aged fifty-three. He received little attention from temperance writers and was only a UKT director for about a dozen years; it seems likely that he was more interested in hospital and university work, though his interest in statistics and efficiency brought him other opportunities. As we return to the theme of improvement, it is worth noting that Thomson's version of progress was a more coercive and repressive one than that suggested by others.

Temperance life assurance as affective technology

Life assurance produced more positive affective returns, principally a sense of security, reassuring the policyholder that future disaster was, to some extent, now guarded against. Until the 1860s, marketing demonstrated a 'ceaseless focus on the death of the breadwinner and subsequent fate of his dependents', as Alborn has shown; life assurance was then offered as the solution.[20] Even Thomson knew that 'one of the most striking features of the [UKT], is the prospect which it holds out to the labouring classes, of acquiring independence, at a period of life when bad health, or the gradual encroachments of age may threaten the gloomy accommodations of a workhouse'.[21] In offering a chance of independence, the UKT created a positive goal, a future state to be achieved through foresight and saving. The firm's two sections also advertised the greater financial value of temperance. In 1881, George Bradley, the Mayor of Wrexham, told a meeting of local Rechabites that he had been a member of the UKT's General section more than thirty years and would have received £50 more in bonuses over that time had he been an abstainer.[22]

This orientation towards the future was built into arguments for both life assurance and total abstinence. Both life assurance and the teetotal pledge dealt in delayed gratification – the loss of money or sociality in the present, in return for future wealth and a longer life. This was noted in a fictitious dialogue between a doctor and his patient, printed as an advertisement for the UKT in 1842. One of the reasons the fictional patient offered to explain why he had not taken out life assurance was that in saving for his children's future he would be denying them assistance in the present.[23] Life assurance looked to the future, promising the prospect of security in return for small sacrifices in the present. In that respect it can be seen as an 'affective technology', producing security and peace of mind alongside prudence and foresight.

The promotion of teetotal temperance faced a slightly different problem, at least until there was wider acceptance of the idea that abstinence might be healthier than moderate drinking. An anonymous reviewer of Charles Wilson's *Pathology of Drunkenness* recognized this problem, noting that 'to *denounce, repress, and render difficult*, are all very well, but unless there be conjoined with these means an attempt to replace the temporary enjoyment you destroy, by something better and more rational, they will be of little avail'.[24] Teetotalers had done a reasonable job of 'denouncing, repressing and rendering difficult' – committing to total abstinence, working towards Local Option to reduce drink consumption – but for this author there had been less discussion of what might replace the 'temporary enjoyment' of alcoholic sociability. The benefits of abstinence in the here and now needed to be made clear.

Thomson had compared 'the bright view of independence, so dear to every British heart' offered by life assurance to 'the alternative of a draught of intoxicating liquid daily, and the horrors of a workhouse', but could only frame this as *economic* independence, freedom from the workhouse – and even that would be deferred until the saver was too old to work.[25] In time the UKT and other firms would use their experience to argue that abstinence extended life; could temperance life assurance offer a more positive sense of abstinence in the present, beyond the relief at having put in place plans for an uncertain future?

The exercise of foresight was certainly presented as having positive consequences in the present. The moral tone of life assurance has been extensively explored by Alborn, Zelizer, Jureidini and White and others, but temperance assurance could also improve a life's business prospects. Samuel Bowly suggested that 'the fact of a man insuring his life gave some respectability and standing to his character. He thought a man was looked upon as more prudent and trustworthy who insured his life than one who did not do so, and that it also gave valuable assistance to his credit'.[26] Other temperance businesses may have also realized that temperance could be productive; Seymour Price was certain that the attitude of the Victorian founders of the Temperance and Permanent Building Society was 'not the purely negative one of denunciation'.

> They sincerely believed, and were not afraid to proclaim as a positive fact, that the life of the abstainer was brighter, better, and likely to be longer than that of the drinker; that the abstainer was mentally and physically the better man; and that, as he did not waste his money on intoxicants, he was able to save and was therefore much the more trustworthy business proposition.[27]

The economic cost of drinking, using money that could be saved, or spent on other things, was a constant refrain in temperance arguments well into the twentieth century. The cover image of the South Wales *Abstainer* of 1926 made the point that 'Prohibition builds houses', showing a man wearing a sash marked 'PROHIBITION', presenting a model of a detached house marked 'HOME'.[28]

Life assurance policies could also be used as security for a loan. Sir Richard Mansel (Chapter 3) had made good use of this, and Sceptre's ledgers record some of the loans established by less privileged individuals. William Scott, a Birstall gardener who was twenty-five when he established his £100 policy in 1865, borrowed £70 from the office, for example; he claimed his policy sometime after 1908, by which time he would also have received over forty years of bonus payments. Henry Newey Moore, a thirty-year-old Aston warehouseman assured for £50 in 1865, also borrowed on his policy, and lived until 1918.[29] Policies could also be surrendered. Surrendered policies established for a short time might return only the premiums paid so far, less costs, making them a poor alternative to other savings schemes, though any bonuses paid to the assured would increase the policy's value. Still, surrendered policies represented a form of capital that could be called upon when needed, and were clearly better value than policies which were allowed to lapse. Policies might have been intended as short-term solutions, too; George Reeves, a twenty-four-year-old Kensington plumber, seems to have surrendered his policy within a few years of establishing it in 1881, but not before using it to establish a loan.[30]

Uneven patterns in the occupations of those who surrendered their policies might support this suggestion, though numbers are small. There are 910 policies in the Sceptre sample where the final outcome is reported; 509 of them (55.9 per cent) were claimed, 264 (29.0 per cent) lapsed and 138 (15.2 per cent) were surrendered. Of the twenty-seven abstainers in that sample who gave their profession as 'agent' – commission or general agents, or selling insurance, coal, or minerals – ten surrendered their policies (38.5 per cent of the twenty-six we know the outcome for). Some would have benefited more than others. Daniel Duckworth, a Leeds commission agent, would have received only a small proportion of the £1,000 policy he established in 1877 when he surrendered it between 1888 and 1893, despite receiving two bonus payments; the £100 policy established in 1877 by Aaron Mobbs, Sceptre's Berkshire district manager, would have greatly appreciated in value by the time it was surrendered sometime between 1923 and 1928, having accrued ten bonuses. The use of policies as collateral for loans might explain what looks like a surprisingly low claim rate for these agents (38.5 per cent). Temperance life assurance promised future security and encouraged prudence in the present, but it also conjured capital out of nowhere in the process.

It is also possible that the security brought by life assurance provided some teetotal lives with the confidence to take on additional risks. Our next temperance life demonstrates how this might have worked.

Temperance lives: Edward Cahill (1833–1911)

Several of the lives in the Sceptre sample sought permission from the firm to travel overseas. Many firms charged extra to cover the additional risks associated with travel; consulting medical and climatological authorities and their own 'experience' of these risks, firms set rates based on latitude, region, or country. Firms compelled policyholders to seek their permission before travelling and would refuse claims from those who had not done this.[31] While firms saw travel and 'foreign residence' as a threat to these lives, the security offered by life assurance may have actually *enabled* their tropical travel and residence by providing reassurance and capital. One Sceptre life, that of the Irish teetotaler, soldier, tailor and shopkeeper Edward Cahill, shows us something of how this might have worked. Cahill's life reminds us that temperance life assurance helped underwrite the expansion of Britain's empire, in ways that further broaden our sense of the multiple meanings of the 'improvement' it promised.

Edward Cahill gave his birth year as 1833 when he established his Sceptre policy in April 1871.[32] It's not clear when he came to England, but he enlisted as a sergeant in the 91st (Argyllshire Highlanders) Regiment of Foot at Westminster in February 1869. He had been born in Limerick city, had no prior military service and was already married.[33] By 1871 he was with his regiment, now the 91st (Princess Louise's Argyllshire Highlanders), at the North Camp, Farnborough, with his wife Ellen and four children under ten years of age. The oldest child had been born in Ireland (suggesting that the family had emigrated between 1862 and 1864), the middle two in St James's parish, Westminster, and the youngest at Dover (implying a recent move from that town, to which the 91st had recently returned following more than a decade's service in India).[34] Sceptre recorded Edward's profession as a master tailor with the regiment, and issued him with a policy for £400 through Nicholson's agency in Southampton.

By 1879 Edward was in South Africa with the 91st, fighting in the Anglo-Zulu war. While there is no record of it in the ledger, Cahill's premiums – £12 3s. 4d. per year – may well have included an additional charge for 'war risk' or active service. The 91st fought at Gingindlovu in April, killing an estimated thousand Zulus. In the following month Sir Wilfrid Lawson, in his speech marking the opening of the new site for the London Temperance Hospital (Chapter 1), noted that this slaughter was partly funded by duties paid to the government by the drink trade – teetotalers like Cahill served in the imperial army while others like Lawson were critics of it. In 1885 Cahill's regiment was sent to Ceylon, Sceptre recording this travel and an additional £4 charge per annum for the risks associated with the tropical climate.

The Highlanders travelled on to Hong Kong in 1888, but Edward Cahill was no longer with them, having sought a discharge in Ceylon in October of 1887.[35] His family joined him and he opened E. Cahill and Sons, a manufacturing tailors' and outfitters' business, in Colombo in that year. By 1902 the firm was employing thirty workers in a two-storey showroom on Chatham Street.[36] Edward died in 1911, Ellen having preceded him in 1894, and his funeral was held at St Philip Neri Catholic church.[37] Bonuses had been paid until 1898, when he would have been sixty-five; with the addition of six bonus payments the policy would have been worth a good deal more than its original value, though the extra payments made for climate risk – which he may have continued to pay after settling in Colombo – would have eaten into that. Edward's policy, presumably established to safeguard his young family after enlisting, might well have provided him with the additional confidence needed to set up in business in Ceylon. The policy might have been used as security for a loan and would have promised a sizeable sum for the family's future. We don't know what this policy meant to Edward, but it seems likely that the security it offered against future loss might well have also become a source of confidence in the present.

Like other firms, the Sceptre assured lives that served in the military or as colonial administrators across the world, or sought work in the colonies, and some of these were teetotalers like Cahill.[38] These travellers may have established these policies as security against the risk of travel or active service, but that did not simply cancel out those risks; it made it possible to take them. The UKT's Reverend Baker told a meeting in Leicester that the firm 'had hundreds of members in Australia; many had emigrated who would not have been able to do so if they had not been members, because they were able to borrow money upon their policies to get abroad'.[39] Sceptre's networks would also have to follow its policyholders, engaging with local temperance societies and agents, just as the Whittington had with Henry Thatcher's application (Chapter 4). Erika Rappaport noted that 'temperance, much like abolitionism and evangelicalism, traveled with missionaries, soldiers, sailors, business people, and reformers'; firms like Sceptre travelled with them.[40]

'The hope of progressive prosperity': The virtuous circle of ethical investment

In his unpublished history of the UKT, James Dawson Burns described the 1855 division of the firm's profits, which first demonstrated that its abstainers lived longer, as a justification of 'the hope of progressive prosperity'.[41] It seems likely that Burns meant the *firm's* hopes, but the phrase also suggests something of the ideals of its members and of other teetotalers. This section considers the potential that temperance life assurance might have offered for progressive prosperity.

Much of this potential came from investing the capital funds amassed by temperance life assurance firms. Those funds guaranteed the future security of the firm's policyholders, but the investment interest they generated could also represented a significant source of income for the company. Sceptre's funds grew by £600,073 during the First World War, for example, and more than a third of that growth was generated by investment income, with the rest derived from premiums.[42] This raised additional complications and possibilities for teetotal investors. In 1851 Robert Charleton had hesitated over investing in a business that drew some of its income from Sunday excursion trains, which encouraged Sabbath-breaking; Quakers like Charleton may have seen the scrutiny of potential investments as an extension of earlier campaigns to boycott sugar grown by enslaved plantation workers.[43] This scrutiny continued into the twentieth century, when the success of large British brewers made their shares attractive to investors, including assurance firms; the temperance column of a Welsh newspaper criticized the Equitable office for holding £65,000 of shares in five breweries.[44]

By the 1860s, though, the UKT had developed a more positive investment strategy, one that provides us with another set of ideas about 'improvement'. In the December of 1867, for example, the company lent nearly £15,000 to Southampton Council at 4.5 per cent interest; the following summer, Portsmouth's Local Government Board borrowed £70,000 to build subsidiary sewers.[45] These loans were mortgaged against the rates, and between 1857 and the early 1870s the UKT's 4.5 per cent loans were cheaper than the 5 per cent interest charged for works of this kind by the Public Works Loan Board, which was also not willing to lend such large amounts over thirty or even fifty years.[46] Some of this borrowing was intended to pay off older loans established at 5 per cent, which had originally funded infrastructural work; the UKT's lower interest rates meant substantial savings for these borrowers. Other life assurance and insurance companies were also active lenders at this moment, as the provision of public health and other amenities by local authorities became mandatory. As Harris and Hinde show, in 1874 insurance companies provided 38.9 per cent of the value of the outstanding loans – around £2.3 million – to urban sanitary authorities which were not also town councils. Only 16.5 per cent of the original value of those loans had been provided by the Public Works Loans Board.[47]

Between 1870 and 1900 the UKT lent significant sums for public works to Merthyr Tydfil's Board of Health; Goole's Burial Board; Ryde Town Council (sewers, esplanade extensions); West Hartlepool's Improvement Commissioners; South Stockton's Local Board (bridge-building); Newry's Local Government Board (at least £60,000, waterworks and markets); Swansea's Board of Guardians; the Local Board at Towey (sewerage works); and Milford Haven's Urban District Council (paving).[48] Harbour improvement works could also be significant – £79,000 for the harbour at Shoreham, for example, or £22,000 at Drogheda, County Louth.[49] The UKT also lent tens of thousands of pounds to Torquay Corporation in 1894, probably through purchasing shares in the company set up to build the new harbour.[50] As the law creating the harbour company had also been the cause of the 'Battle of Torquay' (Chapter 2), this would seem to present a case of the UKT turning the other cheek when it saw an opportunity for investment.

These sums were small compared to the loans offered to sanitary authorities by the Local Government Board, though, which loaned nearly £1.5 million nationally in 1874 and £3–4 million from 1877 to 1879, but they could be *locally* significant, as it became clear when South Stockton incorporated Thornaby-on-Tees to become a new Metropolitan Borough in 1892. The Borough's accounts showed that the UKT was its largest and longest-established single lender, accounting for £6,000 of the £15,000 borrowed and still outstanding since 1883.[51]

The significance of these monies, recorded as 'advances to Local Boards, Corporations, and other Public Bodies on the security of Rates', waxed and waned (Table 6.1). At the end of the 1840s, just under half of the firm's assets were in government stock – the annuities and consols favoured by Robert Warner – and almost all of the remainder was in the form of loans on mortgages.[52] By 1880 loans advanced to local boards and corporations made up a quarter of the firm's assets, though this proportion then declined steadily. UK mortgages remained important until 1900, when UK ground rents became the most valuable asset category.[53] Presumably fewer local authorities needed to borrow money for improvements, and some of the loans established from the 1860s would have been paid off. Other sources of finance were now available, too, particularly from the Public Works Loans Board, which had become the most important source of finance for local government since the 1870s, though towns faced different local challenges as well as borrowing costs.[54] Other investments took the place of these 'advances'. The proportion of the company's funds invested in railway and other debentures and stocks fluctuated over this period but grew to nearly a quarter of the total by 1900, and as we saw in Chapter 1, War Loans were to become increasingly important for the UKT from 1914.

For several decades, though, the UKT, like banks and other insurance companies, was partly in the business of funding *improvement* – not simply the reformation of the

Table 6.1 UKT assets and investments, 1880–1900 (percentage)

Asset	1880	1887	1894	1900
Advances to boards and corporations	25.04	20.17	15.49	8.73
UK mortgages	45.02	25.42	24.55	12.71
UK ground rents	1.10	18.31	25.19	27.78
Railway and other debentures and stocks	17.37	7.33	10.13	23.97
Total value, all assets (£)	2,887,511	4,233,474	5,903,283	7,329,266

Source: United Kingdom Temperance and General provident Institution, Annual Reports and Balance Sheets 1840–1910, Aviva Archives.

self or a section of British society, but the Chadwickian project of cleaning, clearing and building better cities. Samuel Bowly noted at the 1877 Annual Meeting that 'it was a matter of great satisfaction that the funds of the institution were lent to local Corporations for sanitary purposes', because 'such advances also not only benefited communities as a whole, but individual members of this institution, by promoting sanitary improvement, and circumscribing the death-rate'.[55] The UKT had created a virtuous circle. Its members presumably hoped to reap some of the other rewards explored in this chapter, but their collected premiums could also be invested in local authorities, thereby improving the lives of others – including, of course, any UKT policyholders who lived in those areas.

It is tempting to see this as a solution of sorts to the problem identified by Christopher Herbert, who suggested that money acquired an 'incurably paradoxical self-contradicting character' for the Victorians, following 'a perceived shift of influence from traditional structures of wealth based on the massive fixities of landed property to new ones based on the liquidities of manufacturing, commerce, speculation, and credit'.[56] No longer tied to concrete things like land, money acquired an unstable system of values – divinity and excrement, wealth and poverty – which made it a highly productive but taboo concept. Wealth had to be made and displayed, but also hidden away, the knowledge of its origins ignored or repressed. Contemporary political economy was unable to 'decontaminate' the filthiness of money or settle this 'irresolvable conflict of values'. Investing in municipal schemes could be interpreted as another attempt at 'decontamination', using the money generated by individual self-improvement to build a new infrastructure of far wider benefit. If the filthiness of lucre prompted Quaker misgivings about business, this might explain Bowly's satisfaction with finding an improving use for the UKT's growing capital funds, building sewage works to turn excrement into money, while simultaneously 'circumscribing the death-rate'. And of course, this virtuous circle was also generating a return of 4.5 per cent on the investment. More money, more virtue, more money, more virtue – for as long as local boards and corporations needed the money.

The UKT's investment decisions extended ideas of 'improvement' from the individual to the redevelopment of Victorian towns and cities, and in its ability to make money *and* effect these kinds of changes, temperance life assurance seemed to offer an entirely positive form of business.

'A very business-like argument': The laws of mortality and the laws of the market

The success of the UKT and its rivals meant that the statistical arguments examined in Chapter 4 were increasingly taken – by supporters and others – to be proof of the longevity of abstainers. Once this had become a natural 'fact', it changed the tone of arguments made for temperance life assurance. Originally established as a challenge to accepted custom, insurantial practice and medical wisdom, by the end of the century it was possible to present temperance life assurance as simple commonsense, a black box, in Latourian terms, that was becoming increasingly unexamined and therefore harder to open and challenge. Its success was helped by its interaction with two other black boxes: the laws of mortality and the laws of the market. The larger bonuses and longer lives enjoyed by abstainers simply reflected financial and medical realities, acquiring apparently natural values.

This attitude is suggested by newspaper reporting in Britain and North America from the 1880s onwards. Reviewing claims made for total abstinence in 1888, for example, Joseph Cook considered the experience of the UKT and Scottish Temperance, adding 'this assertion is made, not by fanatical agitators, not by partisan temperance organisations, but by business companies governed exclusively by cool commercial prudence'. The commercial success of these firms was proof that their arguments stood up, in other words. Reporting a speech given by Colonel J. L. Green, the President of the Connecticut Mutual Life Insurance Company, which had highlighted the dangers of moderate drinking, Cook concluded that 'this is not the testimony of a temperance agitator, but of an expert in life assurance'.[57] This was, of course, also the understanding that lead William Bingham to say that 'the fact is, those who don't drink don't die so fast'.[58] The *Woman's Signal*, the journal of the National British Women's Temperance Association, took a similar line. It concluded, 'These are not the "statistics of the statistician", and may therefore perhaps be considered free from the charge of dulness [*sic*], nor of the propagandist and rhetorician, but just those of a prosaic insurance office, trading for business purposes on business lines.'[59] Noting that American firms were planning to offer cheaper premiums for policies for total abstainers, while refusing immoderate drinkers, the *New York Tribune* concluded 'the companies have approached this subject without prejudice, as it is merely a matter of dollars and cents with them'.[60] The *Manchester Guardian* noted that 'a very business-like argument for the value of temperance is to be found in the report for last year of the directors of the Sceptre Life Association, Limited'; this argument was 'disappointing the undertakers'.[61] The pithiest summary came from the *Pittsburgh Press* in 1915, in a story titled 'Making the Grim Reaper Hold His Hat And Wait', the author concluding that 'when you get right down to cold facts and figures, life insurance statistics prove that total abstainers live longer than people who indulge in alcoholic liquors'.[62] The coldness, prosaicness, perhaps even dullness of these figures, and the fact that this was a business-like rather than a religious or moral argument for total abstinence, attracted attention in a way that suggests that this was novel but ultimately unremarkable.

Discussions of the personal habits of Samuel Hardy, the UKT's actuary, made a similar point. Dawson Burns reported that 'it has been stated that the Actuary, not himself an abstainer, was exceedingly surprised at the remarkable superiority of the Temperance Section over the General Section' in 1855.[63] Hardy's moderate drinking and the disinterested, expert, nature of actuarial practice helped to distance the board's enthusiasm for abstinence from the story told by the firm's figures. As Timothy Alborn has shown, between the 1820s and 1900 the search for universal 'laws of mortality', which would predict the chance of death at every age, attracted attention from experts in vital statistics, mathematics and life assurance. As firms pooled their experience through their professional centres of calculation, the Institute and the Faculty of Actuaries, and as they engaged with the work of the General Registrar's Office, it seemed increasingly possible that it would be possible to pin down this law, but by 1900 this hope had died.[64]

Taken together, though, the laws of mortality, which seemed to show that drinking reduced life expectancy, and the laws of the market – this product had been tested by supply and demand, after all – presented temperance life assurance as a simple fact of life and business. When Samuel Bowly was asked, at a public meeting for the UKT, whether life insurance showed a distrust in Providence, he answered that 'they were all subject to physical laws, and those laws did not alter without a miracle. It was not a distrust of Providence to provide for those they loved'.[65] Twenty years after Joseph Barker had criticized those who established life assurance instead of trusting God to allow them their allotted time on earth, this pious but business-like Friend provided an answer that united Providence and the 'physical' laws of mortality.

The idea that temperance life assurance was a naturally good thing, producing different kinds of improvement, could also be seen in the changing nature of the UKT's London offices. A survey of the first three buildings is presented in the next section as a form of 'life'.

Temperance lives: Moorgate Street, Adelaide Place and the Strand (1840–1944)

The language of assurance uses the word 'office' to mean 'company' – as in 'the Sceptre office' – but here we are concerned with the building in which a firm was situated. The UKT's first London office, at 39 Moorgate Street, was – like other office space in the city at this time – shared with other businesses. The most important of these, and the reason the UKT chose it, was the New British and Foreign Temperance Society, which held its final meeting in the UKT's offices in 1842; its successor, the National Temperance Society, continued to share the building with the UKT until 1846.[66] The architectural historian John Summerson noted that one early cluster of insurance offices at Blackfriars simply took over terraced houses, housing themselves on 'quasi-domestic lines', and the UKT's first office was no different.[67] When housebreakers attempted to force their way into the Moorgate office in 1842, the board decided that the clerk, Mr Phillips, should live on the top floor rent-free; he was allowed the use of an additional back room to house his family in 1848.[68] These conditions were clearly not ideal, and the firm's growing size and reputation demanded a change of address, away from Moorgate's small and marginal cluster of insurance offices.

The UKT moved to 1 Adelaide Place, its second home, in 1854, remaining there until 1907. Situated on the Thames and erected about 1835 following the opening of the New London Bridge in 1831, Adelaide Place was a far more visible and impressive building.[69] In 1863 the building appeared in a double-page engraving depicting a triumphal arch across the City end of London Bridge, built to mark the marriage of Albert Edward, the Prince of Wales, to Alexandra in 1863 (Figure 6.1). 1 Adelaide Place fills the right-hand side of the image, the words 'Life Assurance' just visible on the wall, with the Monument behind it. The office was in the background of this event, but its position might have reinforced the sense that the UKT's office was at the entrance to the City of London.

The new office also appeared in the firm's marketing. Some UKT policies bore an image of Adelaide Place, while the illustration on the cover of the UKT's pocket prospectuses at the end of the century showed the building from a viewpoint on the other side of Adelaide Place, with the busy Thames behind the office (Figure 6.2).[70]

In Chapter 3 it was suggested that the adoption of grand office buildings like Adelaide Place was prompted by a desire to reassure a public made nervous by life assurance scandal and collapse; for John Summerson, Victorian 'insurance depended, even more than banks, on the wide dissemination of confidence, and, moreover, on the propagation of a sentimental image, the image of upright, prudent men banded together to arrest the cruel hand of fate'.[71] Adelaide Place was a clear statement of the solidity and permanence of the UKT's business. However, while the inclusion of the Monument in the background of Figure 6.2 may have been intended to indicate the location of the UKT's offices, it could also have troubled the image of security that the firm hoped to convey. The Monument is, after all, a marker of the Great Fire of London which had destroyed much of the city. Perhaps the Monument served as a reminder of life's uncertainties – anxiety played its part in the selling of assurance, as the recurring figures of the abandoned widow and orphan in marketing materials makes clear – and perhaps the solidity of the UKT's office symbolized prudent protection against Summerson's 'cruel hand of fate'.

The UKT moved again in July 1907, to a purpose-built office at 196 the Strand, between Milford Lane and Arundel Street and facing the church of St Clement Danes (Figure 6.3). This had been the site of the *Illustrated London News* offices between 1842 and 1905, and *The News* returned here in 1945.[72]

196 was certainly a grand office, fit for the UK's largest mutual life assurance business. The boardroom ceiling featured a large allegorical painting by Gerald Moira, who produced murals and stained glass for the nearby Central Criminal Court, the boardroom of Lloyds, the Wigmore Hall, several town halls and other commercial buildings. Henry Watkins described the UKT's ceiling as follows:

> In the centre Moira painted a dignified figure of a woman, Providence, surrounded by children and the fruits of the earth. Kneeling to her in an attitude of supplication, Motherhood receives her benediction. At one end, Vice and Drunkenness mounted

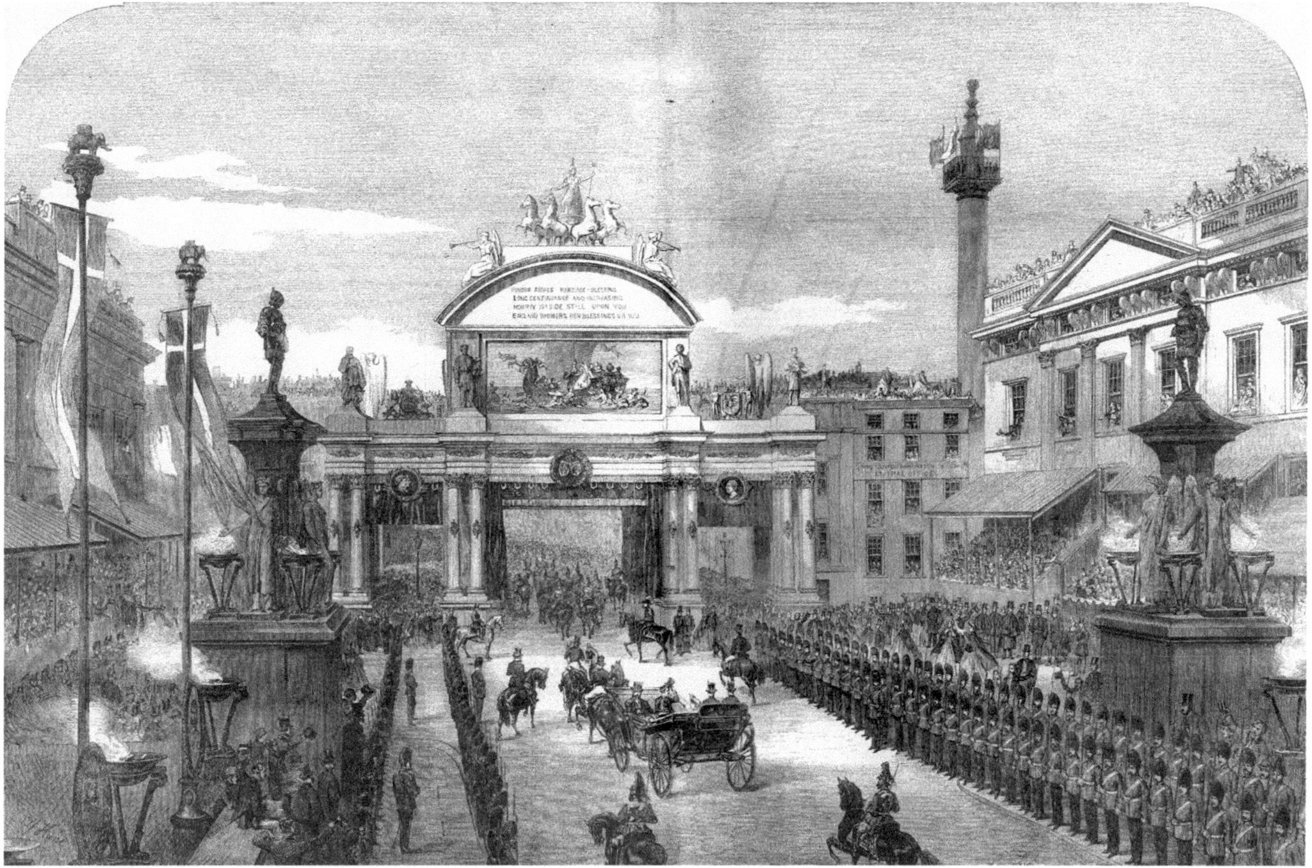

Figure 6.1 The royal procession at the Grand Arch, London Bridge.

Source: *Illustrated London News*, 21 March 1863, 300–1. Courtesy Alamy.

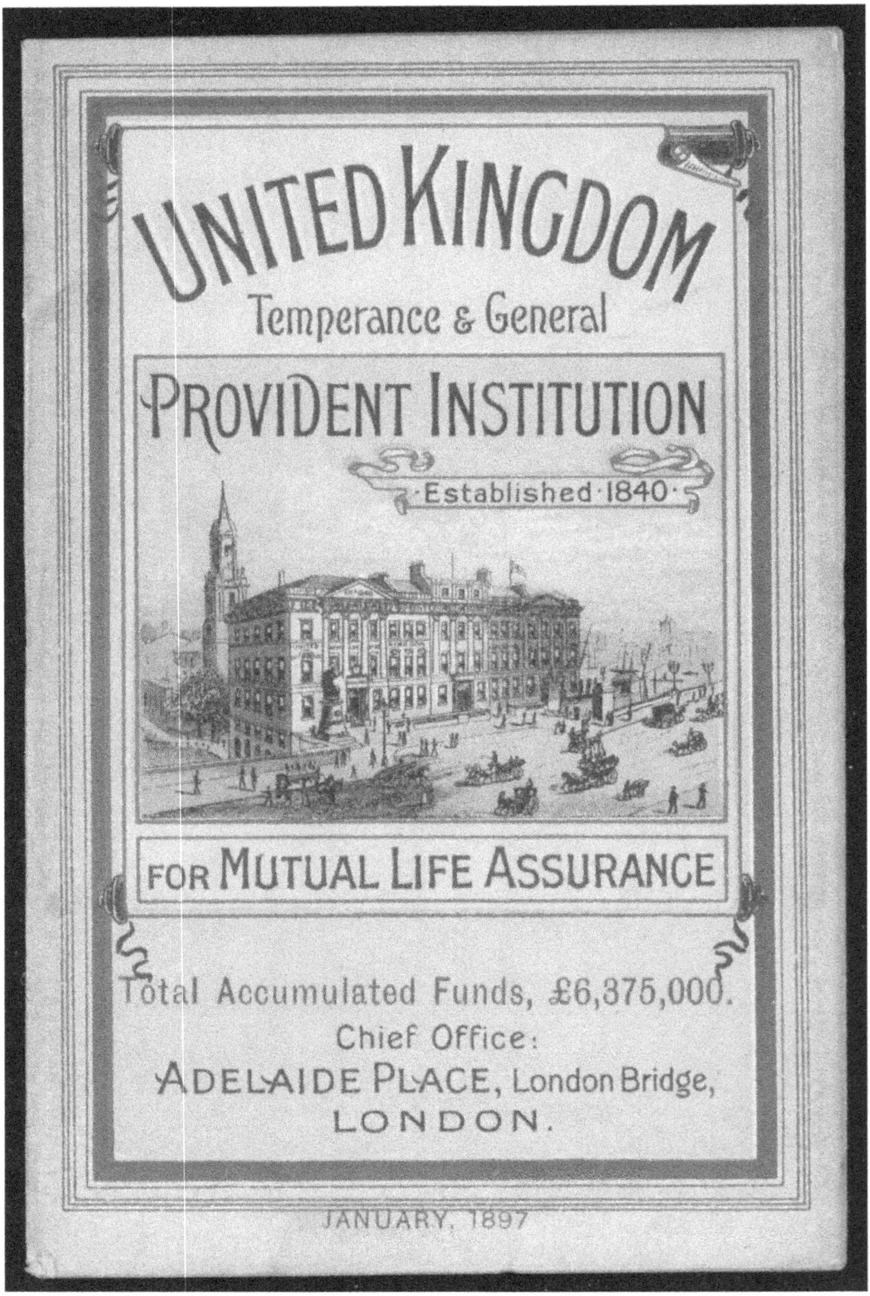

Figure 6.2 UKT prospectus, 1897, showing 1 Adelaide Place.

Source: Aviva Archives.

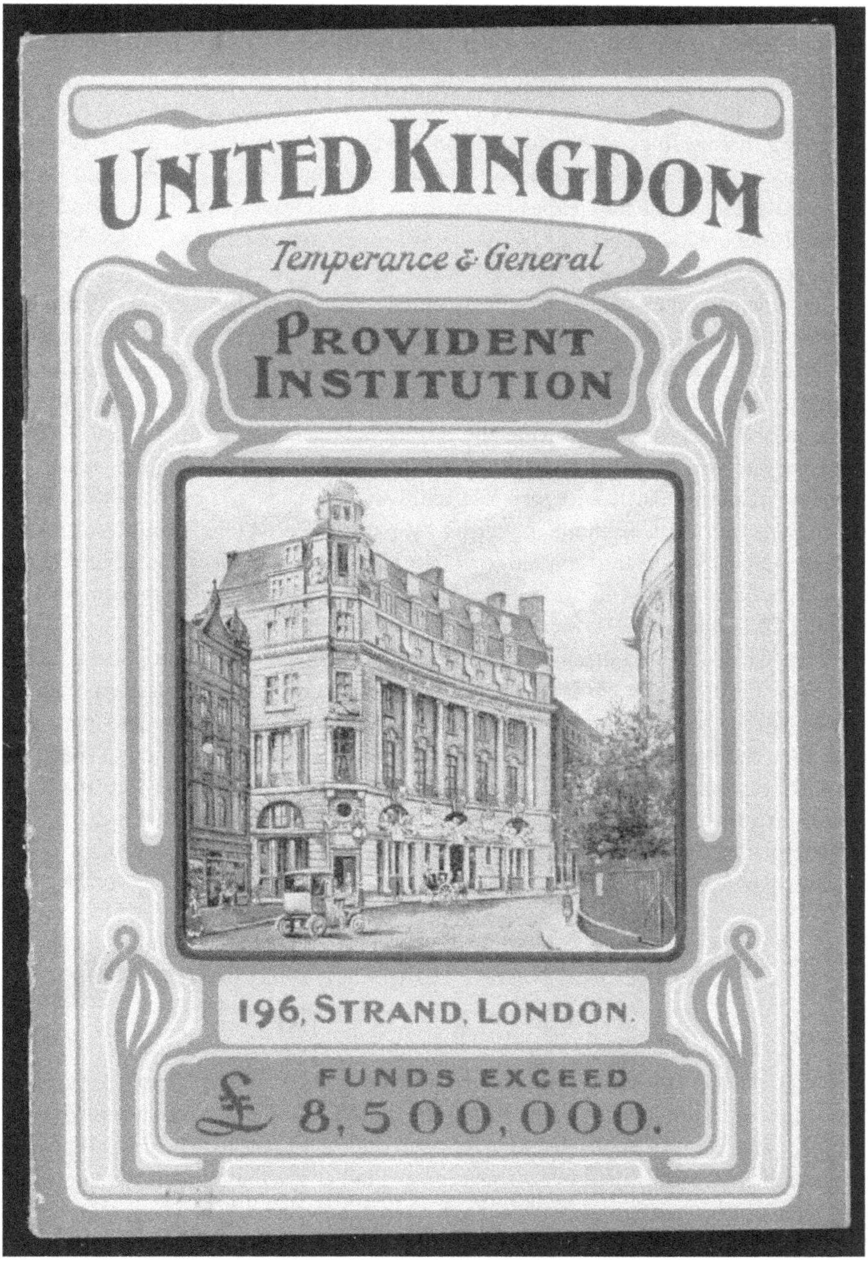

Figure 6.3 UKT prospectus, 1908, showing 196 The Strand.

Source: Aviva Archives.

> on a great-winged eagle, fly before Temperance, who has seized the reins, while Humanity, typified in the stalwart and muscular figure of a man, climbs upwards. Opposite, Knowledge emerges from behind the curtains of the unknown.[73]

Receiving the blessings of Providence and driving out vice and drunkenness, while humanity progresses, and knowledge emerges from ignorance – there could be no better statement of the lofty aims of temperance life assurance. The location and style of the Strand offices served the UKT well until enemy action damaged the building in 1944, necessitating a move to 33 Gracechurch Street.

The new Strand offices were publicly opened in 1907 by the Liberal Chancellor, Herbert Henry Asquith, confirming the importance of the UKT as an economic institution. In his speech at a luncheon at the Hôtel Métropole after the ceremony, Asquith noted that the UKT 'draws its members largely from the thrifty Nonconformist classes which form the traditional backbone of the Liberal Party'.[74] Asquith was widely suspected of alcoholism, acquiring the nickname 'squiff' as wartime prime minister, and even Churchill was embarrassed by Asquith's public drunkenness in the Commons. Asquith's antipathy towards temperance meant that he was unable to resist the temptation to use this speech to declare that governments should avoid managing the drink trade – at a moment when his government was trying to do exactly that.[75]

'Improvement' could mean many things to the UKT's workers and policyholders, and even the messages communicated by its buildings could be misinterpreted or challenged by those hostile to temperance. The firm could not control these meanings after they had been shaped; the grandeur of number 196 meant nothing to men like Asquith, for example. This was also true of the firm's interventions into the built environment, which can tell us something of the relationships between drink and temperance in a world where networks of material things were far harder to shape than images or words.

The multiple (and sometimes unexpected) outcomes of temperance life assurance

The UKT experimented with improvement in other ways. In 1860, probably inspired by the founding of the Metropolitan Drinking Fountain and Cattle Trough Association, the UKT established a public drinking fountain opposite 1 Adelaide Place. This proved popular, but by 1884 it had been replaced by a larger granite fountain, surmounted by a group of bronze figures.[76] Within a few years, however, the new fountain, which weighed 45 tonnes, threatened the integrity of the warehouses below Adelaide Place on Lower Thames Street.[77] The fountain was given to the London County Council, and in 1895 it was transferred to Clapham Common, where it still stands (Figure 6.4).[78]

As Mark Girouard noted, philanthropists who put up drinking fountains 'were, no doubt sincerely, acting on the best Christian principles; but often, one feels … with an eye to their own reputation'.[79] The same was probably true of the UKT, but their intentions were confounded by the material capacities of the environment in which

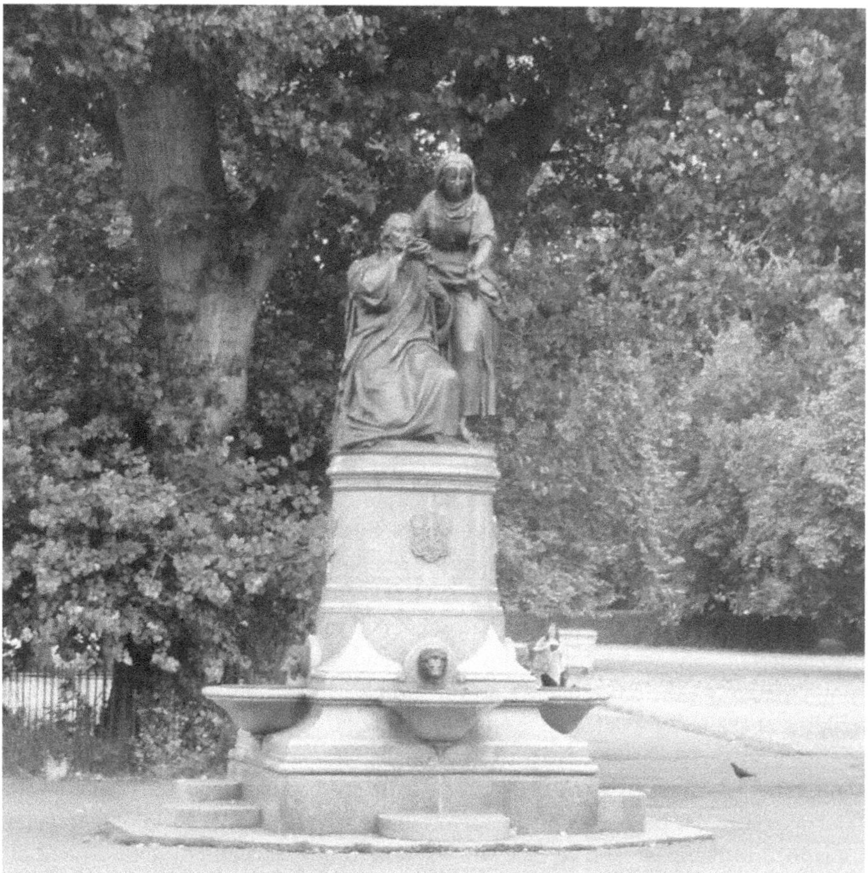

Figure 6.4 The UKT Fountain, Clapham Common.

Source: Author's photo.

they were working. Marble and bronze are very durable, but very heavy; they suited Clapham Common much better than they did Adelaide Place, but the removal of the statue undermined the firm's philanthropic gesture.[80] The fate of the UKT's drinking fountain reminds us that buildings are more than just signs, and that these firms were working in complex social and material environments where their intended outcomes – broadly, 'improvement' – could get tangled up in other arrangements of people and things.

The story of the UKT's fountains is a useful introduction to this section, which explains how the UKT and two of its directors ended up owning several licensed drinking places – a beerhouse, a pub and three hotels. As we will see, one common response to this was to charge them with hypocrisy or inconsistency, but it seems likely that these outcomes reflected, at least in part, the complex environments in which they acted.

In the autumn of 1908 'a London weekly journal' ran a story under the title 'Sir Thomas Whittaker's Public-House', accusing Whittaker – chair of the UKT since 1898, Liberal MP, UK Alliance stalwart and second-generation teetotaler – of being the owner of a pub.[81] The accusation came from Horatio Bottomley, journalist, serial swindler and the then Liberal MP for Hackney South, who had also pointed out that *The Oracle*, a financial paper Whittaker had previously managed, had encouraged readers to invest in breweries and the drink trade; in the Commons Bottomley 'quoted some of this advice amidst roars of laughter, and this comparison of Sir Thomas Whittaker's attitude then with that of his professions to-day was crushing'.[82] Over the summer of 1908 Whittaker had been vocal in discussions of the Licensing Act 1908, insisting that breweries who would lose licensed premises should not receive compensation; Bottomley identified Whittaker as 'the real author of this Bill', which suggests that the timing of the public house story was unlikely to be accidental.[83]

The *Daily Chronicle*'s Parliamentary correspondent reported that the UKT's redevelopment of their new offices on the Strand had caused a nearby public house – the Edinburgh Stores at 1 Milford Lane, just around the corner – to lose air and light. The owner would not accept compensation for this, so instead of 'resorting to costly and doubtful litigation' the UKT bought it from them. They had no control over the pub or the licence, and would simply receive rent from the proprietor until the lease ran out in 1936.[84] In fact Whittaker had suggested to the board that they should sell the property two years before the story broke, and the UKT had already paid £5,000 compensation to their neighbours at *The Graphic* newspaper in 1906, as the new building at 196 had also affected the light of their offices.[85]

This story was probably embarrassing enough, but a week later Whittaker published a response which turned out to concern a different pub altogether, this time in Bournemouth. The corporation had borrowed money from the UKT to buy property it planned to demolish and replace with reading rooms and other public amenities; the problem was that the property included a licensed hotel, the Belle Vue. Whittaker clarified that the corporation, not the UKT, owned the hotel, which would anyway soon be demolished, and that the firm had no control over it.[86] The firm tried to keep to this; when the corporation later proposed a transfer of the existing licence from the Belle Vue Hotel to the new Pavilion, the board minuted that 'the Institution was not prepared to approve or cooperate with the Corporation in any scheme or arrangement which would involve the sale of intoxicants'.[87]

These stories suggest different ways in which a temperance business might acquire land or property associated with licensed premises. Investments of these kinds tied the UKT up in other considerations and obligations, some of which had real legal weight, and it found itself wrapped up in its neighbours' business, or in the plans of those it lent money to. Those new neighbours might well have been the source of Bottomley's story, too. The Edinburgh Stores seems to have been the haunt of a fairly 'fast' set of sporting gentlemen, artists, actors and newspaper men late in the century, when it was called the Milford Arms; a clubby, masculine reminiscence published in 1888 described it as 'a hostelry not unknown to the staffs of the *Illustrated London News*'.[88] *The News* sold its Strand building to the UKT, but retained offices on Milford Lane, sharing the street with *The Graphic*, *The People* and the *Penny Illustrated Paper and Illustrated Times*. The story could easily have been Milford Lane gossip, passed on by journalists who drank in the Stores; Bottomley would have had extensive contacts in this world after twenty years in journalism.

Two of the UKT's directors also acquired public houses. Around 1855 Samuel Bowly found himself the owner of a beerhouse – 'much to his own and friends' amusement' – when he purchased a country estate at Horsepools, Gloucestershire, which included several existing businesses. Bowly persuaded its keeper to give up the trade, providing a 'genteel lodging-house' on the estate in its place.[89] To Bowly this was a minor, amusing incident, but it makes for a productive comparison with the purchase of two fully licensed hotels – the Albion Hotel and the Bath House Hotel – in the North Essex resort of Walton-on-the-Naze by his friend Robert Warner. In 1892 'The Blue Ribbon', writing to the *Essex Standard*, asked:

> Who will answer for or defend the consistency of a leading teetotaller – the Chairman of the United Kingdom Temperance and General Provident Institution who has associated with him on the board such men as W S Caine and Canon Fleming – and yet who is the owner of several large public-houses in our own county – situate in a well-known watering place, say 20 miles from Colchester![90]

Robert's father John Warner had owned three pubs elsewhere in Essex and Suffolk, though he died before the Friends began to collectively question their connections to the trade.[91] Robert developed the land John had acquired at Walton, building a large foundry, cottages for his workers, and larger houses to rent to middle-class visitors and residents. The Bath House was smaller and older, but the Albion Hotel was a substantial building, including excursion rooms which could cater for 600 people; it sold for £1,160 in 1914.[92] The unlicensed excursion rooms were run as 'Temperance Rooms', and the magistrates insisted that a sturdy wall be erected to divide them from the hotel itself.[93] While it is tempting to see that wall as a spatial metaphor for Warner's divided loyalties to temperance, elsewhere in the county magistrates insisted that hotels sell alcohol only to residents, and not to day trippers, so it was probably not Warner's decision.[94]

Unsurprisingly, Warner's interest in these hotels seems to have been largely financial; two days after buying the Albion in 1873 Warner mortgaged it back to the original owner, another of Walton's developers, later mortgaging it to his son-in-law, who ran the Albion until Warner's death.[95] Robert had rivals in the race to develop Walton, however, each of whom also built hotels; it is possible that the Albion also represented Warner's status as a developer, rather than a mere builder. It seems most likely that these sites were investments, but also part of Warner's efforts to develop his part of a fashionable resort and perhaps fund other developments in the town.

Of the six licensed premises discussed in this section, only Warner's Walton hotels really represented the kind of 'inconsistency' that the firm was charged with. The others are best understood as the messy and uncertain outcomes of the actions of the firm's directors, taken in circumstances that were not under their control. Other actors, with different attitudes to temperance – the owner and patrons of the Edinburgh Stores, Bournemouth's Corporation, Horatio Bottomley – had their own plans. On top of this, the material things that the UKT dealt with, like its new offices on the Strand or the marble fountain outside Adelaide Place, did not always play the parts expected of them.

Conclusions

Temperance life assurance represented different ideas of Victorian 'improvement', from paternalism, through the affective and productive value of foresight, to the harnessing of individual contributions to fund public works. At the same time this seems to have been increasingly seen as just 'good business;' these firms prospered, and so did their members, who were also living longer lives. While there were still some who doubted these claims, as we will see in Chapter 8, temperance life assurance was no longer the remarkable thing it had been in 1840. In trying to do the right thing, though, these firms sometimes became entangled with other actors and forces, not all of them human. Teetotalers joined societies because a personal commitment to abstinence was often not enough in itself, and enlisting the help of others made it easier; sometimes, though, the networks they built contained unexpected elements which pushed back, including unfriendly journalists and pubs.

This is a good moment to return to the lives assured by these firms, who were also trying to follow a teetotal path in a world full of snares and obstacles. In Chapter 7 we will get a much closer look at their lives.

Notes

1. Robert Dundas Thomson, *Digestion: The Influence of Alcoholic Fluids on that Function, and on the Value of Health and Life. With a Scheme for Rendering the Working Classes Independent of Parish Relief* (London: John Snow, 1841), 26.
2. Minutes, Manchester and Salford Temperance Society, March 1851, MS M136/2/3/1166, Manchester County Record Office.
3. *Bradford Observer*, 23 March 1854, 8, emphasis added.
4. Samuel Smiles, *Thrift* (London: John Murray, 1875), 112.
5. Bentham, *Works*, vol. 1, 31.
6. 'Sceptre Life Association', *Western Mail*, 15 December 1870, 3.
7. Eagle Star Abstainers' Section Prospectuses, second edition, 1 January 1918, 15, London Archives.
8. Thomas David Lister, *Medical Examination for Life Insurance* (London: Edward Arnold, 1921), 160, emphasis added.
9. Winskill, *Temperance Movement*, vol. 4, 214–15.
10. *Leicester Chronicle*, 19 March 1859, 1.
11. David J. Jeremy, *Capitalists and Christians: Business Leaders and the Churches in Britain, 1900–1960* (Oxford: Clarendon Press, 1990), 330.
12. *The Times*, 4 September 1890, 7
13. W. W. Webb, 'Thomson, Robert Dundas (1810–1864)', rev. Richard Hankins, *Oxford Dictionary of National Biography* (Oxford University Press, 2004), www.oxforddnb.

com/view/article/27322, accessed 17 November 2009; Richard Hankins, 'Pen Portraits of Presidents. Robert Dundas Thomson, MD, CM, FRS', *Weather* 53 (1998).
14. Meeting, 7 December 1840, Minutes of the Standing Committee 1, Aviva Archives; 'Medical Testimonial against Spirits in Medicine', *British and Foreign Temperance Society, Sixth Report* (London: British and Foreign Temperance Society, 1837), appendix, 25, MS T33 C Bri, Livesey Collection.
15. General Board of Health, Medical Council, *Report of the Committee for Scientific Inquiries in Relation to the Cholera Epidemic of 1854* (London: Eyre and Spottiswoode, 1855); Pamela K. Gilbert, *Mapping the Victorian Social Body* (Albany: SUNY Press, 2004).
16. Hankins, 'Robert Dundas Thomson', 267.
17. See, for example 'Health of the Metropolis', *The Times*, 23 March 1865, 12; *Report of the Medical Officer of Health for St. Pancras, Metropolitan Borough*, 1857, 3, Wellcome Library.
18. M. Norton Wise and Crosbie Smith, 'Work and Waste: Political Economy and Natural Philosophy in Nineteenth Century Britain (III)', *History of Science* 28 (1990), 223, fn19 257.
19. Thomson, *Digestion*, 27.
20. Alborn, *Regulated Lives*, 151.
21. Thomson, *Digestion*, 26.
22. *Wrexham Advertiser, and North Wales News*, 3 September 1881, 8.
23. J. Russom, 'Correspondence. Mutual Assurance and Temperance Provident Institution', *British and Foreign Temperance Intelligencer* 6 (1842), 186, MS J Bri, Livesey Collection.
24. 'Review of *The Pathology of Drunkenness* by Charles Wilson MD, Edinburgh 1855', *Monthly Journal of Medical Science* 20 (1855), 247, emphasis added.
25. Thomson, *Digestion*, 26.
26. *Nottinghamshire Guardian*, 24 October 1862, 3.
27. Price, *From Queen to Queen*, 15–16.
28. 'Prohibition Builds Houses', *The Abstainer* 37, 9 (November 1926), 1.
29. Sceptre Life Association Limited Policy Ledger 1, London Archive; *Birmingham Daily Post*, 26 February 1918, 6.
30. Sceptre Life Association Limited Policy Ledger 5, London Archives.
31. On 'foreign residence' and travel risks see Alborn, *Regulated Lives*, 120–1 and *passim*; James Kneale and Samuel Randalls, 'Invisible Atmospheric Knowledges in British Insurance Companies, 1830–1914', *History of Meteorology* 6 (2014), 35–52; Kneale and Randalls, 'Making Climate Risks Work'; and Kneale and Randalls, 'Imagined Geographies of Climate and Race'.
32. Sceptre Life Association Limited Policy Ledger 2, London Archives.
33. WO 97 - Chelsea Pensioners British Army Service Records 1760–1913, Box 2438, Box record number 33, National Archives.
34. WO 12/9310, Commissary General of Musters Office and successors, General Muster Books and Pay Lists, Infantry, 91st Foot 1st Battalion, National Archives; 1871 Census (Class: RG10; Piece: 1232; Folio: 81; Page: 35; GSU roll: 0); John Percy Groves, *History of the 91st Princess Louise's Argyllshire Highlanders* (Edinburgh: W. & A. K. Johnston, 1894), 27.
35. Groves, *History*, 27–8; WO 121 - Chelsea: Pensioners' Discharge Documents 1760–1887, Reference WO 121, Box 0253, National Archives.

36. 'E. Cahill & Sons', in *Twentieth Century Impressions of Ceylon: Its History, People, Commerce, Industries and Resources*, edited by A. Wright (London: Lloyd's Greater Britain Publishing, 1907), 452.
37. 'Limerick Man's Death in Ceylon', *Limerick Chronicle*, 15 August 1911.
38. See Kneale and Randalls, 'Making Climate Risks Work'.
39. *Leicestershire Mercury*, 26 September 1857, 8.
40. Erika Rappaport, 'Sacred and Useful Pleasures: The Temperance Tea Party and the Creation of a Sober Consumer Culture in Early Industrial Britain', *Journal of British Studies* 52, 4 (2013), 1014.
41. Burns, company history, 3, and see Chapter 4.
42. Revenue account for 5 years 1 January 1914–31 December 1918, Valuation accounts and statements of the Sceptre Fund of the Eagle Star & British Dominions Insurance Co. Ltd, 1918, Sceptre Fund, Statements of account, quinquennial valuations and drafting papers, MS SC4/1/7/1/1, London Archives.
43. Letter from Charleton, 15 First Month 1851, cited in Fox, *Memoir*, 40, Library of the Society of Friends; Midgeley, *Women against Slavery*, and 'Slave Sugar Boycotts'.
44. *Llangollen Advertiser, Denbighshire, Merionethshire, and North Wales Journal*, 9 March 1900, 5.
45. Southampton, *Hampshire Advertiser*, 7 December 1867, 6; Portsmouth, *Hampshire Advertiser*, 8 August 1868, 8; *Leeds Mercury*, 23 May 1877, 8.
46. Ian Webster, 'The Public Works Loan Board and the Growth of the State in Nineteenth-Century England', *Economic History Review* 71 (2018), 898.
47. Bernard Harris and Andrew Hinde,'Sanitary Investment and the Decline of Urban Mortality in England and Wales, 1817–1914', *History of the Family* 24, 2 (2019), 347.
48. Merthyr Board of Health, *Merthyr Telegraph, and General Advertiser*, 25 October 1872, 2 and 5 November 1880, 3; Goole Burial Board, *York Herald*, 21 June 1875, 6; Ryde, *Isle of Wight Observer*, 18 June 1881, 5, and 22 October 1881, 5; West Hartlepool, *North-Eastern Daily Gazette*, 18 July 1883, 3; South Stockton, *North-Eastern Daily Gazette*, 7 November 1883, 3; Newry, *Belfast News-Letter*, 23 November 1887, 8 and 3 December 1889, 6; Swansea, 'Finance Report'; *Cambrian*, 22 November 1889, 8; Towey Local Board, *Cambrian News and Merionethshire Standard*, 21 December 1894, 10; Milford UDC, *Pembrokeshire Herald and General Advertiser*, 23 October 1908, 3.
49. Return from Harbour Authorities of Cost of Works, Loans and Scale of Dues, 1883, vol. 62, 302 and 684, 19th Century House of Commons Sessional Papers.
50. Board meetings, 5 and 12 January 1894, Minute Book 12, MS FL119, Aviva Archives.
51. *London Gazette*, 14 June 1892, 3449; Sixteenth annual report of the Local Government Board, 1886–7, C.5131, vol. 36, lXIX.
52. A statement of funds & effects belonging to the institution, 20 November 1847, Ninth Annual Report, United Kingdom Temperance and General Provident Institution, Annual Reports and Balance Sheets 1840–1910, Aviva.
53. Reports of the Directors to the Fortieth, Forty-Seventh, Fifty-Fourth and Sixtieth General Meetings of Members, Annual Reports and Balance Sheets 1840–1910, Aviva.
54. Webster, 'Public Works Loan Board'; Robert Millward and Sally Sheard, 'The Urban Fiscal Problem, 1870–1914: Government Expenditure and Finance in England and Wales', *Economic History Review* XLVIII (1995), 501–35; Johnathan Chapman, 'Interest Rates, Sanitation Infrastructure, and Mortality Decline in Nineteenth-Century England and Wales', *European Historical Economics Society Working Paper No. 218*, October 2021.

55. *Leeds Mercury*, 23 May 1877, 8.
56. Christopher Herbert, 'Filthy Lucre: Victorian Ideas of Money', *Victorian Studies* 44, 2 (2002), 193, 188.
57. *Montreal Daily Witness*, 28 April 1888, 3.
58. *Wings*, 1 July 1893, 219.
59. *Woman's Signal*, 9 September 1897, 169, issue 193.
60. 'Drink Shortens Life: Actuaries so Decide. Big Life Insurance Companies about to Favor Total Abstainers', *New York Tribune*, 23 November 1904, 5.
61. 'Disappointing the Undertakers', *Manchester Guardian*, 17 February 1906, 10.
62. 'Making the Grim Reaper Hold His Hat and Wait', *Pittsburgh Press*, 5 November 1915, 32.
63. Burns, company history, 34.
64. See Alborn, *Regulated Lives*, especially 124–7.
65. *Leicester Chronicle: or, Commercial and Agricultural Advertiser*, 25 October 1862, 3.
66. Winskill, vol. 2, 147, Report of Sixth Annual Meeting, January 1847, 2, United Kingdom Temperance & General Provident Institution Annual Reports and Balance Sheets 1840–1910, Aviva Archives.
67. John Summerson, 'The Victorian Rebuilding of the City of London', *London Journal* 3, 2 (1977), 165.
68. Meeting, 18 April 1842, UKT Minutes of the Standing Committee 1, Board meeting, 6 October 1848, UKT Minute Book 1, Aviva Archives.
69. Henry A. Harben, *A Dictionary of London* (London: H. Jenkins, 1918), www.british-history.ac.uk/no-series/dictionary-of-london, accessed 6 September 2023.
70. See, for example, policy 49203, issued 6 December 1869, Aviva Archives.
71. Summerson, 'Victorian Rebuilding', 165.
72. 'On the Site Where Illustrated Journalism Was Born', *Illustrated London News*, 29 September 1945, 359.
73. Henry Watkins, *The Art of Gerald Moira. With Some Notes and Thoughts on Decorative Art by Gerald Moira* (London: E. W. Dickens, 1922), 21.
74. *The Times*, 11 July 1907, 9.
75. Marvin Rintala, 'Taking the Pledge: H. H. Asquith and Drink', *Biography* 16, 2 (1993), 103–35; David M. Fahey, 'Worrying about Drink', *Brewery History* 166 (2016), 2–19.
76. *Morning Chronicle*, 24 May 1859, 6.
77. *The Standard*, 29 October 1884, 3.
78. The United Kingdom Temperance & General Provident Institution Drinking Fountain, Clapham Common, Public Monument and Sculpture Association National Recording Project, http://pmsa.cch.kcl.ac.uk/CL/CLLH-11.htm.
79. Mark Girouard, 'A Hundred Years of Free Water', *Country Life* 125, 3246 (2 April 1959), 700–1.
80. For buildings as assemblages, see Tim Edensor, 'Entangled Agencies, Material Networks and Repair in a Building Assemblage: The Mutable Stone of St Ann's Church, Manchester', *Transactions of the Institute of British Geographers* 36 (2011), 238–52.
81. '"Sir Thomas Whittaker's Public House" – An Explanation', *Manchester Guardian* 6 November 1908, 14.
82. 'Sir Thomas Whittaker. Another Silly Story about a Public House', *Western Times*, 14 November 1908, 4; 'Comments and Criticisms', *Western Gazette*, 23 October 1908, 12.
83. Licensing Bill, Wednesday 14 October 1908, Hansard, vol. 194, column 341.
84. 'Sir Thomas Whittaker's Public House'.

85. Board meetings, 21 November 1905, 9 January 1906, 1 November 1906, UKT Minute Book 15, MS FL122, Aviva Archives.
86. 'The Attacks on Sir T. Whittaker', *Manchester Guardian*, 13 November 1908, 3.
87. 1910, UKT Minute Book 15, Aviva Archives.
88. *Licensed Victuallers' Mirror*, 1 May 1888, 162.
89. Sessions, 'Samuel Bowly', 12; Taylor, *Memorials of Samuel Bowly*, 29; *Post Office Directory of Gloucestershire, with Bath and Bristol, 1856* (London: Kelly, 1856), 351.
90. *Essex Standard, West Suffolk Gazette, and Eastern Counties' Advertiser*, 16 July 1892, 7.
91. Senter and Senter, *The Warner Story*, 17.
92. 'Sales of Property', *Essex County Chronicle*, 4 September 1914, 7, Valuer's Notebook, MS D/DB B20, Essex Record Office.
93. 'The Albion Hotel and the Victory Inn, Walton-on-the-Naze', Clipping, probably 1893, Becontree Brewster Sessions, 1882, P/B Mc4, Essex Record Office; *Essex County Standard West Suffolk Gazette, and Eastern Counties Advertiser*, 26 August 1893, 6.
94. See, for example, Canvey Island, 12 October 1898, Committees of Quarter Sessions Minutes of Licensing Committee, 1873–1907, Essex County Licensing Committee, 1893–, MS Q/ACm 36, Essex Record Office.
95. Memorandum of Agreement, 14 May 1888, Deeds of Bath House Hotel and Albion Hall, Walton-le-Soken, with correspondence, 1873–1904, MS D/DU 408/11, Essex Record Office.

7

Ordinary lives: The Sceptre sample

Introduction

This chapter examines the records of some of the men and women insured in the Sceptre office, whose ledgers provide detailed information for a sample of nearly a thousand teetotal policies assured between 1865 and 1881, a generation after the UKT had been established. Nineteenth-century alcohol consumption reached its peak in Britain in the 1870s, and this was also the beginning of the end of temperance, as Harrison saw it, with the failure of the Licensing Act 1872 and the election of a Conservative government hostile to temperance in 1874.[1] However, late Victorian temperance seems – on this evidence – to have been healthy. The Sceptre sample lists 967 men and women who would have been members of a teetotal society in this period, and at least 300 of them were still assured between 1901 and 1933, suggesting continued membership of those societies. Even in London – always considered a poor second to the industrial provinces in terms of temperance support – the firm found teetotalers to assure between 1865 and 1881.

The analysis of this material considers general summaries as well as smaller groupings, beginning with the women the firm assured in this period – and the life of one woman, Caroline John, in particular. Examining key occupational groups and dozens of individual lives shows that while Sceptre assured many lower-middle-class lives the sample also contains a significant number of skilled and unskilled workers. The chapter considers what this might tell us about the character of late Victorian temperance and concludes by considering relationships between class and temperance in this period. For now, an examination of the Sceptre sample tells us a little more about who these abstainers were.

Sceptre lives, 1865–81

To what extent do these lives resemble the leaders and activists studied by Brian Harrison in terms of 'age-group, regional background, social class, personality, reforming outlook and religious belief'?[2] Earlier chapters have provided detailed accounts of teetotal lives, and we will see others in a moment. Here, though, we have the opportunity to consider them as a larger group.

Table 7.1 Sums assured, 1865–81

Sum (£)	Numbers of policies					%
	1865	1870–1	1877	1881	Total	
50	5	22	7	5	39	4.0
100	44	190	189	228	651	67.9
101–200	6	41	37	54	138	14.4
201–300	3	10	30	49	92	9.6
301–1,000	3	5	12	19	39	4.0
Total	61	268	275	355	959	100
Average	£134 12s.	£123 7s. 2d.	£149 14s. 1d.	£158 5s.	£143 11s.	

Source: Sceptre sample.

Table 7.2 Policy outcomes, 1865–81

Year	Claimed (%)		Lapsed (%)		Surrendered (%)		Total
1865	52	85.2	3	4.9	6	9.8	61
1870–1	117	43.8	118	44.2	32	12.0	267
1877	147	53.5	86	31.3	42	15.3	275
1881	193	62.9	57	18.2	58	18.9	308
Total	509	55.9	264	29.0	138	15.2	911

Source: Sceptre sample.

The ledgers of the Sceptre office have been used to create a sample of 959 abstainers' policies, covering 967 individuals, from the years 1865, 1870, 1871, 1877. The coverage is rather uneven as a result of the vagaries of the accounting practices of Sceptre's clerks, but the sample provides detailed records of these teetotal lives.[3] We begin by looking at the policies that were recorded in these ledgers before turning to consider what these might tell us about the lives they assured.

The overwhelming majority (89.7 per cent) of the 959 policies in the sample were for 'whole life' polices, which paid out at death. Most of the rest (9.1 per cent) were 'fixed age' policies, to be claimed at a set age – usually sixty – or at death if that came first. While the size of the policy established is not a reliable guide to the situation of the assurer, with additional information it can provide a better sense of their background. Table 7.1 shows that two thirds (67.9 per cent) of these policies covered £100; 24.0 per cent covered sums between £201 and £300; and only 4.0 per cent of all policies were established either for £50 or for more than £300. It might be expected that policies would grow in size as time went on, but in fact their average value fluctuated, dipping in 1870–1, which might reflect the difficulty Sceptre had in recruiting prosperous teetotalers after the first few years.

The outcome was recorded for 911 policies (Table 7.2). Policies established in 1865 were much more likely to be claimed than those from other years, and those in 1870–1 were slightly more likely to lapse than be claimed. Perhaps the first policyholders were determined, and more affluent, and the firm then struggled to

Table 7.3 Age of assured when policy first established, 1865–81

Age at assurance	1865	1870–1	1877	1881	Total	%
Under 10	0	0	0	1	1	0.1
10–19	4	20	17	28	69	7.1
20–29	23	117	145	149	434	44.9
30–39	14	98	81	138	331	34.2
40–49	16	33	31	36	116	12.0
50+	2	6	4	4	16	1.7
Total	59	274	278	356	967	100.0

Source: Sceptre sample.

find others like them, though the proportion of working-class occupations in the sample falls slightly between 1865 and 1881, from 49.2 to 42.3 per cent.

A very large proportion of the lapsed policies in the sample (86.7 per cent) lapsed within five years, which means that nearly a quarter of *all* of the sample polices (23.9 per cent) failed this quickly. It is possible that some policies recorded as lapsed were not 'taken up', but this is noted very rarely in the ledgers.

Almost half (44.9 per cent) of the policies in the sample were established when the assured were in their twenties; about another third (34.2 per cent) in their thirties (Table 7.3). The average age at which policies were established was thirty. Those assuring in 1865 were slightly older than the rest of the sample, with 30.5 per cent aged forty or over (13.65 per cent for the sample), which again might represent established teetotalers taking the opportunity to secure their lives. The youngest life in the sample was six-year-old Mary Elizabeth Grace Hocking (Chapter 2). The oldest was the millwright Thomas Cooke, seventy-eight in 1881, proprietor of the Britannia works at Newark-upon-Trent; he lived until 1892.[4]

The last general pattern to consider is the policyholder's address at the time of assuring (Map 7.1).

Adjusted for population, the most important districts for this sample lie in the East Midlands (Nottinghamshire, Derbyshire, Lincolnshire), western and southern counties (Berkshire, Somerset, Hampshire and Wiltshire) and the Northeast (County Durham and Northumberland). Nottinghamshire and Derbyshire were important for Sceptre, which had close links to local Methodist chapels and ministers like the Antliffs (Chapter 3), and with the lace industry; almost all of the lives in the first county were in Nottingham itself, while the Derbyshire lives were concentrated in Long Eaton and Derby. The relatively large number of lives assured in Somerset is partly explained by the teetotalers of southern Bristol; Hampshire's came from Southampton, Portsmouth, Aldershot and rural towns. Northumberland's lives were almost entirely urban and industrial, though the small town of Hexham provided seven policies between 1877 and 1881 through the local agent, Edward Snowball, a builder active in the North of England Temperance League.[5] The metropolis also accounts for a significant number of lives, with Middlesex bolstered by lives in Surrey and Kent, many of whom would be governed by the London County Council from 1889; there were also Essex lives

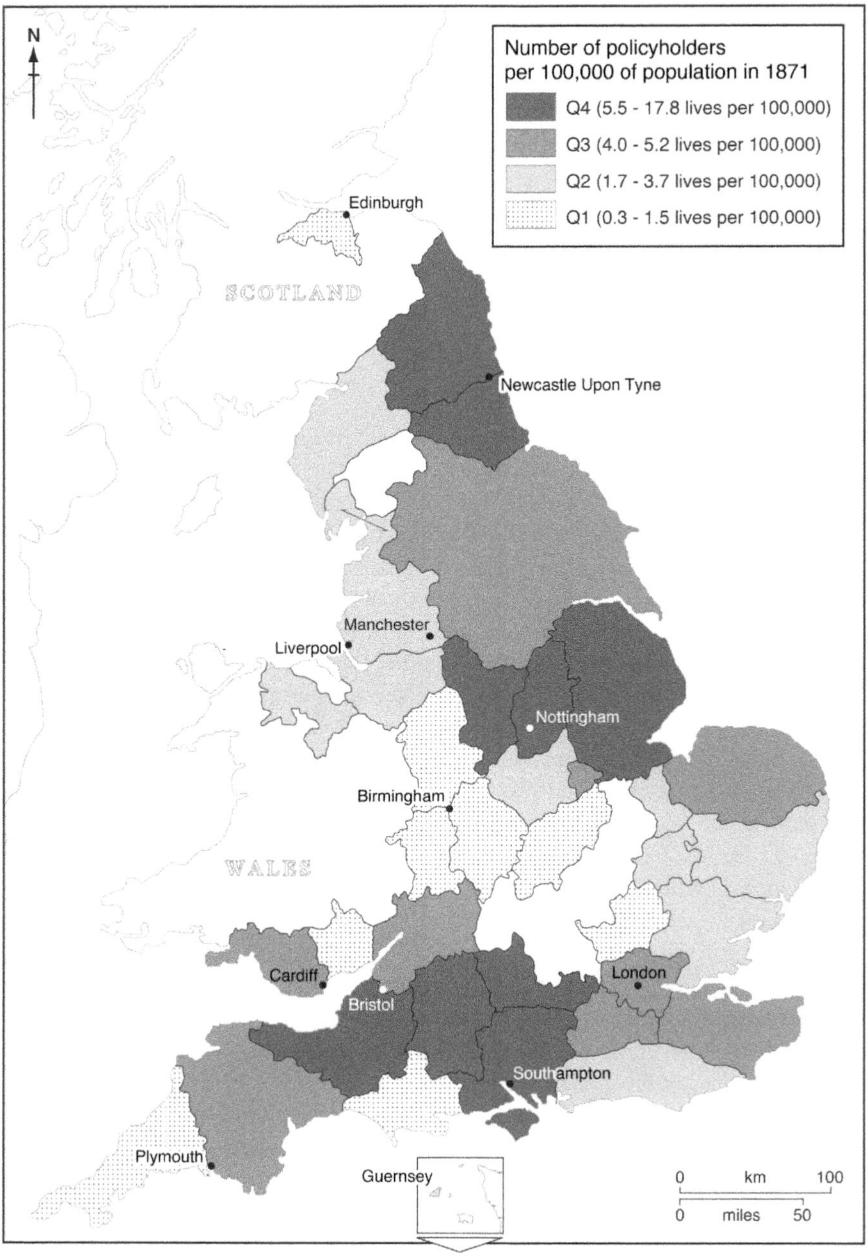

Map 7.1 Sceptre policyholders by county and population, 1865–81.

Source: Sceptre sample. Redrawn by Miles Irving, UCL Department of Geography.

nearby in East Ham, Plaistow and North Woolwich. While Yorkshire was not far behind Surrey and Devon, Lancashire's weighted share of the sample was only the same as Cambridgeshire's, and Cheshire's similar to Essex's, a rather different picture to that drawn by Harrison's sample of Alliance subscribers.[6] Elsewhere – Devon, Lincolnshire – the pattern reflects what might be expected of rural counties with significant temperance populations. Cornwall, Dorset, the West Midlands, Central England and Edinburgh were much less significant, and Central Wales and most of Scotland did not contribute to the Sceptre sample, suggesting strong competition from the UKT and other firms.

Beginning our look at significant groupings within the sample, we turn now to the women who were assured with Sceptre.

Sceptre women

Relatively few British women assured their lives until the last quarter of the century. Timothy Alborn found that the Atlas issued only 13 per cent of its policies to women between 1845 and 1852, and his discussion suggests other firms might have insured a similar proportion of women.[7] The Married Women's Property Act 1882 allowed married women to assure their own lives for the benefit of others, while the policy remained her property; as the Whittington advised its agents in 1889, 'here then is a large field opened for Agents to work in'.[8]

There are only sixty-eight women in the Sceptre sample, which predates the 1882 Act, 7.1 per cent of the policies (Table 7.4). Seven women held joint policies – six with husbands, fathers, or brothers – while the other sixty-one were assured in their own right.

Thirty-two of those women established their policies in connection with a male relative, however, who usually acted as the agent. Only nine of the sixty-one began their policies before marriage, many of the others establishing a policy at the same time as their husbands. Finally, a quarter of the women in the Sceptre sample were forty or older when they began their policies, while only 12.9 per cent of the men were of this age. This might reflect the extra charges companies added to women's premiums to cover the additional risks of pregnancy earlier in life, or unequal earnings, or both.

Table 7.4 Women assured, 1865–81

Year	Women, sole life	Women, as joint lives	Total	% of year's policies
1865	6	2	8	13.56
1870–1	21	4	25	9.12
1877	18	0	18	6.47
1881	16	1	17	4.78
Total	61	7	68	7.03

Source: Sceptre sample.

Sceptre's ledgers also include information about occupation. For five of these sixty-eight women this was simply recorded as 'spinster', and it was left blank for another fifty-three. The other ten were described as two cooks, a domestic help and a housekeeper; two weavers, a dress maker and a tailor and draper; a missionary and a box maker. It is possible to find an occupation for many of these women in censuses and directories, however, and for another forty-five it is possible to at least discover an occupation in the households in which these women were living – from husbands, fathers, mothers, brothers, or uncles. A few women were in service, but they were also to be found teaching, working in shops or as an amanuensis, or managing a laundry.

Their households were as varied as those of the rest of the sample, but the size of the sums assured for suggests many were of relatively modest means. Fifteen (38.5 per cent) of the sample's £50 policies assured the lives of women, with another £50 policy jointly shared by James and Mary Purcell of Nottingham. To put this another way, a quarter of the policies owned by women were worth only £50, though £50 policies make up only 4 per cent of the Sceptre sample. Elizabeth Berryman of Barnstaple, Devon, had one of those policies, which she established in 1870; her husband William, a porter, had another £50 policy. Both were alive in 1911, William now listed as a retired postman, and they had received bonuses on their policies until 1898, when they would have been in their mid-sixties.[9] Other women got much less out of their policies. Amy Edna Raggett, wife of a New Swindon tailor and grocer, allowed her policy to lapse after paying the premiums for at least eighteen years. One of the five £1,000 policies in the sample was established by a twenty-five-year-old woman named Frances Orwin in 1877, but it was also allowed to lapse, possibly because Frances was charged an additional five guineas in the first year to cover the risk of pregnancy. Frances had nine children and lived until she was seventy-three, but those extras may have made the policy too expensive to keep up.[10] Establishing life assurance was not always a straightforward decision for women.

The case of Annie Adelaide Gill provides further evidence of this. At the start of the 1870s, Annie and her second husband Caleb Gill were running a pub in Wellington, Shropshire, after Caleb's watchmaking business had gone bankrupt.[11] The Crown sounds respectable enough, though Caleb was charged with permitting drunkenness there in 1870.[12] They moved their family to Gloucester sometime after 1872, and Caleb, once more working as a watchmaker and jeweller, took out a £100 policy with Sceptre in 1876, with Annie doing the same in 1877. In 1882 the magistrates heard that Caleb had deserted Annie and their daughter, while their servant, Sarah Hanman, had given birth to Caleb's child. Annie sought relief from the Poor Law Guardians, claiming destitution, and Caleb was arrested because it was feared that he, Sarah and their child were leaving for America. In court, after 'a long and painful exposure of the matrimonial differences of Gill and his wife', Caleb claimed he had offered Annie money, though she was not destitute as she owned Co-operative Society cheques. The magistrates dismissed the case, having heard that Annie could cash those cheques for ten or twelve shillings.[13] A few months later Caleb and Annie's Sceptre policies were sold at auction, along with the freehold of a house Caleb owned, and a policy on the life of one of Annie's sons by her first marriage.[14]

Some kind of resolution must have been achieved, though, as Caleb and Annie moved to Romsey, Hampshire, shortly afterwards. One Monday in November 1882 Annie collapsed and died at home while she was washing clothes. The coroner heard Annie had previously suffered a stroke which had left her partially paralysed; apoplexy was given as the cause of death.[15] Caleb and Sarah Hanman married two months later.[16]

It is not entirely clear what happened to Annie's policy, but in the ledger it was noted that it had been established for 'her separate use', and then in November 1881 that it had been assigned to Annie's solicitor, who had arranged the sale of her policy. Annie might have transferred the policy to her solicitor to keep it safe from Caleb or his creditors, just as she had sought to hold onto her Co-operative cheques. In Gloucester she had told the Guardians that Caleb had married her for the money she had from her first husband. Though her policy was claimed, presumably by her solicitor, we don't know where that money went. Annie's life demonstrates the difficulties women might face in holding on to their own property. She also helped run a pub before taking out her abstainer's policy; Annie seems to have showed little interest in temperance in contrast to our next life.

Temperance lives: Caroline John (1821–1903)

Caroline was born in 1821 in Bideford, Devon, to Thomas and Mary Obery; Thomas was a lath maker and labourer.[17] Caroline signed the pledge in 1839, but claimed to be a third-generation life teetotaler, following her great-grandfather's loss of his estate through drink.[18] Bideford had an active teetotal society from 1837, though it encountered strong resistance; at a festival celebrating the Coronation in 1838 the teetotalers successfully fought off a group of 'veterans for the traffic, such as spirit dealers, publicans, and doctors'.[19]

At some point in the 1840s Caroline married a Cardiff man named John, and by 1851 the couple were living in Cardiff with their two daughters and Caroline's widowed father Thomas. John was labouring, and there were three lodgers in the household, all shipwrights; the house was close to the Bute West dock.[20] Ten years later Caroline and John were living around the corner with their daughter Caroline and five boarders – a tailor, two carpenters, a dock policeman and a blacksmith.[21] John died in the first few months of 1870, and at the end of that year Caroline and her daughter, now fifty and twenty-three respectively, assured their lives with the Sceptre office through the local agent, Henry Haynes. Both assured for £50, giving their occupations as 'missionary'. The decision to assure their lives – at what was a relatively late and therefore more expensive age for Caroline senior – may well have been prompted by John's death. In the 1871 Census Caroline was living on another road near the docks with her daughter and two lodgers, another missionary and Henry Bright, a local preacher, who later founded the North London Home for Aged Christian Blind Men and Women.[22] If the Johns' neighbourhood suggests a strongly working-class culture, their lodgers emphasize respectability and piety.

Caroline's involvement with temperance developed after she moved to Bolton with her daughter between 1871 and 1875, working with the British Women's

Temperance Association (BWTA) after 1876. By the 1881 census Caroline was keeping a temperance hotel on Cheapside, in Bolton's commercial district, employing two servants, and in 1891 this was described as a coffee tavern, situated between a pub and a wine merchant.[23] Running temperance hotels could be a good job for women; of the thirty-eight temperance hotels listed in Slater's *Manchester & Salford Directory* for 1895, fourteen are listed as managed or owned by women.[24] Between 1880 and 1893 Caroline addressed dozens of temperance and Rechabite meetings at Leeds, Exeter and Keighley, and BWTA meetings in Lancashire, Hartlepool and Nottingham. Her speeches were often strongly moral and religious in character, and from 1886 she also addressed Gospel Temperance missions.[25] in 1880 she compared complaints made about women's temperance work with the widespread adulation of Sarah Bernhardt's 'acts of questionable morality', asking why women were only acceptable in certain public roles.[26]

In 1895 Caroline was one of about forty women, all abstainers for fifty years or more, celebrated at a meeting of the Women's Total Abstinence Union (WTAU) at Exeter Hall (Figure 7.1). Caroline described herself as 'an old warrior and worker', active for forty

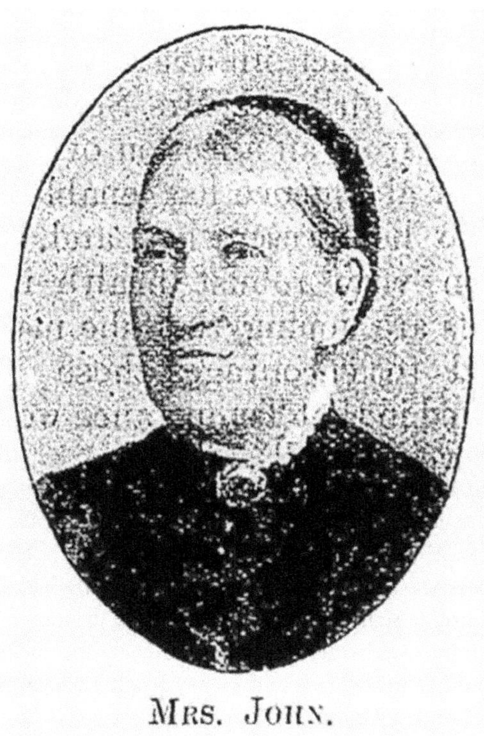

Figure 7.1 Caroline John.

Source: *Wings*, 1 June 1895, 71. Content provided by THE BRITISH LIBRARY BOARD. ALL RIGHTS RESERVED. With thanks to The British Newspaper Archive (www.britishnewspaperarchive.co.uk).

years; 'she had had the great honour of standing in the open streets to be buffeted and stoned as she stood beside some of the old veterans who had gone home'. The WTAU's journal *Wings* described Caroline's earnestness, energy and eloquence, noting that she was an effective speaker.[27] Caroline seems to have been less active after this date and died early in 1903.[28] Her daughter presumably claimed her mother's policy, which would have grown by four bonus payments; her own policy was claimed after 1903, probably when she died around 1908.

While Caroline's sounds like a working-class life, her later temperance work allowed her to share a platform with the great and the good. At an 1886 Temperance Demonstration near Wigan, for example, Caroline spoke alongside James Barlow, the Bolton mill owner (Chapter 2).[29] Temperance created a social space where different classes met, though not necessarily in ways that challenged class divisions. Her life also demonstrates some of the tensions within late Victorian temperance. Arguments about the importance of campaigning for women's suffrage split the BWTA into the National British Women's Temperance Association (NBWTA) and the WTAU, the latter concentrating solely on temperance. Caroline clearly felt closer to the WTAU's definition of the drink problem, working to support Local Veto. A pious and dedicated teetotaler, Caroline John resembled the 'first great advocates' of temperance, as one biographical sketch suggested, and like many of them she had humble origins.[30]

To see how typical that was of the wider sample, we turn now to consider questions of occupation and class.

Occupation and class in the Sceptre sample

The occupations recorded in Sceptre's ledgers when policyholders first assured – supplemented by census and other information on household occupation where necessary – makes it possible to compare Sceptre's assurers with existing studies of the class background of British teetotalers and temperance workers. Considering five registers of teetotalers collected between the 1830s and the 1860s, for example, Brian Harrison concluded they 'were gathering recruits from all social levels below the aristocracy and gentry', including 'some occupations unmistakably at the bottom end of society', with 'a leavening of decidedly respectable individuals'.[31] The Alliance subscribers of 1868–9 he examined for his 1970 prosopographical study were more solidly middle class; 'even the small donations came from quite substantial individuals'. At the same time, 'the "governing class" professions – landowning, law, church, armed services and brewing – are markedly under-represented'.[32]

The 'prohibitionists' analysed by Harrison contained many wealthy industrialists, particularly textile manufacturers and a few dissenting landowners. Below them came the mid-Victorian temperance rank-and-file, who Virginia Berridge characterized as members of the 'labour aristocracy'.[33] Some of the teetotal lives assured by Sceptre and the UKT certainly fit this description. This class fraction also contained some enthusiastic drinkers, though, as the best-paid workers were associated with higher rates of alcohol consumption.[34] The aspirations of this class could be expressed in rather different ways, in other words, and do not reflect a single type; ultimately, as Harrison pointed out, no social class unanimously supported temperance. The less respectable working class were often characterized as unsympathetic to temperance, the source of the 'roughs' who terrorized teetotal meetings. From these studies we might expect the Sceptre sample to contain few aristocrats, some industrialists and many labour artisans, with some individuals from 'the bottom end of society'.

We might also turn to Timothy Alborn's work on British life companies to see how Sceptre compared to other assurance offices (Figure 7.5). Alborn notes that 'most life policies issued by most companies were purchased by middle- or lower-middle-class breadwinners'.[35] The Legal and General and London Life issued around a third of their new policies to professionals (bankers, clergy, lawyers, surveyors) between 1871–90 and 1860–1918 respectively, while the second largest group for each was the gentry (nobles, gentlemen, military officers) for Legal & General, and merchants and manufacturers for London Life. Lower-middle-class policyholders (shopkeepers, clerks) were the third largest category. In comparison, only around 1.5 per cent of the lives in the Sceptre sample could be described as 'gentry', even with the most generous definition of that term; about a tenth were professionals, mostly nonconformist ministers, followed by a slightly smaller number of manufacturers and merchants. Significantly, 30.9 per cent were lower middle class, especially shopkeepers and clerks, and 43.4 per cent of the sample is best counted as 'other' in Alborn's terms, largely because these are industrial or craft workers, or unskilled labour. The average sums assured by Atlas policyholders are also far higher than the Sceptre sample, even for the most modest category of assurers. In this respect the Sceptre lives seem closer to Harrison's sample than Alborn's, though as we will see they are subtly different to both.

The gentry

Only one man in the sample – Horatio Nelson Greenwood, of Nottingham – was described as a 'gentleman'. Nine of the twelve military men assuring with the Sceptre were non-commissioned officers, leaving two lieutenants and a naval cadet; a few farmers and millers established substantial policies but were not significant landowners. One of them, George Harrison Gamble, established a £1,000 policy; there are five of these in the sample, but his was the only one that was claimed. George was a twenty-five-year-old Newark miller when he established that policy in 1877, employing three men and two domestic servants in 1881. He emigrated to Canada with his family in

Table 7.5 Proportion of policyholders in specific occupational groups (%)

Office	Professions	Merchant/ manufacturer	Lower middle class	Gentry	Other
Legal & General (own life, 1871–90)	31.2	5.1	12.7	34.6	16.1
London Life (1860–1918)	34.2	23.8	19.0	5.8	17.2
Sceptre Abstainers (1865–81)	9.9	9.4	30.9	1.5	43.4

Source: Alborn, *Regulated Lives*, Table 5.1, 143, and Sceptre sample

1885, Sceptre charging him an additional £2 10s. for 'sea risk', and settled as a farmer in British Columbia. George lived until 1939, when he would have been around eighty-seven. The policy collected twelve bonuses and had been transferred to his daughter Charlotte in 1902; the office wrote a cheque for £2,310 10s. to honour the claim. George clearly prospered, but he was not a member of the gentry.[36]

The gentry's absence is not surprising, given temperance suspicion of landowners who sat on licensing committees and sold their barley for brewing. The ninth policy Sceptre issued might have confirmed these prejudices. In 1865 the Hercules Insurance Company took out a Sceptre policy for £250 on the life of Sir Alfred Joseph Doughty-Tichborne. The Hercules would have assured Sir Alfred, and they may have feared his life was not a good one, reinsuring with Sceptre to cover potential losses. These came only a year later, as Sceptre's first ever claim. Alfred became the eleventh Baronet of Tichborne on his father's death in 1862, as his older brother Roger was missing, presumed dead. When Alfred died, aged twenty-seven, his infant son Henry succeeded to the title, only for Arthur Orton, the 'Tichborne claimant', to challenge this in 1867.[37] Alfred's role in the sensational Tichborne fraud was a minor one, but Hercules and Sceptre might have seen the establishment of his policy as a similarly deceitful undertaking. Alfred had been declared bankrupt before becoming baronet, and his reported debts included £11 for two dozen bottles of cognac, £65 for a silver tankard and £93 for tobacco. The baronet proved to be a bad life.[38]

Professionals

Apart from ministers, who make up the largest single occupation in the sample with seventy-four policies covering seventy-two individuals, and two doctors, a solicitor and a surveyor, there are comparatively few professionals in the Sceptre sample. The distribution of sums these professionals assured for is also close to the sample as a whole, though claim rates were higher (76.4 per cent as opposed to 55.9 per cent). Most, though not all, of the larger sums were claimed. Joseph Manton Smith had one of the four minister's policies worth more than £300, for example, assuring his life for £400 in 1881. A Methodist turned Baptist, Smith was close to the popular London preacher (and teetotaler) Charles Haddon Spurgeon.[39] Alfred Rhodes Pearson, who assured his life for £100 in 1865 at Pendleton, Lancashire, was an important part of the Methodist New Connexion and its president in 1889.[40] He died in 1890, aged only fifty-four, though four bonuses had been paid and a loan had been made on the policy. Henry Alcock, the son of a Buckinghamshire farm labourer, and a farm boy himself at twelve, presents a striking contrast to these lives (Chapter 2). He established the only £50 minister's policy in the sample in 1870, when he was thirty-one and a Primitive Methodist Minister at Teignmouth, Devon; the policy lapsed within a few years.

Many of the Methodist ministers assured by Sceptre had three things in common. First, they travelled widely, from circuit to circuit, possibly taking temperance convictions with them. Samuel Beavan ministered for the United Methodist Free Churches in Cheshire, Yorkshire, Northumberland, Somerset, Lancashire and Staffordshire from 1855 to the early years of the twentieth century; his policy was claimed sometime around 1900, when he would have been about seventy, and he lived until 1916.[41] The Primitive Methodist minister Arthur Beavan also had a long life, claiming his policy eight years before his death in 1922; he served at nineteen chapels in Wales and England and was made Secretary of Conference in 1912.[42] Second, these men moved in a thoroughly Methodist world. Arthur Beavan's first wife was the daughter of a Primitive Methodist preacher, and other Sceptre ministers married the daughters of Methodist preachers. Third, beyond their Sceptre Abstainer's policies, there is little sign of any temperance activism amongst these men, apart from Samuel Beavan's 1890 paper on 'The Bible and Total Abstinence', which would have sounded old-fashioned compared to contemporary medical research.[43]

However, the Sceptre office did have a special attraction for these men. By the 1860s actuaries had noticed that the mortality of the clergy was better than that of other occupations, saving firms perhaps 30 per cent in claims, and it was suggested that their premiums should be reduced to reflect this.[44] Sceptre reached this conclusion in 1866, establishing the 10 per cent 'minister's discount' by 1880. This was extended to missionaries who had not been ordained, allowing Thomas Cope Deeming, a Leicester engineer, and Ann Bacon, the wife of a Primitive Minister, to receive this discount, presumably as lay preachers.[45]

While numerous, these ministers were not necessarily typical of Sceptre or temperance. They were a varied lot, and while they may have been active within temperance, few appear in histories of the movement.

Merchants and manufacturers

Of the ninety sample policies assuring lives in this group, thirty were insurance, coal, commission or estate agents. There were also many dealers, and some manufacturers – of nails, sewing machines, or watches – with substantial policies. This category's policies tended to be larger than others in the sample, in fact; three of the five £1,000 policies belonged to these merchants and manufacturers, and the average policy was worth £234 3s., as opposed to £143 11s. for the whole sample. Evington Dalby of Long Eaton, Derbyshire, established a £250 policy in 1870 and by the 1880s was manufacturing silk lace at the Harrington Mills.[46] He died in 1919, aged seventy-nine, but collected the policy, with four bonus payments, around 1900, when he would have been about sixty. George Henry Drewery, who established a £900 policy in 1881, was a Nottingham hosiery manufacturer employing sixty-nine hands, though his policy lapsed after a few years.

None of the three £1,000 policies in this category were claimed, in fact. Daniel Duckworth, a Leeds commission agent, surrendered his policy; a United Methodist, he was closely associated with the York Temperance Club and Cocoa and Coffee Rooms.[47] Frances Orwin, the Newcastle woman mentioned above, allowed her £1,000 policy to lapse within a year. In fact, the claim rate is lower for this category than it is for the sample as a whole, at 41.1–55.9 per cent, while a larger proportion of policies were surrendered (24.4 compared to 15.2 per cent), suggesting some use was made of the sums invested in them.

Joseph Haines Stiles's assured life, the third £1,000 policy in this group, is perhaps one of the more unusual. A tinware manufacturer, Joseph and his wife Helen also established homes for destitute boys in South London and Surrey. Stiles's philanthropic National Working Boys' Home Company, training boys to make and sell tin items door to door, was floated on the stock exchange in 1881; the Homes would be 'conducted on Temperance principles'.[48] The company was wound up two years later, around the time that Stiles surrendered his policy, possibly to pay off debts.[49] In 1892 Stiles appeared in court, in much reduced circumstances, to defend some of his 'boys', who had been arrested selling tinware on behalf of the Home, which no longer existed.[50] Stiles then somehow became the British Commissioner to the highly successful California Midwinter Fair in San Francisco in 1894, going on to promote a similar 'British Empire Exposition' at Montreal.[51] The Exposition did not happen, though, and Stiles seems to have disappeared. Would-be exhibitors claimed he owed them thousands of dollars and applied for a warrant for his extradition.[52] It is not clear what happened next, but Stiles surfaced in London in 1901, describing himself as 'an exhibition agent'. He lived until 1921, when he was seventy-one.

Stiles remains a mysterious character – philanthropist, booster, fraud? – but he was certainly nothing like the great men of the Alliance. More generally, the Sceptre sample does not contain businessmen of the same rank as Harrison's prohibitionists.

Lower-middle-class lives

The lower middle class was important for both life assurance and temperance, and so was likely to be a significant category for Sceptre. The sample's lower-middle-class lives were made up of two main groups: shopkeepers, with 170 of the 296 policies in this category, and clerks and other white-collar workers like bookkeepers, accountants, secretaries and collectors, who made up the other 126. There's little difference between these subgroups in terms of the size of their policies or outcomes. White-collar lives were more likely to be in their twenties when they arranged their policies (55.6 compared to 44.9 per cent for the sample as a whole), and 75.9 per cent of the fifty-eight clerks were in their teens or twenties, compared to 52.0 per cent of the whole sample.

We will deal with these groups in turn.

Shopkeepers

The shopkeepers' group is dominated by forty-nine grocers, but also contains seventeen drapers, sixteen bakers, sixteen butchers and smaller numbers of confectioners, chemists, ironmongers, stationers, booksellers, clothiers, greengrocers and others. Nine commercial travellers have also been considered in this group, as have smaller dealers who did not seem to fit the 'merchants' category. Some of the leaders of the British temperance movement came from this particular background, including Joseph Livesey, and Harrison found grocers, drapers and other retailers among the Alliance's donors in the 1860s.[53] Sceptre's shopkeepers were no more successful than the rest of the sample of lives, however. Having already examined the life of one UKT draper-agent, John Laverock (Chapter 1), we will concentrate here on grocers, as the largest and in some ways most typical group of shopkeepers in the sample.

Grocers represented a solid market for temperance assurance firms, and they made good agents for them too. In the 1860s Joseph Theobald, the UKT's agent for Bath and treasurer of the city's Temperance Society, was a tea and coffee dealer and grocer. Tea and coffee were appealing alternatives to alcohol, encouraging the development of what Erika Rappaport describes as a 'sober consumer culture' of temperance teas from the 1830s or 1840s.[54] By the 1880s Theobald & Son were also selling temperance beverages, including unfermented wine.[55]

Many grocers sold alcoholic beverages, however, and in fact Christopher Hosgood suggested that 'an off-licence was often a necessity for business success'.[56] Sceptre treated this as an additional risk. By 1900 the firm was charging an additional annual charge of £1 per £100 assured for 'Grocers selling Wines and Spirits in bottle' – the same rate charged for residence in India or the Caribbean.[57] This was reduced to 15s. for a grocer named Williams, as he 'does not sell spirits and keeps his place of business entirely closed on Sundays'.[58] In 1910 B. W. Outred challenged this extra premium, but 'it was resolved to decline to remove this, medical examination at Head Office eliciting that the life had been permanently damaged by association with the Liquor Trade'.[59] It seems likely that this was Benjamin William Outred, a grocer in Hersham, Surrey, in 1911; he would have been a grocer for twenty years when he was called in to Sceptre's office, and the board was certain his health had suffered as a result.[60]

As businesses, though, grocers were more or less typical of the sample. A slightly higher proportion of grocers surrendered their policies (23.4 per cent, compared with 15.2 per cent for the whole sample), however, which suggests policies might have been valued as investments that could be surrendered for cash. James Austin, a Birmingham grocer and chemist, assured his life for £500 in 1865, and his policy was claimed sometime around 1895, after receiving six bonus payments and establishing a loan. In contrast, Weston-Super-Mare grocer Henry Huyton Harris established a £500 policy in 1877, but allowed it to lapse; the 1881 census lists him as a master carpenter, so the lapse might reflect the failure of his original business. Others, like Frederick John Shilling, of Faversham, Kent, also abandoned grocery and their policies, but prospered anyway. Taking out a £250 policy in 1877, when he was only twenty-two, Frederick reduced the sum to £100, but the policy lapsed all the same. Frederick was listed as a butcher and Wesleyan local preacher in the 1881 and 1891 Censuses, leaving over £2,000 to his wife and children when he died in 1932.[61] Perhaps he established the policy too early, before his business had become established.

That may also have been true of Ebenezer Beavan, a grocer and coal merchant in the heart of Cardiff's docks – a near neighbour of Caroline John – who assured his life for £200 in 1870, at the age of twenty-nine.[62] A Methodist preacher at fifteen, Beavan had 'been in the [temperance] van for years', as Winskill put it, and he was the Alliance agent for South Wales and honorary secretary of the Cardiff Temperance and Prohibition Association.[63] He was closely involved in the agitation for Sunday Closing in Wales, which had significant working-class support in Cardiff, and his wife Harriet Ann was an important temperance figure in her own right, as author of the well-known poem 'Alice Lea: or the Lips that touch Liquor shall never touch Mine'.[64] A Liberal described by the *Western Mail* as 'not afflicted with any painful lack of assurance', Beavan was active in Cardiff politics as a councillor, alderman, J.P. and mayor.[65] Martin Daunton

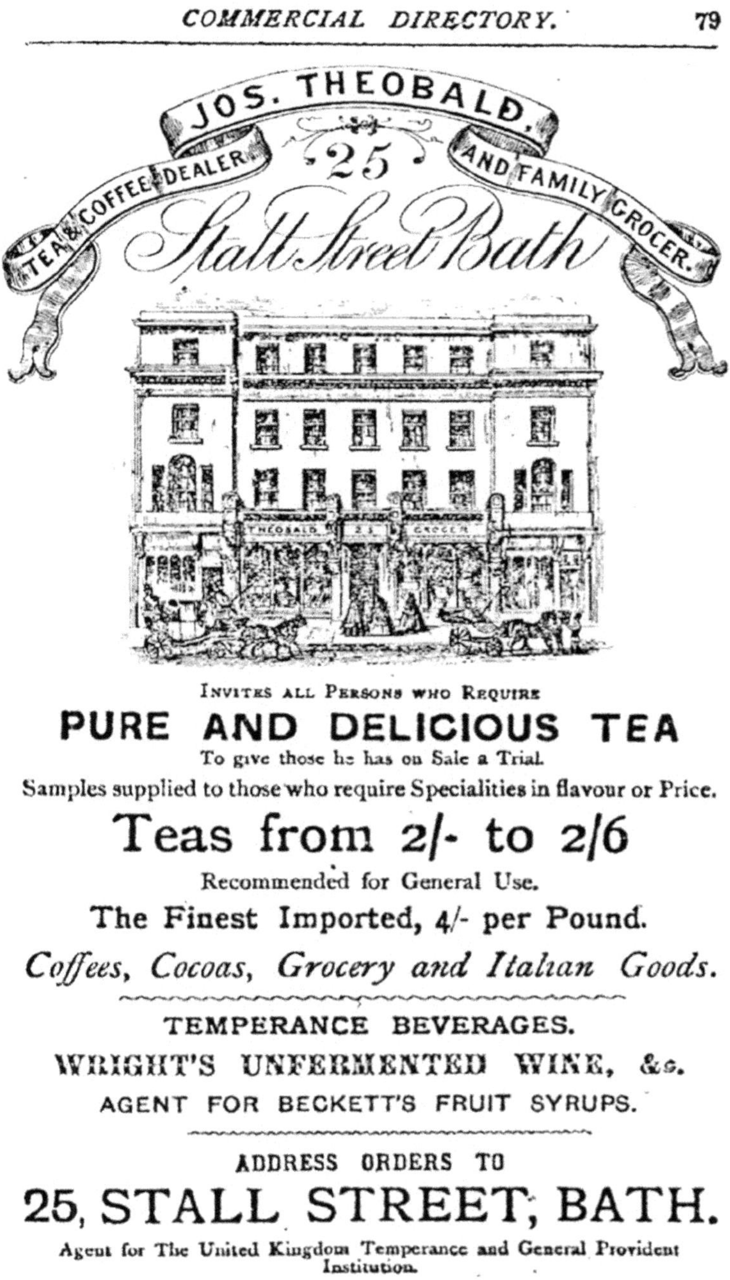
COMMERCIAL DIRECTORY. 79
JOS. THEOBALD,
TEA & COFFEE DEALER
25
AND FAMILY GROCER.
Stall Street Bath
THEOBALD 25 GROCER
INVITES ALL PERSONS WHO REQUIRE
PURE AND DELICIOUS TEA
To give those he has on Sale a Trial.
Samples supplied to those who require Specialities in flavour or Price.
Teas from 2/- to 2/6
Recommended for General Use.
The Finest Imported, 4/- per Pound.
Coffees, Cocoas, Grocery and Italian Goods.
TEMPERANCE BEVERAGES.
WRIGHT'S UNFERMENTED WINE, &c.
AGENT FOR BECKETT'S FRUIT SYRUPS.
ADDRESS ORDERS TO
25, STALL STREET, BATH.
Agent for The United Kingdom Temperance and General Provident Institution.

Figure 7.2 Advertisement, Joseph Theobald.

Source: Post Office Bath Directory, 1884–5 (Bath: Lewis, Sons & Tyte, 1884–5), 752, Historical Directories of England & Wales. Courtesy of University of Leicester Special Collections Online.

describes Ebenezer and his brothers as 'old' Liberals within Cardiff's political world, interested in moral rather than welfare reform.[66] Ebenezer had retired by 1911 but lived until 1925, when he was eighty-three.[67]

Ebenezer Beavan would seem to be the model of a good Sceptre life: a nonconformist with the requisite temperance zeal, commercial nouse and political ambition. However, as an assured life he was much less successful, surrendering his policy within three years. He later concentrated on coal dealing and temperance work, so was perhaps not a typical grocer. In other ways, though, Ebenezer was atypical, because few other shopkeepers showed much temperance zeal or political activity.

White-collar workers

The size of the policy was no guarantee of its outcome for white-collar workers either. No information is given about what happened to the fifth £1,000 policy in the sample – the only one in this subgroup – which was issued to Edward Eden Hanslow, a London banker's clerk living in Wokingham, Berkshire, in 1881.[68] Another forty-one lives in this group were assured for more than £100, reminding us that being a clerk, accountant, secretary, schoolmaster, or auctioneer could be the basis for a decent middle-class life. These lives could still be uncertain, though. In 1865 John William Cooke, a London shorthand writer, established a £500 policy which received one bonus payment and was used to borrow £60, but then lapsed. George Wilson, a Post Office clerk from Woodford, Essex, established a £500 policy in 1877, two days after his marriage to Alice Molyneaux. He died less than four years later, aged twenty-nine, leaving £592 to Alice and their two young sons.[69] The policy probably made up most of his estate, and George's story could well have been drawn straight from Sceptre's marketing.

More modest policies might have made a bigger difference to lower-middle-class lives. Bristol provision merchant's clerk Frank Goldsworthy was seventeen when he assured his life for £100 in 1871. He went on to be a commercial traveller, an occupation whose 'brotherly' ethos was so closely bound up with drinking that some insurance examiners classified them as undesirable lives.[70] Thirteen bonus payments were added to Frank's policy, however, and it was claimed in 1940 when he died aged eighty-five.[71]

This group also contains one of the smaller policies in the sample, belonging to the forty-four-year-old London messenger and clerk John Maynard, who took out a £50 policy in 1877. His occupation, age and modest policy all suggest he was an office errand boy and general factotum; he had been employed as a porter in 1871. Bonuses were paid on the policy until 1888, and it was claimed before 1893.[72]

Other lives

Nearly half of the Sceptre sample – 464 policies – do not fit the categories explored above and are a mix of industrial and craft workers, skilled trades and unskilled labour. One large subgroup of 215 policies covers weavers, stationary engine drivers and other factory workers, smiths and tailors and makers of everything from boots to coaches or cabinets. There is then a smaller subgroup of 130 policies covering the building trades – builders, joiners, carpenters, fitters, plumbers, painters, plasterers and bricklayers. Smaller subgroups include labourers and those in domestic service. The outcomes of these policies seem to follow a broadly similar pattern to the rest of the sample, though their average size is slightly smaller than the sample as a whole – £117 10 s. compared to £143 11s. – while the averages for the labour and service subgroups are both just under £100.

Industrial workers

Sceptre's industrial lives are unevenly distributed across England and Wales. There are forty lives in this subgrouping in Derbyshire and Nottinghamshire, and twenty-two of them were employed in the region's lace industry – lace makers or designers and framework knitters. Ironworkers and shipbuilders made up twelve of the twenty-two industrial workers in County Durham. Ten of the thirty workers in Lancashire worked in textiles, including the Pennines weavers examined in Chapter 2; another ten seem likely to have been employed in factories rather than small workshops. In Middlesex there are fewer lives so clearly involved in factory work; thirteen of the twenty-eight policies in this subgrouping covered older trades – smiths, coopers, saddlers, shoemakers, tailors, ropemakers, binders and upholsterers, printers, box- and bag-makers – though some of these may well have become industrialized by this point. Another three engine drivers could be found in Plaistow and Canning Town, and an iron moulder in Camberwell, but lives in metropolitan Essex, Kent and Surrey also included printers, tailors, watchmakers and other longer-established trades. Yorkshire's twenty-three policies in this subgrouping divide more or less evenly between newer and older trades: moulders, engineers and glassblowers, on the one hand, and cabinet-makers, smiths, tailors and dressmakers on the other. This suggests this industrial subgrouping included different kinds of workers, not all of whom might not have counted themselves members of the labour aristocracy.

This subgrouping also included eleven of the thirty-nine £50 policies in the sample, assuring a mix of trades: a joint policy for a Nottingham lacemaker and his wife, James and Mary Purcell; two of the Sabden weavers; and Samuel Jarmin Voysey Churchill, who was only a twenty-two-year-old tailor's cutter when he assured in 1870, but went on to own a substantial Teignmouth business. We know less about Bromley's Samuel Hayhoe, who paid an extra five shillings a year, probably for the additional risk he faced as a railway platelayer, who seems to have died shortly after establishing the policy. George Samuel Pinfold, a Limehouse shipwright, surrendered his policy within a few years, as did Benjamin Hemingway, a Yorkshire hurdle-maker, and Emily Walker of Bradford, who assured her life before marrying a milliner.

Building

The distributions of sums assured and outcomes of the 130 policies covering building workers resemble those of the sample as a whole. The builders seem to have been a little older, too. Two Portsea teetotalers assured with Sceptre; George Damon was fifty-two – the seventh oldest life in the sample – and his £50 policy came with a 'truss clause', meaning his policy would be invalidated if he did not wear a surgical truss, while Joseph Damon, a carpenter, was thirty-seven when he assured his life for £250. George's business was liquidated and Joseph was declared bankrupt, but despite his apparent disadvantages, George's policy was claimed after receiving four bonus payments, while Joseph's lapsed before bankruptcy proceedings began.[73] Two other builders, Frederick Beilby, of Hull, and William Webb, of Chippenham, established £300 policies, in 1877 and 1881 respectively, receiving five or six bonuses on their policies, which were claimed when they were both around sixty. None of these men seem like natural teetotalers, but our next life is a better fit. When he assured in 1865, William Bott of Wrexham, North Wales, was fifty, advertising himself as a general contractor for excavations, roads and railways.[74] His policy was claimed after two bonus payments, when William would have been around sixty, but by then it had been transferred to another owner, perhaps to settle debts. William was very active in temperance and Methodism around Wrexham.[75]

Lives in other building trades were slightly younger than the builders, and their average policies slightly smaller. It is also hard to find a public teetotaler amongst them, despite P. T. Winskill's claim that 'plastering, slating, painting' produced 'earnest, useful temperance advocates'.[76] Robert Townson may have been one of them, though. He was twenty-eight when he assured his life for £100 in 1877 and his policy would have been claimed at fifty-five, around 1904; he spent his whole life in Morecambe, Lancashire, dying in 1915, aged sixty-five. Robert's father had been a joiner, and Robert was described as a joiner in every Census from 1871 to 1911, except in 1881, when he was listed as the manager of a coffee tavern in Morecambe.[77] Besides that, though, there is little sign of Robert's temperance activity, and in that he is typical of these men.

Labouring

Not all of the fifty policies in this subgroup are unskilled workers, but they do include eight of the sample's thirty-nine £50 policies, and there are only three policies for more than £100. The largest occupational group here was warehousemen, with sixteen policies, then nine coachmen, three car men and a horse driver, six labourers, five porters, several mariners and railway workers, and a bell-hanger, stablehand and sweep. The metropolitan character of this subgroup is striking – nineteen of the fifty policies assured lives in Middlesex, with another five in contiguous parts of Essex and Surrey, making up almost half of this subgroup between them.

Traces of temperance activity can be found. Frank Clarke, a coachman, assured his life for £100 in 1881, when he was living in Jays Mews near Kensington Gore, London; his son assured with Sceptre earlier that year. Frank then took a position at a house at Warblington, Hampshire, joining eight other servants. By 1891 Frank and his wife were running a coffee tavern in nearby Farlington, and they went on to run a Havant refreshment and lodging house in 1901 and 1911.[78] Another coachman, Thomas Palmer, took a different path. He assured with Sceptre in Newcastle upon Tyne in 1870, but his ledger entry is marked with the word 'Publican'. In 1881 Thomas was a barman at the Eldon Arms, and he went on to manage the Butchers Arms at Byker; he was still a licensed victualler in 1901. Thomas's policy was claimed around 1905, and he died in 1907, aged sixty-three.[79] Sceptre allowed him to keep the policy, though he paid an additional £2 every year for it, which almost doubled his premiums. If we compare Thomas to John Samuel Horsham (Chapter 5), who lost his policy because he drank, it seems likely that John's deception was felt to be more serious than Thomas's occupation. The firm treated him in the same way they dealt with grocers.

Others in this subgroup allowed their policies to lapse, including Benjamin Willoughby Down, a Rotherhithe dock labourer (£50, 1877); Francis Coates, a Stockton porter (£50, 1870); Edward Coverdale, a Middlesbrough horse driver (£100, 1871); and Thomas Clayton, a London sweep, who – at fifty-seven – was one of the oldest lives in the sample when he assured in 1881. John Hicks, a Poplar carman, paid the premiums on his £50 policy long enough to garner two bonuses, before surrendering it sometime after 1883. Others were more successful. Henry Warren, a labourer in Canning Town in 1877, worked as a grocer from 1891 to at least 1911; his £100 policy was claimed sometime around that date, when he would have been about fifty-six, having benefited from seven bonus payments.

These are clearly working-class lives. Again, there is little to suggest that they were particularly active within temperance, but they must have been members of a society that would vouch for their abstinence. Even the £50 policies are larger than the sums an industrial office like the Prudential would pay their working-class policyholders, so these are men and women to make Samuel Smiles proud. At the same time, they clearly show that businesses like Sceptre – and therefore the temperance societies they depended upon – extended below the lower middle class and the 'labour aristocracy'.

Conclusions: Class, Sceptre, temperance lives

The lives of Sceptre's policyholders are more modest than those found in Alborn's or Harrison's samples. The higher social positions were held by nonconformist ministers, non-commissioned officers, smallish manufacturers and dealers, and successful tradesmen, while there was a sizeable lower-middle-class group of shopkeepers, clerks and other office workers. The largest group is made up of working-class lives, however: industrial workers, building tradesmen, labourers and those in service. Some in this group, like the builders, could be considered to be lower-middle-class lives, and all could afford to pay Sceptre's premiums, perhaps a shilling a week for a thirty-year-old compared with the thruppence a week paid by Edwin Newton, a Birmingham drayman assured with the Prudential for a sum of £21 3s. in 1864.[80] Others, in London at least – lightermen and carmen, painters and porters – might well have been threatened by casualization in the last decades of the century.[81]

The group that seems most important here, though, is the lower middle class. This class has received some attention from historians, and this work throws some light on the sample and on temperance. First, this is not a single class, nor one that can be simply divided into shopkeepers and small businessmen on the one hand, and white-collar workers and clerks on the other. Geoffrey Crossick and others argued that the British petit bourgeoisie was too heterogeneous to share even a divided social position or political identity; 'lower middle-class consciousness remained more cellular than either stratified or bifurcated', as Peter Bailey put it.[82] This also explains the difficulties historians and historical geographers have had trying to locate this class in census records. Armstrong's influential classification of nineteenth-century social strata placed a third class of skilled workers between the upper two (professional and intermediate) and lower two (semi-skilled and unskilled.) 'Class III' provided temperance with many recruits, and historians and historical geographers suggested it made up between 42 and 68 per cent of the population of a dozen industrial towns and cities. However, as Richard Dennis pointed out, this class 'embraces several quite distinct types of occupation: skilled manual workers who comprised the elite among factory workers, small shopkeepers and ... junior non-manual workers such as clerks. It is unlikely that all these groups thought of themselves as a coherent social class or even behaved at all alike'.[83]

Using Armstrong's classifications, the Sceptre sample looks a little like another industrial town in terms of the proportions within each class, with class III making up around half of the sample. In this case, though, these men and women may well have shared a consciousness characterized by the principles of temperance and life assurance, by the need for forethought, thrift and prudence. This was not necessarily a *class* consciousness, though, as it may well have cut across other forms of identification. The fact that some benefited from that prudence while others let their policies go suggests that material circumstances were also important, though differences in outcomes do not neatly map onto occupations.

Still, the political loyalties of the lower middle class seem to have been more complicated than a split between radical artisans and conservative shopkeepers or clerks.[84] Christopher Hosgood suggested small grocers defended their working-class customers from temperance campaigns against grocer's licences, for example.[85] It is quite possible that this reflects the development of working-class Toryism over this period. As Jon Lawrence pointed out, 'the Tories' deliberate identification with key aspects of masculine urban popular culture, such as the pub, football, and racing, was intended to distinguish them from the "moral reforming" style of Liberal politics'.[86] Late Victorian temperance was thought to exemplify a Liberalism that had been 'hijacked' by nonconformist fanatics, abandoning its libertarian traditions in favour of 'coercive "moral reform"' and placing the interests of party above those of nation and empire.[87]

This complicates our understanding of the political trajectory taken by this class, summarized by Bailey as shifting from a role as the 'lightning conductors' of social change to the 'shock absorbers' who channelled it into reformist channels.[88] Is this the story of temperance? Another Sceptre life suggests that the rise of popular Toryism has to be taken into account. The Chester salesman James Theophilus Davis assured with the firm for £50 in 1870, and he went on to run a substantial business as a tailor, hatter and outfitter, also becoming the manager of a local savings bank and director of a building society. A member of the Methodist New Connection and Rechabite treasurer, he was well known in Chester temperance, with connections to the Alliance and local nonconformity.[89] In 1892 Davis was part of a deputation which quizzed parliamentary candidates on their position on temperance. The supportive responses of the Liberal candidate, Baron Halkett, 'had fallen on their ears like rain on the thirsty ground'.[90] Halkett said 'I wish to prevent the plutocrat brewer from forcing his liquor upon the people at every corner', and attacked his Conservative rival's 'enormous cheque-book', which bought votes through his friends in the drink trade.[91] Halkett lost the election, though Home Rule may have been more significant than temperance. Chester's middle classes abandoned the Liberals, and the Conservative and Unionist share of the vote remained above 50 per cent until 1906.[92]

Davis may have personified the three problems of late Victorian Liberalism – its nonconformist 'fanaticism', its plans for coercive moral reform, and its preference for party machinery, like Chester's temperance deputation, over the Union. Other members of the lower middle class may well have been caught up in this populist Toryism; Liberals, Tories and socialists all drew their recruits from the same lower-middle- and working-class strata. But while Davis was clearly a successful capitalist, he does not sound like a 'shock absorber', even if what might have been described as 'radicalism' earlier in the century was now recast as 'fanaticism'. Elsewhere there were also elements of progressive activism within the lower middle class, some of it related to temperance, for example within the London County Council, or the socialist cyclists and ramblers associated with the *Clarion* newspaper.[93]

This complex grouping was also described by Bailey as 'a class of mimics and dissemblers', reminding us of his earlier study of the performance of respectability as Bill Banks, the 'self-improving artisan', was revealed to be an 'English workman on a spree', full of bank holiday beer.[94] Some of Sceptre's lives appear to be something other than the occupations described in the ledgers, or reveal the problems we now have classifying them. Would a farm labourer like Henry Alcock ever be regarded as a 'professional', even as an ordained minister? Can we count Joseph Stiles as a 'manufacturer', when his business seems to have relied at least in part on sales skills he would later put to good use as an exhibition promoter? Other Sceptre lives include merchants who turn out to be small dealers, manufacturers who are makers and so on. The precarity and fluidity of trades like building and shopkeeping further complicate these questions of identity. Perhaps some of the members of this class were also fooling *themselves*, if we think of all of those lapsed policies, victims of optimism over experience. Thrift and self-transformation had uncertain outcomes. And of course, life assurance almost *encourages* dissembling, in this case applicants hiding their drinking from the Board, as Benjamin Outred and Sir Alfred Doughty-Tichborne remind us.

The Sceptre sample presents many examples of this class, especially if it is broadened out to include some of the artisans in the 'industrial' grouping. Peter Bailey concludes his survey of the historiography by making an important claim for people like these abstainers: 'socially and politically marginal, the lower middle class was in many ways culturally central, perhaps the closest we get to "ordinary" people'.[95] If there is anything to this claim, then Sceptre's abstainers – including 'fanatics' like James Davis – should certainly be considered to be 'ordinary'.

Notes

1. George B. Wilson, *Alcohol and the Nation: A Contribution to the Study of the Liquor Problem in the United Kingdom from 1800–1935* (London: Nicholson and Watson, 1940); Dingle, 'Drink and Living Standards'.

2. Harrison, 'The British Prohibitionists', 377.
3. See the appendix for discussion.
4. 1881 Census (Class: RG11; Piece: 3377; Folio: 77; Page: 3; GSU roll: 662); Advertisement, *Nottinghamshire Guardian*, 1 October 1886: 1. England & Wales, Death Index, 1837–2005, first quarter 1892, Volume: 7b; Page: 298.
5. *York Herald*, 25 September 1895, 6.
6. Harrison, 'British Prohibitionists', 380, 382.
7. Alborn, *Regulated Lives*, 142.
8. Whittington, 'Instructions to Agents'.
9. 1871 Census (Class: RG10; Piece: 2183; Folio: 35; Page: 25; GSU roll: 132); 1911 Census (Class: RG14; Piece: 13323; GSU roll: 205).
10. 1911 Census (Class: RG14; Piece: 30440; GSU roll: 339).
11. 1871 Census (Class: RG10; Piece: 2806; Folio: 101; Page: 2; GSU roll: 6); 'Bankrupts, &c.', *Liverpool Mercury*, 20 April 1868, 8.
12. 'Fortnightly Petty Sessions', *Shrewsbury Chronicle*, 13 May 1870, 7.
13. 'District News. Gloucester. Charge of Deserting a Family', *Bristol Mercury and Daily Post*, 25 March 1882, 8; Advertisement, *Gloucester Citizen*, 20 March 1882, 1; 'The Supposed Disappearance of a Servant Girl in Gloucester', *Gloucester Citizen*, 17 February 1882, 4; 'Charge against a Gloucester Jeweller of Neglecting to Support His Family', *Gloucester Citizen*, 22 March 1882, 4; 'Gloucester County Court', *Gloucester Journal*, 22 April 1882, 7.
14. *Gloucester Journal*, 12 August 1882, 4; 'Extraordinary Application', *Gloucester Journal*, 25 March 1882, 6.
15. 'Sudden Death', *Southampton Herald*, 25 November 1882, 7.
16. Volume 2A, page 328, England & Wales Marriages 1837–2005.
17. Devon Baptisms, Birth, Marriage, Death & Parish Records, 1841 Census (Class: HO107; Piece: 242; Folio: 7; Page: 9; GSU roll: 1168).
18. 'Reception to Veteran Abstainers', *Wings*, 1 June 1895, 79.
19. *History of Teetotalism in Devonshire*, 48–51, 52, 56.
20. 1851 Census (Class: HO107; Piece: 2455; Folio: 330; Page: 46; GSU roll: 169).
21. 1861 Census (Class: RG09; Piece: 4034; Folio: 90; Page: 52; GSU roll: 236).
22. 1871 Census (Class: RG10; Piece: 5363; Folio: 131; Page: 61; GSU roll: 375); Henry J. Wagg, *A Chronological Survey of Work for the Blind* (London: Pitman and Sons, 1932), 58.
23. 1881 Census (Class: RG11; Piece: 3846; Folio: 96; Page: 11; GSU roll: 647); 1891 Census (Class: RG12; Piece: 3124; Folio: 129; Page: 6; GSU roll: 21).
24. *Slater's Manchester & Salford Directory, 1895* (Manchester: Slater's and London: Kelly's, 1895), 283.
25. *Leeds Mercury*, 4 May 1880, 5; 'The Rechabites Jubilee', *Trewman's Exeter Flying Post or Plymouth and Cornish Advertiser*, 12 August 1885, 5; *British Women's Temperance Journal*, 1 November 1886, 123; 'Bolton', *British Women's Temperance Journal*, 1 April 1886, 41; 'The Women's Temperance Crusade', *Northern Echo*, 9 April 1888, 3; 'Nottingham', *British Women's Temperance Journal*, 1 January 1891, 2–3; 'Darwen', *Blackburn Standard*, 19 February 1887, 8.
26. Letter to the editor, *The Cambrian*, 9 December 1881, 8.
27. 'Reception to Veteran Abstainers', and F. Forsaith, 'Biographical Sketches', *Wings*, 1 June 1895, 79, 71.
28. Civil Deaths & Burials, Volume 8C, Page 318, England, England & Wales Deaths 1837–2007.

29. 'Record of Work', *British Women's Temperance Journal*, 1 October 1886, 7–8.
30. G. A. Jervis, 'Farnworth', *British Women's Temperance Journal*, 1 February 1890, 15.
31. Berridge, *Demons*, 132.
32. Harrison, 'British Prohibitionists', 383, 386.
33. Berridge, *Demons*, 38.
34. See James Kneale, 'Consumption', in *Alcohol in the Age of Industry, Empire and War*, edited by Deborah Toner (London: Bloomsbury, 2021), 49–50 and 53.
35. Alborn, *Regulated Lives*, 142.
36. 1881 Census (Class: RG11; Piece: 3375; Folio: 106; Page: 31; GSU roll: 940); Canadian Censuses, 1901, 1911, 1921, 1931.
37. Board Meetings, 28 March and 29 June 1866, Sceptre Minute Book 1, LMA; see Rohan McWilliam, *The Tichborne Claimant: A Victorian Sensation* (London: Continuum, 2007).
38. 'An Extravagant Baronet', *Royal Cornwall Gazette, Falmouth Packet, and General Advertiser*, 20 February 1863, 3.
39. Winskill, *Temperance Standard Bearers*, 458–9.
40. 'Methodist New Connexion', *Huddersfield Chronicle and West Yorkshire Advertiser*, 16 June 1877, 3; *Leeds Mercury*, 9 August 1890, 5.
41. *The Methodist's Who's Who* (London: Charles H. Kelly, 1912), 25.
42. My Primitive Methodists, www.myprimitivemethodists.org.uk/page_id__2184.aspx?path=0p3p78p139p.
43. 'Temperance Convention', *Daily Gazette for Middlesborough*, 25 February 1890, 3.
44. Alborn, *Regulated Lives*, 117–18.
45. Board meetings, 16 February 1866, Sceptre Minute book 1; 13 May 1880, Sceptre Minute book 2; 12 November 1891, Sceptre Minute book 3; 2 June 1898, Sceptre Minute book 4, London Archives.
46. *Kelly's Directory of Derbyshire, 1895* (London: Kelly, 1895), 233, 235.
47. 'Opening of the York Temperance Club and Coffee House', *York Herald*, 4 December 1878, 6.
48. 1881 Census (Class: RG11; Piece: 820; Folio: 32; Page: 57; GSU roll: 244); *The Standard*, 28 February 1881, 1; 'London Gossip', *Worcestershire Chronicle*, 31 December 1881, 6.
49. *Manchester Courier and Lancashire General Advertiser*, 26 May 1883, 7.
50. *The Times*, 23 November 1892, 3.
51. *Daily Inter Ocean*, 27 October 1893, 3; 'Stiles Sure of Success', *Atchison Globe*, 26 December 1895, 2.
52. 'Looking for Stiles', *Daily Inter Ocean*, 19 March 1896, 1; *Boston Daily Advertiser*, 20 March 1896, 12.
53. Ian Levitt, ed, *Joseph Livesey of Preston: Business, Temperance and Moral* Reform (Preston: University of Central Lancashire, 1996); Hannah Barker, *Family and Business during the Industrial Revolution* (Oxford: Oxford University Press, 2016); Harrison, 'British Prohibitionists'.
54. Rappaport, 'Sacred and Useful Pleasures'.
55. *Post Office Bath Directory 1884–5* (Bath: Lewis, Sons & Tyte, 1884–5), 752.
56. Christopher P. Hosgood, 'The "Pigmies of Commerce" and the Working-Class Community: Small Shopkeepers in England, 1870–1914', *Journal of Social History* 22, 3 (1989), 452.
57. Board meeting, 13 December 1900, Sceptre Minute book 4, London Archives.
58. Board meeting, 2 June 1892, Sceptre Minute book 3, London Archives.

59. Board meeting, 4 and 11 August 1910, Sceptre Minute books, London Archives.
60. 1911 Census (Class: RG14; Piece: 2989; GSU roll: 250); 1891 Census (Class: RG12; Piece: 630; Folio: 6; Page: 6; GSU roll: 32).
61. England & Wales, Index of Wills and Probates, 1853–1943; 1881 Census (Class: RG11; Piece: 968; Folio: 115; Page: 7; GSU roll: 943); 1891 Census (Class: RG12; Piece: 936; Folio: 98; Page: 3; GSU roll: 10).
62. *The Post Office Directory of Monmouthshire and the Principal Towns and Places in South Wales* (London: Kelly & Co., 1871), 239; Winskill, *Temperance Movement*, vol. 4, 159.
63. Ibid., 102; *Owen & Co.'s Cardiff Directory, 1887* (Cardiff: Owen, 1887), 30.
64. Ebenezer Beavan, *History of the Welsh Sunday Closing Act* (Cardiff: Daniel Owen, 1885); Winskill, *Temperance Movement,* vol. 4, 159; Daunton, *Coal Metropolis*, 221.
65. 'The Bute Dock Bill', *Western Mail*, 28 July 1882, 3; John Hobson Matthews, ed., 'Cardiff Council Minutes: 1879–81', *Cardiff Records: Volume 5* (Cardiff: Cardiff Records Committee, 1905), 46–62; *British History Online*, 7 August 2017, www.british-history.ac.uk/cardiff-records/vol5/pp46-62.
66. Daunton, *Coal Metropolis*, 51, 175, 180.
67. England & Wales Deaths 1837–2007, vol. 11A, p. 339.
68. 1881 Census (Class: RG11; Piece: 1310; Folio: 48; Page: 1; GSU roll: 1241318).
69. London Archives, Reference Number: p93/dun/111, Calendar of the Grants of Probate and Letters of Administration made in the Probate Registries of the High Court of Justice in England.
70. De Havilland Hall, *Medical Examination*, 178–9; see Christopher P. Hosgood, 'The "Knights of the Road": Commercial Travellers and the Culture of the Commercial Room in Late-Victorian and Edwardian England', *Victorian Studies* 37, 4 (1994), 519–47.
71. *Western Daily Press and Bristol Mirror*, 9 February 1940, 1.
72. 1871 Census (Class: RG10; Piece: 221; Folio: 53; Page:15; GSU roll: 112); 1881 Census (Class: RG11; Piece: 199; Folio: 54; Page: 37; GSU roll: 509); 1891 Census (Class: RG12; Piece: 130; Folio: 68; Page: 9; GSU roll: 66).
73. *Post Office Directory of Hampshire, Wiltshire & Dorset, 1875* (London: Kelly, 1875), 185; *Kelly's Directory of Hampshire & Isle of Wight, 1898* (London: Kelly's, 1898), 316, 329, 698.
74. *The Wrexham Advertiser*, 21 May 1864, 1.
75. 'Cefn-Mawr', *Wrexham Advertiser*, 23 April 1864, 6; 'Presentation to Mr Lester at Sarn Bridge', *Wrexham Advertiser*, 23 October 1875, 6; 'Annual Meeting of the Wrexham Temperance League', *Wrexham Advertiser,* 28 October 1871, 5.
76. Winskill, *Temperance Movement*, vol. 2, 262.
77. *Lancashire Evening Post*, 17 September 1915, 4; 1881 Census (Class: RG11; Piece: 4262; Folio: 75; Page: 19; GSU roll: 914).
78. *Kelly's Directory of Hampshire & Isle of Wight 1911* (London: Kelly's, 1911), 255.
79. 1881 Census (Class: RG11; Piece: 5059; Folio: 88; Page: 9; GSU roll: 734); England & Wales Deaths 1837–2007, Durham, vol. 10A, p. 564.
80. Policy 94, 11 December 1864, Life Policies, 1855–, MS 3545. Prudential Archives.
81. Gareth Stedman Jones, *Outcast London: A Study in the Relationship between Classes in Victorian Society* (London: Penguin, 1992), 56–65.
82. Geoffrey Crossick, ed., *The Lower Middle Class in Britain, 1870–1914* (London: Croom Helm, 1977); Peter Bailey, 'White Collars, Gray Lives? The Lower Middle Class Revisited', *Journal of British Studies* 38 (1999), 275.

83. W. A. Armstrong, 'The Use of Information about Occupation', in *Nineteenth-Century Society*, edited by Edward A. Wrigley (Cambridge: Cambridge University Press, 1972), 191–310; Richard Dennis, *English Industrial Cities of the Nineteenth Century* (Cambridge: Cambridge University Press, 1984), 189, 188.
84. Gareth Stedman Jones, 'Working-Class Culture and Working-Class Politics in London, 1870–1900: Notes on the Remaking of a Working Class', in *Languages of Class: Studies in English Working Class History 1832–1982* (Cambridge: Cambridge University Press, 1984), 179–238.
85. Hosgood, 'Pigmies of Commerce'.
86. Jon Lawrence, 'Class and Gender in the Making of Urban Toryism, 1880–1914', *English Historical Review* 108, 428 (1993), 638.
87. Lawrence, 'Class and Gender', 635.
88. Bailey, 'White Collars', 277.
89. 'Death of J. Theophilus Davis', *Cheshire Observer*, 5 October 1895, 5; *Kelly's Directory of Cheshire, 1896* (London: Kelly's, 1896), 214; *Cheshire Observer*, 25 June 1892, 1; 'Local and District News', *Cheshire Observer*, 12 October 1895, 6.
90. *Cheshire Observer*, 16 April 1892, 8.
91. 'Baron Halkett on Mr. Yerburgh', *Cheshire Observer*, 2 July 1892, 5.
92. Henry Pelling, *Social Geography of British Elections 1885–1910* (London: Macmillan, 1967).
93. Susan D. Pennybacker, *A Vision for London, 1889–1914: Labour, Everyday Life and the LCC Experiment* (London: Routledge, 1995); Chris Waters, *British Socialists and the Politics of Popular Culture, 1884–1914* (Stanford, CA: Stanford California Press, 1990); Pearce, 'A Landscape of Dissent'.
94. Bailey, 'White Collars', 289; Peter Bailey, '"Will the Real Bill Banks Please Stand up?" Towards a Role Analysis of Mid-Victorian Working-Class Respectability', *Journal of Social History* 12, 3 (1979), 341.
95. Bailey, 'White Collars', 290.

8

Medicine: An institution for educating the medical men

Introduction: Medicine, alcohol and life assurance

When the UKT issued its first policy, life assurance practice took its cue from established medical opinion, which assumed moderate consumption was safe, and perhaps even necessary for life. In the 1830s the first temperance societies, which were largely anti-spirits organizations, persuaded some doctors to sign medical declarations stating, for example, 'that distilled spirit is not only unnecessary, but injurious to health; that it contains no nutritive quality; that its daily use is a strong temptation to drunkenness … and that its entire disuse except for purposes strictly medicinal, would powerfully contribute to the health, morality, and comfort of the community'.[1] The British and Foreign Temperance Society claimed more than 1,500 physicians and surgeons had signed similar declarations since 1834. However, spirits were not the only thing in a doctor's medicine bag – or his cellar. The Cheltenham physician Henry Charles Boisragon organized a medical declaration against spirits to present to James Silk Buckingham's 1834 Select Committee on Drunkenness, for example, though someone in his household was certainly drinking, his diary recording that he paid for £80 of sherry and more than £100 of wine in October and November 1830. Boisragon's description of one dinner in May 1831 illustrates why some teetotalers included doctors alongside Anglican clerics as supporters of the drink trade: 'That everlasting old Tuxbelly, Jossietti, brought his infamous fat friend to dine, a cleric with one leg, and key volume of the *Encyclopaedia*, and drank six bottles.'[2]

Medical abstainers were rare. Dawson Burns thought it unlikely that there were more than fifty in the late 1830s.[3] In 1842 William Batchelor, the UKT's referee for Dunstable, lost his position as the medical officer to the Luton Poor-Law Union because he refused to administer alcohol to patients; he published a pamphlet entitled *Trials and Persecutions of a Teetotal Surgeon* to defend his position.[4] The opposition the UKT encountered shifted only gradually. Though Grindrod and Mudge (Chapter 5) joined another 2,000 doctors in signing a medical declaration stating that 'perfect health is compatible with total abstinence from all intoxicating beverages' in 1847, this remained a controversial issue in medicine for decades.[5] In 1871 the eminent hygienist Edmund Alexander Parkes helped the National Temperance League organize a medical declaration supporting total abstinence, publishing signatories' names in the *British*

Medical Journal; while opinion was beginning to shift Parkes was still criticized by other doctors, as we will see.[6] By 1907, in contrast, it was the doctors who still believed alcohol had a place in medical treatment who had to take to the pages of *The Lancet* to make their case.[7] It seems likely that mainstream medical opinion had more or less accepted that total abstinence could be healthy by 1900. It also seems plausible that the experience of temperance life assurance firms helped persuade doctors that teetotalers could live long and healthy lives. The statistics they collected presented a new form of evidence, which, alongside other developments in medical science, offered new ways of engaging with alcoholism and alcohol's effect on the body.

In this way the examination rooms of medical officers and examiners became significant 'spaces of diagnosis', in David Livingstone's terms, alongside better-studied sites like hospitals, dispensaries and workhouses.[8] In 1854 the fourteen assurance offices in Scotland conducted nearly 9,000 examinations between them, paying examiners around £6,000 in fees, which demonstrated 'the extent of the duties in connection with Life Assurance now devolved on medical practitioners – duties which scarcely existed twenty years ago'.[9] Marguerite Dupree suggests that 'a substantial proportion of the medical profession gained valuable part-time appointments which helped to alter the diagnostic techniques of the profession more generally', a welcome supplement when competition forced many doctors to develop what M. Jeanne Peterson described as 'medical entrepreneurship' in the search for additional income.[10] The UKT had originally paid up to a pound for policies worth £500 or more, but settled on a fee of ten shillings for policies of £100 or more, while smaller policies were covered by the Industrial section.[11] These examinations made up a relatively small part of a firm's costs; in 1871 Sceptre paid £378 11s. in medical fees, compared to £525 for Director's fees and £707 10s. for the salaries of the London office staff.[12]

Between the medical declarations of the 1830s and 1870s, teetotalers faced opposition from medical authorities who continued to use alcohol in their practice, arguing it served as both medicine and food. The German chemist Justus von Liebig argued that alcohol was a food, and in the 1830s the British and Irish doctors Robert Bentley Todd and Robert J. Graves drew on this work to develop systems of treatment that used set doses of alcohol to 'feed' fever patients. Unsurprisingly, teetotal doctors welcomed F. R. Lees's translation of the 1860 research of the French researchers Lallemand, Perrin and Duroy, who rejected Liebig's argument.[13] Rather than settling the debate once and for all, however, Lallemand et al.'s conclusions prompted further research; Sarah E. Williams concluded that 'by the end of the 19th century, the medical literature on alcohol as medicine was voluminous' in the United States.[14] This chapter examines some of the work conducted in Britain in this period, concentrating on the places where there were connections and tensions with understandings of drink produced by life assurance.

In doing so it challenges Brian Harrison's assertion that temperance stifled British medical research on alcohol in the 1860s and 1870s. Harrison argued that the Alliance's refusal to broaden its focus beyond Local Option explains why it was the Swedish scientist Magnus Huss who made the most important contribution to studies of alcoholism in these decades. 'In England', he suggested, 'the temperance and prohibitionist movements had so advertised the moral dimensions of the problem that its scientific aspects could be effectively studied only on the continent'.[15] Notwithstanding the fact that it was Lees, one of the more moralistic teetotalers, who brought those continental ideas to England, Harrison's argument misses two key things. The first is that medical work was being done in these decades, sometimes by doctors like Mudge and Grindrod, and sometimes by doctors provoked by temperance arguments; if this work is hard to see now that probably reflects the attitudes of contemporary medicine, which had yet to be convinced that work like Huss's was worth conducting. The second is that medical research – of a kind – was also being done in other sites, like the offices of life assurance companies. Doctors had to be persuaded that alcohol might be harmful, and it seems very unlikely that they felt excluded from the debate about drinking – in fact some, like Francis Anstie, were much provoked by temperance arguments, and some of this work was influenced by the experience of life assurance firms like the UKT. For this reason, Jean-Charles Sournia's history of alcoholism dated the medicalization of alcohol from the UKT's founding in 1840, rather than the publication of Huss's *Alcoholismus chronicus eller chronisk alkoholssjukdom* in 1849–50.[16]

This chapter will show that the success of temperance assurance influenced arguments about the risks associated with alcohol and abstinence in medicine. The evidence collected by these firms provided new ways of knowing and representing the dangers of drinking, rivalling both medical practitioners' existing experience and new experimental research. Attempts to use medical research to establish a safe daily limit for alcohol consumption then became part of insurance practice in the US, UK and elsewhere, suggesting not only broad agreement between actuaries and doctors about the risks of drinking, but also the dissemination of this understanding through insurance networks. By the beginning of the twentieth century this suspicion of excessive drinking was widely shared by doctors, though scepticism remained in more conservative quarters. Tracing these developments, this chapter will also consider the lives of the royal physician Sir Thomas Barlow and the doctor and health writer Joseph Mortimer Granville. It begins, though, with an institution every bit as experimental as the UKT had been at its founding.

Educating the medical men: The Temperance Hospital and temperance life assurance

At the eleventh annual meeting of the board of the National Temperance Hospital in 1884 the Somerset shoemaker James Clark described the hospital as 'an institution for educating the medical men', going on to say 'they had educated the insurance offices by the work of the United Kingdom Temperance Life Office, and they had as great a work to do with the doctors in this hospital'.[17] For Clark both the Hospital and the UKT had important roles to play as the first institutions of their kind; their success would prove the claims made by teetotalers for the healthfulness of abstinence. The two institutions shared many directors and patrons; Thomas Cash, a director of the UKT since 1852, its secretary since 1861, and the chair of the board and managing director following Warner's death, was also the chair of the Hospital board from 1873. Its patrons included James Barlow, the Bolton mill owner and father of Thomas Barlow, who would become the UKT's medical officer in 1876, Samuel Bowly and Drs Grindrod, Mitchell and Mudge. The Hospital's donors and subscribers were drawn from the same people and places that had supported the UKT: wealthy nonconformists like Barlow and the Backhouses, Barclays and Cadburys, as well as theatres and missions, Good Templar Lodges and temperance societies.[18]

As Clark suggested, like the UKT the Hospital encouraged new ideas about drinking. The Hospital had been established to treat patients without alcohol, except where absolutely necessary, to demonstrate that this was safe and effective. In other hospitals drink was used as a stimulant, to treat illness – especially fevers – or to relieve pain, and drugs were given to patients in wine; in-patients were given daily rations of alcoholic beverages too, as they were in workhouses and asylums.[19] At the Temperance Hospital, in contrast, doctors would 'give nature an opportunity of showing what she can do in the absence of alcohol', as J. James Ridge, one of the visiting physicians, put it in 1888.[20] Ridge founded the British Medical Temperance Association and its *Medical Temperance Journal* with the Hospital's other visiting physician, James Edmunds, in 1876; membership was restricted to teetotal qualified medical practitioners interested in researching 'the physiological action of alcohol'.[21] The Medical Temperance Association, like the Hospital and the UKT, was designed to examine the consequences of drinking, regardless of the Alliance's definition of the drink problem. Laying the memorial stone for the Hospital's new site in 1879 (Figure 8.1), Wilfrid Lawson said 'I have no right to say whether alcohol is a useful or a deleterous [*sic*] drug, but … I want to see the question have a *bona fide*, fair, straight-forward, practical trial'. He continued that those leading this enterprise 'are but one branch of the great army which is

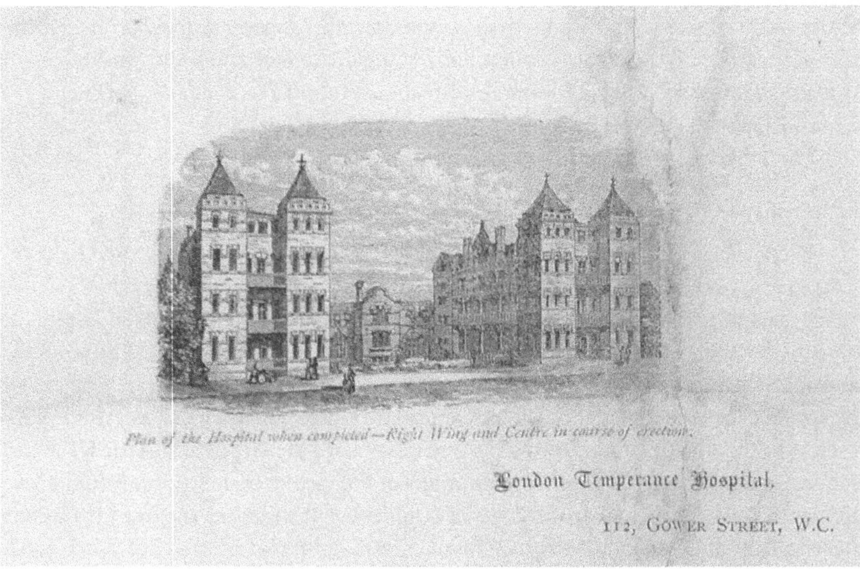
Plan of the Hospital when completed—Right Wing and Centre in course of erection.
London Temperance Hospital,
112, Gower Street, W.C.

Figure 8.1 The London Temperance Hospital, 1879.

Source: Author's photo.

attacking our national intemperance'.[22] Lawson, responsible for leading the charge for Local Option as the Alliance's Parliamentary spokesman, did not restrict temperance to that narrow definition.

Both institutions approached alcohol in a new way, creating new forms of evidence in the process. As the senior institution, the UKT's experience provided support for the founding of the Temperance Hospital. Mr Dunn, the Hospital's vice-chair, told its first meeting of patrons, governors and supporters that 'the fact was that total abstainers were freer from disease than other persons', supplying proof of this in the form of figures from the UKT's records.[23] Before long, though, the Hospital was creating its own evidence, as the treatment and recovery of in- and out-patients was recorded, along with the occasional (and very rare) use of alcohol, as well as the treatment and outcome of cases of alcoholism, in Huss's sense of the action of alcohol on the body.

Contemporaries often misunderstood the point of the Hospital, assuming it was a specialist institution for teetotalers rather than a general hospital operating on temperance principles. The humorous newspaper *Fun* reprinted an advertisement for a house surgeon for the Hospital ahead of its opening in 1873, drily noting that 'we should think it would be an easy situation, as, according to their own doctrine, teetotallers are never ill'.[24] That in itself suggests that arguments made for the healthiness of abstinence had become familiar to the public, even if they were not necessarily believed. As it treated both abstainers and non-abstainers, though – nearly 1,400 of each as in-patients in its first twelve years, plus another 19,000 out-patients – the Hospital could claim to be just like any other hospital, but with one key difference, just as the UKT's abstainers were presented as typical apart from their abstinence. The Hospital's experience seemed to show that it was possible to treat patients for a wide range of problems without using alcohol.

The Temperance Hospital was a diagnostic space testing arguments about alcohol-free treatment. The contribution of life assurance offices was perhaps less obvious but still important.

A rival source of evidence

By the 1870s other life assurance firms began to share the UKT's suspicion of heavy drinkers and those in the licensed trade, and in the 1880s some offered abstainers' policies too (Chapter 1). The practice of rating up workers in the drink trade was well established by the 1880s, as we can see in the medical handbooks written for assurance examiners, which were designed to summarize medical and insurantial knowledge for ordinary practitioners. While their authors were often prestigious men, associated with the great London teaching hospitals, we cannot know if their opinions on different risks were necessarily believed; they do offer useful surveys of industry practice, however. In 1876, for example, Francis Moinet suggested that some offices always added an extra charge for publicans.[25] By 1882 Edward Sieveking was noting that 'it is the *custom* to add 10 to 20 per cent to the premium for innkeepers, for their trade alone', because publicans were 'constantly surrounded by an atmosphere of alcohol'. While he felt it was unfair to exclude them altogether, he thought a 25 per cent addition was just.[26] James Edward Pollock and James Chisholm's handbook concluded that '*intemperance* is perhaps the most formidable enemy to the safe assurance of life', though 'the moderate use of stimulants does not tend to shorten life'. Like Sieveking, they thought a 10 per cent addition for publicans was not enough to cover the extra risk, though most firms charged only a little more; they added that 'some offices will not have them on any terms, and they are not far wrong'.[27] Life assurance records and statistics from the GRO both demonstrated the higher mortality of licensed victuallers; the UKT's statistical experience had become part of the discussion of the risks associated with drinking. Sieveking mentioned the UKT's data on longevity, quoting their actuary Samuel Brown and a paper Dr James Edmunds presented to the Society for the Medical Officers of Health in 1877.[28]

Between 1850, when 55 per cent of Alborn's sample of assurance offices asked whether the applicant's drinking was intemperate, and the 1870s, when definitions of what might be counted as 'moderate' drinking tightened sharply, British life assurance firms became increasingly suspicious of those working with alcohol, while instructing their examiners to scrutinize all applicants for signs of hidden intemperance, and to check that abstainers were not reformed drunkards.[29] Significantly, though, life assurance was also beginning to influence medicine, and the dialogue between the two grew closer over the second half of the century, though important tensions remained.

In 1845 Francis Neison, the actuary of the Medical, Invalid and General Life Office, published *Contributions to Vital Statistics*, which drew upon the records of life assurance companies to investigate social questions, including 'the rate of mortality among persons of intemperate habits'.[30] Several years before the UKT could compare its two sections, Neison calculated the longevity of 'decidedly intemperate' and temperate lives. Neison's work was influential within life assurance, but it was also read by the hygienist Edmund Parkes, who cited it in the first edition of his *Manual of Practical Hygiene* in 1864, concluding that 'the effect of intemperance in any alcoholic beverage is to cause premature old age, to produce or predispose to numerous diseases, and to lessen the chance of living very greatly'.[31] Parkes was also struck by the paper that Edward Vivian (Chapter 2) read before the British Association at Bristol in 1875, which showed that the UKT's abstainers enjoyed better longevity. In the final edition of his *Manual* Parkes noted that 'very striking evidence of favour of total abstinence, as contrasted with moderation, is given by the experience of the United Kingdom Temperance and General Provident Institution'.[32]

Significantly, though, Parkes also later cited the work of Francis Anstie, whose experimental research in the 1860s suggested that alcohol could not be considered to be a poison, food or medicine in and of itself, because its effects depended upon the quantity consumed. Anstie began trying to assess the upper limit that could be safely consumed in 1862, and by 1870 he had established that this dose was an ounce, or an ounce and a half, of absolute alcohol.[33] Inspired by Anstie, and working with Count Cyprian Wollowicz, Parkes published four papers on the effects of alcohol on the temperature, pulse and health in the Royal Society's *Proceedings* between 1869 and 1873.[34] His popular *On Personal Care of Health* contained detailed descriptions of how much alcohol, of different kinds, could be consumed by those wishing to remain below Anstie's 'limit of moderation'.[35]

Combining life assurance statistics and experimental medical research, Parkes sought a meeting point for different approaches to studying alcohol's effect on the body, one that suggested that moderation was an acceptable alternative to abstinence. Other medical writers refused to reconcile these different ways of doing medicine, sometimes rejecting them for a third form of practice associated with the 'gentleman physician' who 'resisted the wholesale conversion of bedside practice into a science'.[36] Christopher Lawrence saw this attitude as part of an attempt to protect elite physicians, who dominated the Royal Colleges and London teaching hospitals, from attempts to define medical professionalism as a question of scientific progress. Work on the history of Anglo-American medicine between 1850 and 1914 has shown that professionalization was not a consequence of the adoption of contemporary medical science by doctors, not least because there were different kinds of 'science' available to them.[37] It has also explored what Lawrence described as 'the peculiarly difficult passage of continental experimental science, notably physiology, into the British medical curriculum'.[38] Lawrence's gentlemen physicians resisted specialization, put great store in personal experience and believed that medicine was an art that took decades to acquire and was 'personal to the possessor of it [and] incommunicable by word or letter', to quote Sir Dyce Duckworth, who also had plenty to say about alcohol and the use of insurance statistics to assess its effects on drinkers, as we will see later in this chapter.[39]

The tension between gentlemanly, physiological and statistical approaches to alcohol can be seen in the reception given to William Howship Dickinson's 1872 paper on 'Alcohol as a Cause of Renal Disease' in the *British Medical Journal*. He argued that the relationship between alcoholism and renal disease was not as strong as was often imagined, supplementing statistics from the GRO with post-mortem records from St George's Hospital, London.[40] His conclusion lead to a bad-tempered debate in the *Journal*, not least because an anonymous editorial article in the same issue criticized similar arguments Dickinson had made in a paper presented to the Royal Medical and Chirurgical Society, based on records of post-mortem analyses of nearly 300 subjects, half in the liquor trade and half 'not known to have been drunken'.[41] While the leading article touched on questions of method, it also cast doubt on the value of the wider approach, dismissing the utility of the returns of the Registrar General and stating that 'the best field for observing the morbid effects of alcohol is neither the *post mortem* theatre nor the hospital ward, but the daily round of private practice, where, the reticence of the patient being supplemented by the candour of his friends, habits of intemperance can rarely be concealed from the medical attendant'.[42] This perfectly captures the attitude of Lawrence's gentlemen physicians and may explain why Dickinson's reply said the editorial 'savours of the bar rather than the bench' – of learned sophistry rather than laboratory research.[43]

The hostile response to Dickinson's study demonstrates that the tensions explored by Lawrence have important consequences for the history of medical research on alcohol in Britain. The resistance of many clinicians to laboratory science could be seen as 'a failing, a lagging behind the continent, a stiff-upper-lipped insularity', as Lawrence put it, much as Harrison saw the neglect of work on alcohol as the outcome of the Alliance's influence, when it seems more likely to have been the outcome of a struggle between rival approaches to medicine.[44] Laboratory work on the effects of alcohol on the body continued through the 1860s and 1870s, and was suppressed not by the Alliance, but by gentlemanly physicians wary of this rival definition of medicine.

Medical practitioners considering the consequences of drinking had at least three approaches to choose from in the second half of the century: the gentlemanly art of Duckworth; the laboratory medicine of Anstie or Dickinson; and what we might now describe as a 'public health' approach, which drew conclusions from statistical evidence – the returns of the GRO or life assurance 'experience'. This mixture of approaches can also be seen in the life of Thomas Barlow.

Temperance lives: Sir Thomas Barlow (1845–1945)

Thomas Barlow was born in Edgworth, to James and Alice Barlow (Chapters 1 and 2). Thomas read medicine at University College London from 1868, acting as William Jenner's house physician before being appointed medical registrar at the Hospital for Sick Children, Great Ormond Street, London, in 1874, where he remained as assistant and then full physician until 1899, working also at the Charing Cross, London and University College Hospitals before retiring in 1910. A fellow of the Royal Society and president of the Royal College of Physicians, Barlow made his name through his clinical research on scurvy and other diseases of childhood and in neurology. As he increasingly concentrated on private practice, though, he 'ministered to an ever more elevated circle of private patients', including Randall Davidson, the archbishop of Canterbury, and in 1896 he became physician to the royal household, acting as physician-extraordinary to the Queen in her final years. Barlow was created a baronet in 1901. Originally a Methodist like his father, Barlow became an Anglican at around the time of his royal appointment.[45]

Barlow made his name as a medical scientist but became a gentleman doctor. In 1877 a testimonial from Dr Wilson Fox described Barlow as 'both in scientific knowledge and personal character a gentleman'.[46] When James Reid wrote from Balmoral to offer Barlow the post of Physician to the Household in 1896, he noted that the Queen acknowledged Barlow's 'high position in the Profession and your high character in every respect', adding 'the only thing she has against you is your wishing to admit women to the College, which she disapproves of!!'[47] Thomas did not lose his parents' temperance convictions, however, an obituarist noting that 'total abstinence from alcohol had early been accepted by him as a good rule for a man in life, and he never abated his open support of tee-totalism'.[48] He was president of the National Temperance League from 1923–30 and had been offered the role of Chief Physician of the Temperance Hospital in 1896, though he declined.[49] The materials collected in his archive suggest that Thomas kept up with research on alcohol into the 1920s.

Thomas also worked for the UKT as their medical officer from 1876 and as a director between 1904 and 1943.[50] When Joseph T. Mitchell, the firm's first physician (Chapters 4 and 5), died in February 1876, his son – also Joseph Thomas, and also a medical practitioner – immediately wrote to offer his services as a replacement, reminding Thomas Cash that he had covered his father's duties in 1867 and 1871 when Joseph senior was unwell. Joseph junior admitted that he was not a teetotaler but 'would readily sign the pledge, if required to do so'.[51] He lost out to Barlow, however, whose impressive referees included William Jenner at University College Hospital; Dr Charles West at the Hospital for Sick Children, who was president of the Medico-Chirurgical Society; William Howship Dickinson of St Georges and the Hospital for Sick Children; and Julius Pollock at the Charing Cross Hospital.[52] Thomas's father James also wrote to Cash to recommend his son, 'who has been many years in London at the Hospitals & has the highest Diplomas of the London University. He is a Life Abstainer & is thoroughly sound & conscientious in every respect'.[53]

Thomas Barlow's life traces one of the paths taken by temperance over the period covered by this book, from his father's Methodist philanthropy to the heart of the British establishment. At the beginning of Victoria's reign Lord Melbourne told her that all teetotalers were Radicals; at the end of her life, a teetotaler served as her physician and was at her deathbed. A well-known medical scientist who successfully adopted the trappings of the gentleman while simultaneously working for a life assurance company, Barlow brought together all three of the styles of medicine described above, though he did not draw upon them to study alcohol.

We return now to a doctor who was much less sympathetic to temperance, though his work was adopted by life assurance firms eager to protect themselves from immoderate drinkers.

Anstie's limit: Quantifying moderation in life assurance

Francis Edmund Anstie (Figure 8.2) was born into a liberal nonconformist family in 1833 in Devizes, Wiltshire. Training at King's College, London, he became Robert Todd's clinical clerk and watched Todd prescribe alcohol to fever patients who could not eat solid food. Once qualified, Anstie worked at several London hospitals before becoming Physician at the Westminster in 1873. He was the editor of *The Practitioner* and became a member of *The Lancet*'s editorial team.[54] Specializing in diseases of the nervous system, Anstie developed an interest in the effects of alcohol and other drugs in the early 1860s. He also assisted in the production of *The Lancet*'s reports on the state of workhouse infirmaries in 1865 and supported the founding of both an association for Poor-Law Medical Officers and the London School of Medicine for Women. If it had not been for his early death in 1874, Anstie would have been the school's first dean.[55]

Perhaps because of his training with Todd, Anstie resisted the idea that alcohol was one simple thing – poison, food, or drug. In two early pieces he wrote anonymously for the *Cornhill Magazine*, on the encouragement of his friend William Makepeace Thackeray, Anstie suggested that there was a limit to how much alcohol the body needed; above that point the drinker became intoxicated.[56] Anstie returned to this emphasis on the quantity of the dose administered in his subsequent research, but it is also worth noting that in the second of these two papers he argued that 'there should not be a total silence on the part of those members of the profession who do not see themselves called upon to yield to the mere force of agitation, and become the obsequious mouthpiece of the teetotal party'.[57] Given everything else he wrote about

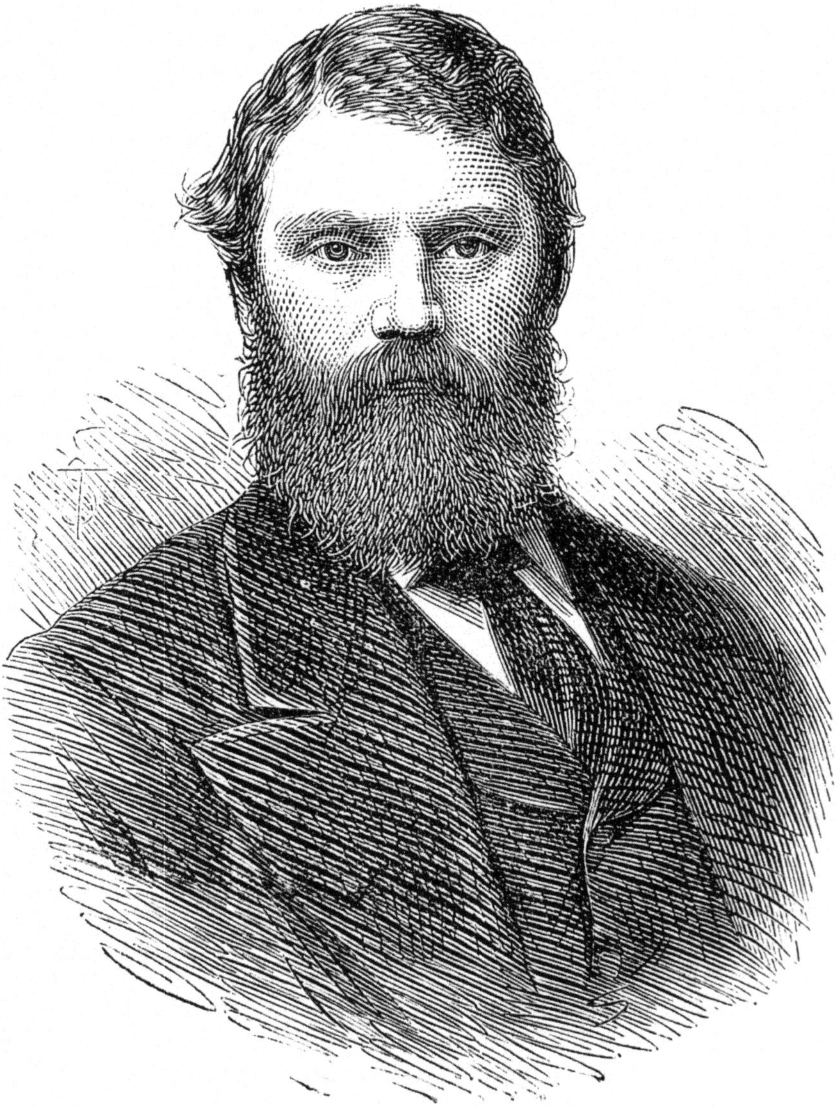

Figure 8.2 Dr Francis Anstie.

Source: *Illustrated London News*, 26 September 1874, 305. Courtesy Getty Images.

this question, it seems most likely that Anstie took exception to the pressure exerted by organizations like the Alliance; but in his case it seems to have *encouraged* his research.

Anstie's *Stimulants and Narcotics*, published in 1864, examined the state of work in the field and reported on the results of his own experimental research, inspired by Edmond Baudot's discovery that the chromatic test used to detect alcohol was capable of very fine measurements.[58] His experiments convinced him that 'a moderate or non-intoxicating' dose of alcohol produced only tiny quantities of eliminated alcohol, while large doses made large quantities of alcohol appear in the breath, sweat, blood and urine of the drinker. He concluded that the body appeared to benefit from alcohol, but *only up to a certain dose*, beyond which it ceased to be a food or stimulant, beginning to act as a sedative, with narcotic and harmful effects, while excess alcohol began to be eliminated from the body.[59] Anstie continued to refine this method, testing animal and human subjects and improving methods for collecting and analysing eliminated alcohol, as well as using Marey's new sphygmograph to study the drinker's pulse.[60]

All of this work indicated that most bodies began to eliminate alcohol after one or one and a half ounces of absolute alcohol had been consumed. By 1870 Anstie was referring to this as a 'daily allowance' of 1 or 1½ ounces of absolute alcohol, 'about the limit of what can be habitually taken by persons leading a not very active life, without provoking symptoms of chronic malaise indicative of actual alcoholic poisoning'.[61] This became known as 'Anstie's Limit', and after being taken up by Parkes and others would be widely recognized and discussed within and beyond British medicine.[62] Reviewing work on drinking in the United States at the turn of the century, the Committee of Fifty referred to Anstie's limit to settle 'the question as to the amount of alcoholic drinks which can be used freely by the average adult without producing bad results'.[63] Harry G. Levine suggested that the Committee defined the ideal of moderate drinking that replaced Prohibition, so it seems likely that Anstie's influence was highly significant in the US.[64]

Anstie's work illustrates the importance of experimental physiology in shaping understandings of the effects of alcohol on the body, part of a European-wide dialogue with other researchers. Diagnostic tools – the chromatic test and the sphygmograph – replaced the experience of the gentleman physician. The idea that moderation could now be quantified was something of a breakthrough, and the limit found its way into unexpected places – including life assurance practice. While examiners' handbooks attempted to provide guidance about how much alcohol might safely be consumed by an applicant, this tended to be vague and hedged with qualifications. When Pollock and Chisholm told their readers that moderate drinking did not shorten life, they defined that as 'small quantities – with the meals – and not more frequently than twice in the day', without specifying those quantities.[65] Jonathan Adams Allen cited Anstie's work, but not the limit, in 1870, and it was not until Edward Mansfield Brockbank's handbook was published in 1908 that 'the physiological amount of one and a half ounces of absolute alcohol' was referenced.[66] By 1927 James Paterson MacLaren's handbook could confidently define 'a "*sober* and *temperate*" person in the insurance sense' as one drinking less than one and a half ounces of alcohol.[67]

Perhaps the most significant adoption of Anstie's Limit was its use in the analysis of the Medico-Actuarial Investigation of the Mortality of American and Canadian Life Assurance Companies, which began in 1909 and was published between 1912 and 1914. A synthesis of the experience of dozens of North American companies with respect to many risks, including alcohol consumption, in the hands of Arthur Hunter, actuary at New York Life, the Investigation also became an opportunity to replace the subjective assessments of examiners with a series of readings and measurements that could be converted into a quantitative assessment of an applicant's overall risk. The Investigation was also an assessment of industry practice. In terms of alcohol, Hunter divided firms depending on whether they used a 'conservative' or 'liberal' definition of moderate drinking, with Anstie's limit marking the division between the two. While lives drinking below the limit still suffered 18 per cent more deaths than expected, those drinking at or above Anstie's limit experienced 86 per cent more deaths than expected. Hunter also noted that more than 70 per cent of the lives investigated were assured under the riskier 'liberal' definition, leading him to conclude that 'anything but a very moderate use of alcohol is detrimental to longevity'.[68] Returning to this question in 1922 with his colleague Oscar Rogers, Hunter described Anstie's limit as 'far too liberal', adding 'there appears to be no limit within which alcohol may be entirely harmless'.[69]

Hunter's caution was prompted by business instincts. As the author Eugene Lyman Fisk described the authors of the Investigation 'these men were fairly saturated, not only with scientific, but with business conservatism, for their main purpose was *to ascertain facts from which principles of business action could be derived*'.[70] Medical and insurantial writers participated in a dialogue about the usefulness of physiological research in life assurance, and though this dialogue could be incomplete and inconclusive, it did shape assurance practice, particularly in North America, while life assurance continued to provide an alternative source of knowledge for medical practitioners.

Anstie remained critical of organized teetotalism until his death. In 1871, when the *British Medical Journal* published Parkes's medical declaration supporting abstinence, Anstie wrote to *The Lancet* to protest, before writing an editorial in *The Practitioner* accusing the *BMJ*'s editor of assisting the National Temperance League's 'terrorism' of the profession, suggesting that doctors had been forced into signing.[71] His opposition seems likely to have been the result of his determination to provide an answer to this question through experimental science.

Our next Life – not, it has to be admitted, a very temperate one – was also opposed to temperance, and it suggests that by the 1890s, those who made a spirited defence of the necessity of alcohol for life were taking a rather marginal position in relation to mainstream medicine.

Temperance lives: Dr Joseph Mortimer Granville (1833–1900)

Joseph Granville was born in Devonport in 1833, before training as a doctor, probably in London.[72] He became a member of the Royal College of Surgeons in 1856, before moving to Bristol, where he founded the Free Institution for the Treatment of Diseases Peculiar to Women and Children in 1857, later part of the city's Hospital for Children. Until 1867 Granville combined general practice with work at the Institution, the Royal Infirmary and the Clifton workhouse. He married Mary Ellen Ormerod, the daughter of his partner in practice, in 1858, and the family were living in a prestigious Bristol neighbourhood in 1861, the year that he was admitted to the Royal College of Physicians.

Granville then seems to have suffered some kind of crisis: his partnership dissolved in 1866, he was declared bankrupt in 1867, and the family broke up. Granville surfaced in London, and somehow became – perhaps through West Country connections – the personal physician of Sir Stafford Northcote, later Lord Iddesleigh, First Lord of the

Treasury. Through Northcote's patronage Granville also became the editor of *The Globe* newspaper between 1871 and 1874, and while he proved to be an unpopular editor the role gave him a taste for journalism. As a medical writer and general practitioner, Granville began to accumulate markers of medical respectability, joining the staff of *The Lancet* and publishing books on nervous illness and gout; his practice moved from Savile Row to Hanover Square, where his neighbour was Sir James Paget, and finally to Cavendish Square.[73]

In 1891 Granville joined a discussion of the drink problem in the letter columns of *The Times*. He stated that moderate drinkers were healthier than abstainers, and that teetotalism had been entirely iniquitous; while life expectancies might be growing, general health was worsening because resistance to illness was weakening.[74] His letter attracted much criticism, the *British Medical Journal* describing it as 'thoughtless and inaccurate ... so extravagantly worded, so devoid of evidence, and it may fairly be said so contrary to fact, that it is deplorable that any educated medical man should have been willing to append his name to it'. The editorial concluded, in what could be taken as a statement of mainstream late Victorian medical opinion on drinking, that 'it is not only presumptuous, but mischievous, for any man to assert – as has been done in this discussion – that abstinence from alcoholic drink is, except perhaps in an infinitesimally small number of cases, injurious to health and likely to lessen the strength of the individual or to shorten life'.[75]

Undeterred, Granville then published an essay in which he insisted that 'the drinking of fermented or alcoholic liquors is a matter of duty and right'.[76] He acknowledged Anstie's limit, but added that

> I think there are very few persons over the age of puberty who do not require a stimulant and would not be the better for taking it, and, so far from abstinence being the rule and drinking the exception, I have no hesitation in saying that the organism needs the alcohol, and that it should be the rule to supply the this need, no exception being made without medical advice.[77]

He said he knew many doctors would disagree with him, but his experience in practice had convinced him that teetotalers suffered from neuralgia, heart disturbances and indigestion, all ailments that could be cured by 'rational drinking'.[78] Granville also dismissed the value of the UKT's experience, saying, 'No one who has much to do with statistics, and at the same time mixes in society so that he is not figure-mad, can put his faith in them.'[79]

Granville's hostility to temperance may also reflect his own politics and his desire for publicity. In the preface to his gout book Granville wrote that his apparently old-fashioned views had 'outlived in my mind the changes of a revolutionary epoch in science (for I am a Tory in Science as in Politics)'.[80] Northcote's *Globe* was a Conservative paper, and Granville even contributed an essay on drink to the first number of the anti-Socialist periodical the *Liberty Review* in 1893.[81] Granville may have seen temperance as a form of liberal coercion (Chapter 7).

His desire to provoke might also have been shaped by his earlier failure as a surgeon in Bristol. Many of Granville's activities – founding Bristol's children's hospital, popular health writing, arguments for drinking – exemplify what Anne Digby described as the 'medical entrepreneurialism' of doctors trying to find a place in an overcrowded market.[82] These developments were not necessarily unscientific – Granville's 'percuteur', or mechanical massager, was one of several developed at this time and was intended to be of real therapeutic value – but they were often driven by faddish currents in popular thinking.[83] Granville contributed to *The Lancet*, but he also published many popular one-shilling health books like *Common Mind Troubles* or *Minds and Moods: Gossiping Papers on Mind-Management and Morals*, as well as essays like 'Worry' and 'Fish as food and physic'.[84] His peculiar advice – prescribing the wearing of nightcaps as protection from bad dreams, taking snuff to alleviate colds – were reported by serious and comic papers alike.[85]

In fact it seems significant that the *Leeds Times* described the *BMJ*'s criticism of Granville as the sort of treatment they might give an 'enterprising American quack'.[86] The British medical press was hostile to quackery and 'puffing' – doctors' endorsements in advertisements – because they undermined the independence of medicine, allowing the medical market to decide which treatments were best. Granville's opinion that port from the wood was better for invalids than that from the bottle was used in advertisements, as it was for Yates's wine lodge in Blackburn, for example.[87] At the same time these activities allowed Granville to demonstrate what Peterson called 'medical individualism', making him stand out.[88] This may well reflect Granville's earlier precarity – criticism from the *BMJ* was preferable to bankruptcy, after all – but it also puts his position on drinking into wider perspective. While this did remain consistent over several decades, it also allowed him to mark himself out as different from the medical establishment. His insistence that alcohol might be a daily requirement had commercial implications, with one observer predicting that '[society] will flock to a medical man who will not cut off their liquor, and presumably also reduce their other enjoyments, as is now the custom of most of our great doctors'.[89]

Granville became ill in 1898 and died in November 1900.[90] His life allows us to identify different medical attitudes to drinking in the 1890s. The *BMJ* was clear that alcohol was not a necessary element of diet, which meant that abstinence was not a threat to health, and the wider response to Granville's sally suggests that his opinion was a marginal one by this point. However, his popular medical writing and flirtation with quackery indicates that he may have felt that the market, rather than the *BMJ*, was best placed to answer this question. Even though he was a Fellow of the Royal Statistical Society, Granville also rejected statistical reasoning as a way of knowing alcohol. The controversy he stirred up in 1891 allows us to see the different positions taken by those in and beyond medicine with regard to the drink question, but it was also good marketing for Granville's practice as a society doctor who allowed patients to continue their drinking.

Conclusions: Twentieth-century acceptance and scepticism

Granville's argument may have been unusual by the 1890s, but moderate drinking was still being defended by elite doctors. Sir Dyce Duckworth startled delegates at the Fourth International Congress on the Abuse of Alcohol at The Hague in 1893 by telling them that he thought that 'a moderate consumption of alcoholic liquid taken with other food' was not harmful to health, defining moderation as one or one and a half ounces of alcohol. The audience was largely but not entirely committed to total abstinence. Duckworth finished by saying that 'he offered no apology for statements which controverted much teaching now prevalent', and insisted that alcohol was a food, 'whatever the physiologists might say to the contrary'. He was hissed as he left the stage.[91] While it seems likely that many doctors would have agreed with Duckworth, given that Anstie's limit was still being discussed in the twentieth century, this opinion opposed the temperance argument that moderation was harmful.

Duckworth was physician and lecturer in medicine at Barts, and physician to the Prince of Wales, holding a number of senior positions at the Royal College of Physicians; he was knighted in 1886 and would become a baronet in 1909.[92] Another gout specialist, he had made his opposition to total abstinence clear in 1877 and remained convinced that alcohol in moderation could be safe or even healthy; it was reported that he claimed that abstinence was not suitable for everyone, and Duckworth was one of the doctors who signed the 1907 medical declaration supporting the use of alcohol as medicine.[93] For Duckworth drinking was really only a problem as either a public nuisance or a form of insanity afflicting a minority, and should be treated accordingly. He had called for corporal punishment for occasional drunkenness and the loss of the right to vote for repeat offenders, though he did later support the UK Alliance's Local Option scheme.[94] Interestingly his brother, Canon Robinson Duckworth, supported the temperance work of Dr Norman Kerr, who was one of his parishioners at St Mark's church, Maida Vale.[95] Dyce Duckworth's opinion on the drink question was complicated, in other words; he was keen to keep it in the doctor's inventory and rejected temperance attacks on moderate drinking, but was also prepared to support moderate temperance efforts, and, in time, the Alliance.

What is telling here, though, is Duckworth's emphasis on the *evidence* available to those who were trying to decide what to do about drinking. He cautioned against physiological studies that undermined the arts of prognosis, telling the annual meeting of the British Medical Association in 1896 that 'we must, if we are to be great in medicine, sometimes lift our eyes from the microscope, and away from the engrossing researches of the laboratories'.[96] He made a similar argument in 1909, saying, 'I greatly fear that [in listening to laboratory experts] we run the risk of crowding out a good deal of soundly acquired, and proved experience … and of becoming medical scientists rather than expert medical practitioners.'[97] At the Hague in 1893 Duckworth had also been challenged by speakers drawing on other forms of evidence. Joseph Malins, head of the Good Templars teetotal fraternal society, asked Duckworth to 'name any hospital other than the London Temperance Hospital that had a larger percentage of recoveries from diseases of every kind and from operations of the most dangerous character?' Malins also noted that he would pay cheaper life and accident insurance premiums than a moderate drinker like Duckworth, which might have sounded strange to delegates unfamiliar with British arguments that alcohol could be assessed through these other forms of evidence.[98]

Duckworth was quite closely connected to life assurance, however, advising three different companies. Addressing the Life Assurance Medical Officers' Association as their president in 1904, he insisted that drink could be beneficial, stating that 'no statistics should shake our convictions or efface our carefully gathered experience in regard to this matter. They will most certainly not shake mine'.[99] An anonymous correspondent in the *Journal of the American Medical Association* had criticized an earlier version of Duckworth's argument, noting that 'the weak point in his argument is that he offers nothing but his own authority for all he says, and bases his opinion only on his personal general observation and experience'.[100]

In the 1890s and 1910s a range of medical opinions about the risks of drinking existed in Britain, informed by and informing work in Europe and North America. If a spectrum of opinion can be imagined, stretching between complete opposition to medical support for drinking at one end and complete tolerance at the other, then Granville's position would be closer to the tolerant end; abstinence could be dangerous, and drinking daily, but moderately, was recommended to most adults. While it was less consistent, Duckworth's position was broadly tolerant, though closer to the centre than Granville. Anstie might have been placed between Duckworth and the centre, as he argued that drink was safe until the Limit was reached. A middle point, represented by the *British Medical Journal*'s response to Granville, might be described as remaining convinced of the healthfulness of both total abstinence *and* moderate consumption, the latter defined by Anstie's Limit. It is impossible to establish what Barlow's position might have been, but the staff of the Temperance Hospital and other members of the Medical Temperance Association were clearly at the end of the spectrum opposed to alcohol's use in medicine or diet.

As we have seen, doctors involved with life assurance could hold very different opinions about alcohol, but if the firms that employed them had been doctors, they might have been located somewhere between complete opposition and the *BMJ*'s halfway point. The North American actuarial investigation showed that lives assured by firms who used a liberal definition of 'moderate consumption' suffered greater mortality than those who were conservative in that definition, but also that the 'liberal' definition was far more commonly used. Firms using that definition were perhaps close to the centre, while those with a more 'conservative' interpretation were closer to temperance. The UKT would of course also be somewhere between the opposition end and the more conservative American firms.

While a sketch of this spectrum of opinions is helpful in reminding us that there was no single medical response to temperance, or even a division into 'temperance' and 'mainstream' medical camps, it needs to also consider the kind of work these positions depended upon, and the forms of evidence and argumentation they employed. These questions of method and argument do not neatly map onto tolerance or suspicion, but they are suggestive. The 'tolerant' end of the spectrum was much more closely associated with the gentlemanly style of Duckworth, but Granville's attempts to carve a niche for himself saw him explore physiological and experimental work, complicating that assessment. The 'oppositional' position was more likely to be inspired by physiological work, the data produced by life assurance and the GRO, or both. It is also worth pointing out that the 'tolerant' position on drinking was strongly conservative politically; Duckworth's writing on social questions criticized socialism, women's employment and the abandonment of the cane in schools.[101]

All of this suggests two things: first, that life assurance definitions of the risks of drinking tended, perhaps unsurprisingly, to be more cautious than those of many doctors, and second, that these firms played some role in encouraging medical caution about alcohol, along with the experimental research of Anstie, Parkes and others. The combination of those two developments, drawing on forms of research, evidence and reasoning alien to the gentlemanly style of medicine practiced by Duckworth, further sharpened the attention of life assurance firms to the quantity of alcohol consumed by moderate drinkers who sought policies with them.

At the turn of the century, medicine was no longer so obviously 'averse to the promulgation of total abstinence principles, and in favour of the use of alcoholic liquors as beverages', as Peter Winskill had described earlier attitudes.[102] At the same time moderation had become more acceptable, or perhaps defensible, as a result of Anstie's work, and this had been influential within life assurance as well as medicine. For firms with Abstainers' sections, like the UKT and Sceptre, this was a mixed blessing. It is hard to imagine an abstainer being refused assurance in the 1890s, unless they were suspected of being a reformed drunkard. At the same time, though, while assurance experience showed that abstainers lived longer, a stronger case was now being made for moderate drinking – a much less appealing development.

Chapter 9 explores the working out of these trends in the first decades of the twentieth century, complicated somewhat by the rise of new questions, like those associated with the eugenics movement, but still returning to this more clearly defined opposition between moderate drinking and total abstinence. In time this would become the 'new moderationism', which defined twentieth-century attempts to regulate alcohol. Arguably temperance life assurance played a role in developing that consensus.

Notes

1. 'Medical Testimonial against Spirits in Medicine', *British and Foreign Temperance Society, Sixth Report*, appendix, 24, Livesey Collection.
2. Medical declaration, Cheltenham, 112. Report from the Select Committee on Inquiry into Drunkenness, with minutes of evidence, and appendix, 1834, House of Commons Papers, 1834 (559). Boisragon in George Arthur Cardew, *Echoes and Reminiscences of Medical Practitioners in Cheltenham of the Nineteenth Century* (Cheltenham: E. J. Burrow, 1906), 42.
3. Burns, *Temperance History*, vol. 1, 127.
4. Winskill, *Temperance Movement*, vol. 1, 254; *Standard Bearers*, 94; Burns, *Temperance History*, 212.
5. Winskill, *Temperance Movement*, vol. 2, 172.
6. 'Medical Declaration Respecting Alcohol', *British Medical Journal* 2, 573 (23 December 1871).
7. Thomas McCall Anderson, Alfred G. Barrs, William H. Bennett, James Crichton-Browne, W. E. Dixon, Dyce Duckworth, Thomas R. Fraser, T. R. Glynn, W. R. Gowers, W. D. Halliburton, Jonathan Hutchinson, Robert Hutchinson, Edmund Owen, P. H.

Pye-Smith, Fred. T. Roberts and Edgcombe Venning, 'The Use of Alcoholic Beverages', *The Lancet* 169, 4361 (30 March 1907).
8. David N. Livingstone, *Putting Science in Its Place: Geographies of Scientific Knowledge* (Chicago: University of Chicago Press, 2003), and see Graham Mooney, 'Diagnostic Spaces: Workhouse, Hospital, and Home in Mid-Victorian London', *Social Science History* 33, 3 (2009), 357–90.
9. Alborn, *Regulated Lives*, 239–41; 'Statistics. Medical Examinations in Scotland for Life Assurance Companies', *Edinburgh Medical Journal* 1, 6 (1855), 553, 554.
10. Marguerite W. Dupree, 'Other than Healing: Medical Practitioners and the Business of Life Assurance during the Nineteenth and Early Twentieth Centuries', *Social History of Medicine* 10, 1 (1997), 102; M. Jeanne Peterson, *The Medical Profession in Mid-Victorian London* (Berkeley: University of California Press, 1978), 253.
11. Board meetings, 3 November 1843; #1025, 3 September 1848; #1036, 6 October 1848, UKT Minute Book 1, Aviva Archives.
12. 1872 (7th Annual Report), Reports of Directors to Annual Meetings of Shareholders, 1872, 1886–90, 1903–4, 1914–17, SC 1/8/1/1 London Archives.
13. Joanne Woiak, '"A Medical Cromwell to Depose King Alcohol": Medical Scientists, Temperance Reformers, and the Alcohol Problem in Britain', *Social History* 54 (1994), 337–65; Cheryl L. Krasnick, '"Because There Is Pain": Alcoholism, Temperance and the Victorian Physician', *Canadian Bulletin of Medical History/Bulletin canadien; histoire de la meďecine* 2 (1985), 1–22.
14. Sarah. E. Williams, 'The Use of Beverage Alcohol as Medicine, 1790–1860', *Journal of Studies on Alcohol* 41, 5 (1980), 562.
15. Harrison, *Drink*, 354, emphasis added.
16. Jean-Charles Sournia, *A History of Alcoholism*, trans. Nick Hindley and Gareth Stanton (Oxford: Basil Blackwell, 1990), 25.
17. Clipping, *Temperance Record*, 31 May 1884, n.p., in Minute Book Two, National Temperance Hospital Board of Management Minutes 1885–8, MS NTH/1/1, University College London Hospital Archives.
18. First Annual Report of the London Temperance Hospital, National Temperance Hospital Annual Reports, 1874–84, 2, 18–30, MS NTH/11/1 UCLH, University College London Hospital Archives.
19. Niall McCrae, 'The Beer Ration in Victorian Asylums', *History of Psychiatry* 15, 2 (2004), 155–75.
20. J. James Ridge, 'Medical Declarations re Alcohol', *British Medical Journal* 1 (1888), 1033.
21. Winskill, *Temperance Movement*, vol. 4, 6.
22. 'Laying of the Memorial Stone of the New Hospital Building', Sixth Annual Report of the London Temperance Hospital, 1879, 38–9, National Temperance Hospital Annual Reports, 1874–84, MS NTH/1/1, University College London Hospital Archives.
23. Cutting, 'Opening of the London Temperance Hospital', *London Mirror*, 11 October 1873, 235, in Minute Book One, National Temperance Hospital Board of Management Minutes 1873–85, MS NTH/1/1, University College London Hospital Archives.
24. *Fun*, 14 June 1873, 252.
25. Moinet, *Guide to Medical Examination*, 50.
26. Edward Henry Sieveking, *The Medical Adviser in Life Insurance*, second edition (London: J & A Churchill, 1882), 66, emphasis added; 62, 110, 111.
27. Pollock and Chisholm, *Medical Handbook*, 61, original emphasis; 65, 163, 66.
28. Sieveking, *Medical Advisor*, 68, 116.

29. Alborn, *Regulated Lives*, 225.
30. Neison, *Vital Statistics*, 201–29.
31. Edmund Parkes, *Manual of Practical Hygiene*, first edition (London: John Churchill and Sons, 1864), 229.
32. Edmund Parkes, *On Personal Care of Health* (London: Society for Promoting Christian Knowledge, 1876), 63–5; Parkes, *Manual of Practical Hygiene*, eighth edition (London: J. A. Churchill, 1891), 333.
33. Francis Anstie, 'Alcohol. Is It Food, Medicine, or Poison?', *Cornhill Magazine* 5, (1862), 713; Francis Anstie, *On the Uses of Wines in Health and Disease* (New York: J. S. Redfield, 1870), 12.
34. See, for example, Edmund Parkes and Cyprian Wollowicz, 'Experiments on the Effect of Alcohol (Ethyl Alcohol) on the Human Body', *Proceedings of the Royal Society London* 18 (1869–70), 362–93.
35. Parkes, *Personal Care*, 63.
36. Lawrence, 'Incommunicable Knowledge', 505.
37. Samuel E. D. Shortt, 'Physicians, Science, and Status: Issues in the Professionalization of Anglo-American Medicine in the Nineteenth Century', *Medical History* 27, 1 (1983), 51–63; Gerald Geison, *Michael Foster and the Cambridge School of Physiology: The Scientific Enterprise in Late Victorian Society* (Princeton, NJ: Princeton University Press, 1978).
38. Lawrence, 'Incommunicable Knowledge', 504.
39. Dyce Duckworth, 'An Address on Collective Investigation of Disease', *British Medical Journal* 1, 1201 (5 January 1884), 4.
40. William Howship Dickinson, 'Alcohol as a Cause of Renal Disease', *British Medical Journal* 2, 621 (23 November 1872), 572–5.
41. 'The Morbid Effects of Alcohol', *British Medical Journal* 2, 621 (23 November 1872), cited 583.
42. Ibid., 584.
43. William Howship Dickinson, 'The Morbid Effects of Alcohol', *British Medical Journal* 2, 622 (30 November 1872), 605.
44. Lawrence, 'Incommunicable Knowledge', 510.
45. Richard Aspin, 'Barlow, Sir Thomas, First Baronet (1845–1945)', *Oxford Dictionary of National Biography* (Oxford University Press, 2004), www.oxforddnb.com/view/article/30595, accessed 5 February 2013; Anon., 'Obituary: Sir Thomas Barlow', *Manchester Guardian*, 16 January 1945, 3; T. R. Elliott, 'Thomas Barlow. 1845–1945', *Obituary Notices of Fellows of the Royal Society* 5, 14 (1945), 158–67.
46. Fox, testimonial (1877), Testimonials, Thomas Barlow Letters, MS BAR/K33, Wellcome Library Special Collections.
47. James Reid to Barlow, 30 May 1896, original emphasis, Professional and other correspondence, Thomas Barlow Letters, MS C/107b, Wellcome Library Special Collections.
48. Elliott, 'Thomas Barlow', 166.
49. Letter from Grosvenor, Duke of Westminster, 6 December 1896, Professional and other correspondence, Thomas Barlow Letters, MS C/129, Wellcome Library Special Collections.
50. Withers, *Pioneers of Life Assurance*, 93.
51. Mitchell's letters survive in Barlow's archive, Joseph T. Mitchell to Thomas Cash, 7 and 16 February 1876, Testimonials, Thomas Barlow Letters, MS BAR/K/23, BAR/K/27, Wellcome Library Special Collections.

52. Printed booklet, 'Testimonials in Support of the Candidature of Dr Thomas Barlow, for the Post of Assistant-Physician to the London Hospital', February–July 1877, Testimonials, Thomas Barlow Letters, MS BAR/K34, Wellcome Library Special Collections.
53. James Barlow to Thomas Cash, 23 February 1876, Testimonials, Thomas Barlow Letters, MS BAR/K/28, Wellcome Library Special Collections.
54. 'In Memoriam: Francis Anstie', 427, and 'Obituary: Francis Anstie', 433–4, *The Lancet* 104, 2664 (19 September 1874); Arthur D. Baldwin, 'Anstie's Alcohol Limit. Francis Anstie 1833–1874', *American Journal of Public Health* 67, 7 (1977), 679–81; M. P. Earles, 'Anstie, Francis Edmund (1833–1874)', *Oxford Dictionary of National Biography* (Oxford University Press, 2004), www.oxforddnb.com/view/article/583, accessed 12 August 2013.
55. Anon., 'Poor-Law Medical Officers' Association and the Late Dr. Anstie', *The Lancet* 104, 2668 (17 October 1874), 568–9; E. Moberly Bell, *Storming the Citadel: The Rise of the Woman Doctor* (London: Constable, 1953).
56. Anstie, 'Alcohol' and 'Does Alcohol act as Food?' *Cornhill Magazine* 6 (1862), 319–29.
57. Ibid., 329.
58. Francis Anstie, *Stimulants and Narcotics, Their Mutual Relations: With Special Researches on the Action of Alcohol, Aether, and Chloroform, on the Vital Organism* (London: Macmillan, 1864).
59. Francis Anstie, 'On the Physiological and Therapeutical Action of Alcohol', *The Lancet* 86, 2195 (23 September 1865), 344. This was later summarized in Anstie, 'Final Experiments on the Elimination of Alcohol by the Body', *Practitioner* 13 (1874).
60. Francis Anstie, 'On the Diurnal Fluctuations of the Pulse-Form, and on Certain Cautions Necessary to Be Observed in Sphygmography', *The Lancet* 68, 2267 (9 February 1867), 170–2; 'Lectures on the Prognosis and Treatment of Certain Acute Diseases, with Special Reference to the Indications Afforded by the Graphic Study of the Pulse', *The Lancet* 90, 2289 (13 July 1867), 35–6, and *The Lancet* 90, 2294 (17 August 1867), 189–91.
61. Anstie, *On the Uses of Wines*, 12.
62. For more on responses to this work see James Kneale and Shaun French, 'Moderate Drinking before the Unit: Medicine and Life Assurance in Britain and the US c.1860–1930', *Drugs: Education, Prevention and Policy* 22, 2 (2015), 111–17.
63. J. S. Billings, C. W. Eliot, H. W. Fortune, J. L. Greene and F. G. Peabody, *The Liquor Problem. A Summary of Investigations Conducted by the Committee of Fifty 1893–1903* (Boston: Houghton Mifflin, 1905), 32.
64. Levine, 'The Committee of Fifty'.
65. Pollock and Chisholm, *Medical Handbook*, 65.
66. Jonathan Adams Allen, *Medical Examinations for Life Insurance*, sixth edition (New York: J H and C M Goodsell, 1870), 162; Edward Mansfield Brockbank, *Life Insurance and General Practice* (London: Henry Frowde, Hodder and Stoughton, 1908), 181.
67. James Paterson MacLaren, *Medical Insurance Examination: Modern Methods and Rating of Lives, for Medical Practitioners, and Insurance Officials* (London: Baillière, Tindall and Cox, 1927), 157, original emphasis.
68. Arthur Hunter, 'The Medico-Actuarial Investigation of the Mortality of American and Canadian Life Assurance Companies', *Journal of the Institute of Actuaries* 48, 2 (1914), 190.

69. Arthur Hunter and Oscar H. Rogers, 'Ratings for the Principal Impairments', *Proceedings of the Association of Life Insurance Medical Directors of America* 8 (1922), 167.
70. Eugene Lyman Fisk, *Alcohol: Its Relation to Human Efficiency and Longevity* (New York: Funk and Wagnalls, 1917), 21, emphasis added.
71. Francis Anstie, 'The Medical Declaration Respecting Alcohol', *The Lancet* 98, 2522 (30 December 1871), 931; Francis Anstie, 'The Medical Declaration Respecting Alcohol', *The Practitioner* 8 (January 1872), 45–8; Letter from Dr Parkes, re 'The Medical Declaration Respecting Alcohol', *The Practitioner* 8, February 1872; Anstie, 'Final Experiments', 15–28.
72. See James Kneale, 'Dr Granville's Thunderbolt: Drink and the Public in the Life of One Nineteenth-Century Doctor', *Social History of Alcohol and Drugs* 28, 2 (2014), 120–42.
73. Joseph Mortimer Granville, *Nerve-Vibration and Excitation as Agents in the Treatment of Functional Disorder and Organic Disease* (London: J. & A. Churchill, 1883) and *Gout in Its Clinical Aspects: An Outline of the Disease and Its Treatment for Practitioners* (London: J. & A. Churchill, 1885); Frederic Boase, *Modern English Biography*, vol. 5 (1912, reproduced London: Frank Cass, 1965).
74. Joseph Mortimer Granville, 'Drinking and Drunkenness', *The Times*, 15 September 1891, 8.
75. 'Drinking and Drunkenness', *British Medical Journal* 2, 1604 (26 September 1891), 702.
76. JosephMortimer Granville, 'Drink: Ethical Considerations, and Physiological', *National Review* 18, 104 (1891), 164.
77. Granville, 'Drink', 166.
78. Ibid., 167.
79. Ibid., 169.
80. Granville, *Gout*, vi.
81. *Birmingham Daily Post*, 23 November 1893, 5.
82. Anne Digby, *Making a Medical Living: Doctors and Patients in the English Market for Medicine, 1720–1911* (Cambridge: Cambridge University Press, 1994).
83. Granville, *Nerve-Vibration*, 15, 18.
84. Joseph Mortimer Granville, 'Worry', *Nineteenth Century* 10, 55 (1881), 423–9; Joseph Mortimer Granville, 'Fish as Food and Physic', *Good Words* 22 (1881), 676–7.
85. Joseph Mortimer Granville, *Common Mind Troubles* (London: David Bogue, 1878); *Minds and Moods: Gossiping Papers on Mind-Management and Morals* (London: Renshaw, 1878); 'Nightcaps', *Huddersfield Daily Chronicle*, 12 December 1883, 4; 'Seasonable Wish', *Moonshine*, 12 January 1884, 24.
86. *The Leeds Times*, 3 October 1891, 7.
87. *The Blackburn Standard*, 20 March 1886, 1.
88. Peterson, *Medical Profession*, 253–8.
89. *Devon and Exeter Daily Gazette*, 19 September 1891, 5.
90. *Morning Post*, 13 June 1898, 7; and 27 November 1900, 2.
91. 'Congress about Alcohol. Attitude Taken by the Doctors. Extraordinary Debate', *Auckland Star* 24, 250 (21 October 1893), 4; 'An Anti-Alcohol Congress. Extraordinary Debate', *Birmingham Daily Post*, 17 August 1893, 8.
92. A. E. Garrod, 'Duckworth, Sir Dyce, First Baronet (1840–1928)', rev. Patrick Wallis, *Oxford Dictionary of National Biography* (Oxford University Press, 2004), www.oxforddnb.com/view/article/32912, accessed 27 July 2012.

93. Dyce Duckworth, 'On the Medical Injunction of Stimulants in Disease and in Health', *British Medical Journal* 2, 880 (10 November 1877), 660–2; 'Moderate Drinking and Total Abstinence', *Journal of the American Medical Association* 37, 21 (1901), 1396; Anderson, 'The Use of Alcoholic Beverages'.
94. Anon., 'A Novel Punishment for Drunkards', *Manchester Guardian*, 14 August 1891, 6; Dyce Duckworth, *Views on Some Social Subjects* (London: George Allen & Unwin, 1915).
95. 'Temperance Notes and News', *Quiver* 908 (January 1902), 207.
96. Dyce Duckworth, 'Address in Medicine. The Prognosis of Disease', *British Medical Journal* 2, 1857 (1 August 1896), 251.
97. Dyce Duckworth, 'An Address on Some Insufficiently Recognized Points in the Diagnosis of Disease', *British Medical Journal* 1, 2516 (20 March 1909), 701.
98. 'The Anti-Alcohol Congress', *Leeds Mercury*, 17 August 1893, 8.
99. Dyce Duckworth, 'Some Observations on Medical Examinations for Life Assurance: Being the Presidential Address Delivered before the Life Assurance Medical Officers' Association on January 27th, 1904', *The Lancet* 163, 4197 (6 February 1904), 356.
100. 'Moderate Drinking', *Journal of the American Medical Association.*
101. *The Western Times*, 2 July 1894, 4; *Hull Daily Mail*, 20 March 1928, 5; Duckworth, *Social Subjects.*
102. Winskill, *Temperance Movement*, vol. 4, 1.

Part 4

Conclusions

9

Temperance life assurance and the new moderationism

Introduction: The 'new moderationism'

An emphasis on prohibition has encouraged historians to date the end of the temperance movement from the end of the First World War. This final chapter will suggest, instead, that this period represents not the end, but the beginning of a new way of thinking about alcohol and temperance – one that perhaps had its origins in temperance life assurance.

The problems that made up the 'drink question' had certainly changed profoundly since the 1840s. Per capita alcohol consumption and the number of both drinking places and arrests for drunkenness all fell steadily from the 1890s, and consumption would not rise again until after the Second World War.[1] Temperance now enjoyed the support of the Church of England Temperance Society (CETS) and Wesleyan Methodism. Women were more active and visible in temperance work, including aristocratic leaders like Rosalind Howard, Countess of Carlisle, Lady Isabella Somerset and Lady Elizabeth Biddulph, a sign of the growing respectability of the movement.[2] They were joined by women doctors like Mary Darby Sturge and by Nancy Astor, the first woman MP to take her seat.

These developments reflected, in part, the fortunes of the Alliance's campaign after the Peel Commission had explored alternative solutions to Local Option in the 1890s. As David Fahey put it, 'though Lord Peel's Report promised the Veto in the future, it focused on reduction [of licences] in the present'.[3] In the first decade of the new century proposals for licensing reform remained divisive, but there was a growing acceptance in Parliament of the desirability of reducing licences, a feeling shared by Conservative ministers ready to contribute to the cause of 'reasonable temperance' and magistrates prepared to use the 1891 legal ruling of Sharp *vs.* Wakefield to close pubs.[4] Encouraged by wartime controls, the trade developed the 'improved' pub in response to these pressures.[5]

Anglophone life assurance and medicine also seemed to have reached a broad consensus by the beginning of the new century. As the American teetotalers John Woolley and William 'Pussyfoot' Johnson put it:

> The insurance men of to-day are in agreement with the medical profession as to the effects of the use of alcohol and of abstinence therefrom. The medical men have reached their conclusions by investigation and experiment in individual cases and by scientific reasoning; the insurance men by the simpler method of statistics. Since the statistics used are unimpeachably correct, the endorsement of the medical theories by the insurance men is a valuable confirmation.[6]

Woolley and Johnson may have exaggerated the strength of the 'agreement' between assurance and medicine – not least over what constituted moderate use – but the convergence of work in physiology, the 'unimpeachable' statistics of life assurance, and the prior convictions of teetotalers suggested something like a triangulation of research on alcohol. Perhaps the high point of the UKT's influence in Britain was reached in 1904, when its experience informed not only the reports of the Inter-Departmental Committee on Physical Deterioration, which was concerned about the effects of alcohol on public health, but also the content of a syllabus of temperance lessons for teachers in public elementary schools.[7] It's not clear how extensive or influential this was, but it suggests support for the conclusions drawn by the UKT.

However, the first decades of the twentieth century also saw the rise of what Joanne Woiak called 'the New Moderationist paradigm' in alcohol research and policy.[8] The shift towards a more positive attitude towards moderate drinking was shaped by the Central Control Board (Liquor Traffic), established in 1915 to manage wartime alcohol production and consumption. The far-reaching powers of the CCB and success in minimizing the disruptive effects of drinking on wartime industry and public order offered an alternative to prohibition or nationalization of the drink industry, both of which had been considered by the wartime government. While the CCB did not speak with one voice and was criticized by both temperance and the trade, it encouraged a new approach to the sale of drink in Britain, from 'improved' drinking places to shorter opening hours.

Woiak argues that post-war medical research in Britain approached the study of alcohol 'with the express intent of supporting certain proven state alcohol policies'; the results 'provided a clear scientific justification for the continuation and extension of the successful wartime measures'.[9] While wartime necessity was clearly significant, some within temperance were already sympathetic to arguments for alternatives to Local Option – the Wesleyan minister Henry Carter, a member of the CCB, supported 'constructive' reforms that provided alternatives to the pub and resisted calls for prohibition, for example. As a result, it is only possible to support Woiak's argument that this 'new moderationism' represented 'a clean break with the ideology of the temperance movement' if we take that movement to exclude men like Carter – in other words to continue to equate 'temperance' with 'prohibition'.[10] It seems more likely, as Ryosuke Yokoe has recently argued, that this new moderationism 'pacified the divisions between the temperance movement and the Trade through the idea that alcohol was both harmless and harmful depending on how it was consumed'.[11]

This concluding chapter examines temperance life assurance in this early twentieth-century context. These decades saw some qualification of the claims made for abstinence by the experience of the UKT and other firms, while moderate drinking was judged to be safe for most people. On the other hand, the style of reasoning used by these firms, and the forms of evidence produced to support their arguments, became increasingly dominant through the twentieth century and remain important in Britain today. Rather than marking the end of temperance this period represents the beginning of a new way of thinking about alcohol, one that remains influential today. The first part of the chapter examines three reports issued in the first three decades of the twentieth century: the CCB's 1918 report, and two more bracketing it in 1910 and 1926. Statistical reasoning became increasingly important, though this was framed by new perspectives and suggested new conclusions. The second part of the conclusion summarizes the book's arguments and provides an assessment of temperance life assurance over the period 1840–1918 and a conclusion.

Moderation and the CCB

Between 1915 and 1921 control over drink and drinking places was placed in the hands of the Central Control Board (Liquor Traffic). In 1918 the board's Advisory Committee published a 'review of the existing state of scientific knowledge regarding the action of alcohol on the human organism'.[12] The Committee was comprised of two men from the CCB, its chair Lord D'Abernon and Sir George Newman, Principal Medical Officer to the Board of Education, plus experts in physiology, pharmacology, psychiatry, psychology and medical statistics. The report's eight chapters reviewed the current state of medical thinking on eight topics. While the first seven were informed by 'direct experimental, pathological or clinical researches', the last, 'Alcohol and Longevity', was different. The report explained that the relationship between alcohol and sociological or economic problems 'can rarely be subjected to the process of isolation and intensive study which is the essence of experimental science. Hence arises the appeal to other kinds of evidence. In popular discussions a good deal of use has, for instance, been made of statistics', acknowledging that life assurance companies, and particularly the UKT, had been 'partially successful' in collecting useful records.[13]

The board considered three sources of evidence: the UKT's records from 1848 to 1901, the statistics of the General Register Office and the Prudential on the mortality of those employed in the licensed trade, and F. G. P. Neison's 1889 report comparing the Rechabites to non-abstaining friendly societies. The UKT's records showed that 26.4 per cent fewer deaths occurred amongst male abstainers with whole life policies than would have been expected if they had died at the rate experienced by lives in the General section. The General section did not contain 'bad' lives, but its average moderate drinker was expected to die three and a half years earlier than the average Abstainer. The UKT had assured far fewer women, though, and the difference in mortality between the sections was only 3 per cent.[14]

While these results seemed clear enough, the interpretation required more attention, the report suggesting 'it would not be scientific to attribute the result solely to the fact of abstinence from alcohol without further analysis'.[15] Questions of selection had to be considered. The UKT's argument in favour of abstinence assumed that there was only one difference between their two sections. At the start of the century Sir

Thomas P. Whittaker described the UK's abstainers and moderate drinkers in this way: 'When we see these men ... no one could detect any difference between them in appearance. They live in the same towns, are engaged in the same occupations, have similar incomes, and, *with the exception that one class abstains and the other does not*, there is no difference whatever between them.'[16]

This argument could be challenged, though. In 1891 T. E. Young, a vice-president of the Institute of Actuaries, cast doubt on the value of Sceptre's records as proof of their abstainers' longevity, suggesting that they 'live long, not because they abstain, but because, on the whole, they possess a more than usually prudential, self-preserving, and moderate nature, of which the feature of abstinence is simply a manifestation in one special form'.[17] Young doubted that abstinence alone could explain their greater longevity; temperance life assurance could not establish a *general* relationship between abstinence and longevity. The author of the *British Medical Journal*'s dismissal of Granville's 'thoughtless and inaccurate' letter (Chapter 8) had made a similar point; while the research of Drysdale had made persuasive use of temperance life assurance experience, the abstainers assured by those companies 'are prudent, self-controlled people, and their life expectation is likely to be longer because they have a tendency to regulate their lives in everything with wisdom and moderation'.[18]

The CCB's Committee made similar comments about the UKT's experience. The report confirmed that abstainers assured by temperance life offices lived longer than their moderate drinkers. However, it went on to note that while adopting a practice of abstinence in order to lengthen life might be 'a sound rule of conduct', it could not be considered 'a scientifically established conclusion', because it was impossible to isolate abstinence as the sole cause of longer life.[19] Worse, the Committee concluded that 'the temperate consumption of alcoholic liquors ... may be considered to be physiologically harmless in the case of the large majority of normal adults', with a few minor caveats. No definition of a safe limit was offered, though toxic doses were quantified. At the same time the report was equally clear that 'it is certainly true that alcoholic beverages are in no way necessary for healthy life' and in fact 'are harmful or dangerous if the above-mentioned precautions are not observed'.[20]

The Advisory Committee's report did not seem to provoke much comment, though it had been intended to be a popular, one-shilling introduction to the scientific aspects of the drink question. *The Times* noted that many of the questions raised in the report's introduction were left unanswered; the *Western Times* wondered if it had been worth printing.[21] The report was reissued in 1924 by the Medical Research Council and again in 1939.

Still, the report is significant, for a number of reasons. First, its conclusions were clearly not far from the 'mainstream' position of the 1890s identified in Chapter 8, acknowledging the safety of both total abstinence and moderate drinking. Second, the UKT's experience was the most important source of evidence assessed in the chapter on longevity. That is important, as Yokoe has shown, because the report anticipated much of what was to come in alcohol research through the twentieth century: a strengthening focus on the safety or otherwise of both abstinence and moderate drinking, and the increasing importance of statistical work as the methodology best suited to answer those questions. This reflected the growing significance of these questions as matters for state action, first in educating citizens as to how to proceed in terms of consuming alcohol, and second in setting out how the state might assess this problem. In both cases life assurance, and its temperance variations, might be said to have served as an initial guide.

We now turn to two other reports, published eight years before and eight years after the CCB's, to develop our understanding of this new focus on moderation in two main ways. The first is the growing significance of statistical, epidemiological work, and the second is the political context and consequences of these trends, which were rather different to those of the UKT.

Moderation and eugenics

In the early years of the twentieth century statistical research played an important role in the study of alcohol, as researchers concerned with health, epidemiology and sanitation turned to increasingly sophisticated forms of statistical analysis. Research on the effects of drinking on childhood health conducted at the Francis Galton Laboratory for National Eugenics at University College London offers a good example. In 1910 Ethel Elderton and Karl Pearson published a report concluding that the children of 'alcoholic parents' – by which they meant drinkers, not 'addicts' – were taller and stronger than those of abstainers.[22] Pearson, one of Francis Galton's protégés, would become head of UCL's Department of Applied Statistics and director of both the Biometric and Galton Laboratories on Galton's death in 1911.[23] Elderton, a gifted mathematician, had been Galton's assistant since 1905, becoming Galton Fellow and then Assistant Professor in the Galton Laboratory until 1933.[24] The 1910 study examined the relationship between parental drinking and the health of 'defective' children, using two samples from Edinburgh and Manchester, presenting a good example of the working methods of Pearson's laboratories. Elderton and Pearson concluded that heredity was far more important than environment, though they were probably lead, as Lyndsay Farrall suggests, by their pre-existing convictions.[25]

Theories of heredity and medical and social 'degeneration' predated eugenics, and the idea that alcoholism – understood as both 'harm' and, as the disease theory of alcoholism became more popular, 'addiction' – might be inherited could be found in scientific and commonsense understandings of the effects of drinking.[26] The implications of this were not clear, however. Norman Kerr, the president of the British Society for the Scientific Study of Inebriety, may have anticipated eugenicist arguments when he suggested that 'no uncured inebriate should have children' in 1888, but he did at least believe they might be cured.[27] Inheritance was commonly assumed to be an issue for life assurance, too, as medical examiners' handbooks warned from the 1860s into the twentieth century.[28] Assurers may well have been predisposed to accept this idea because they had been examining applicants' family histories since the 1840s, looking for signs of tuberculosis in particular. British actuaries became increasingly cautious of eugenic arguments, however, as Timothy Alborn has shown; after 1900, companies were prepared to accept that there might be a relationship between family history and the incidence of tuberculosis, but were not convinced that this meant the disease was inherited.[29]

Elderton and Pearson's methodological choices provoked hostility. The Cambridge economists Alfred Marshall and John Maynard Keynes criticized their sampling strategy and interpretations of correlation coefficients in *The Times* and the *Journal of the Royal Statistical Society*, for example; Pearson and Elderton's responses seized on statistical errors in this criticism.[30] Others like Victor Horsley and Mary Darby Sturge were critical of Elderton and Pearson's conclusions.[31] Horsley was a physiologist and surgeon at University College London and later at the National Hospital, Queen Square, now the National Hospital for Neurology and Neurosurgery, who adopted temperance 'on scientific grounds', as one memoir noted.[32] Mary Sturge was physician to the Birmingham and Midland Hospital for Women, having graduated from the London School of Medicine for Women before teaching at the New Hospital for Women, later the Elizabeth Garrett Anderson. A member of the Society of Friends, her great-uncle was the abolitionist, teetotaler and pacifist Joseph Sturge (Chapters 1 and 4). Horsley and Sturge's 1907 *Alcohol and the Human Body* was largely a review of physiological work, though the final chapter, written by Arthur Newsholme, later the principal medical officer of the Local Government Board under the teetotaler John Burns, drew upon the UKT's experience. The book's final conclusion was in line with the argument made by temperance life offices: 'what is commonly described as moderate drinking has a most injurious influence on health and life ... the best practice, both in the interests of health and morality, consists in the avoidance of all alcoholic drinks as a beverage'.[33] Newsholme would later speak on temperance and life assurance while lecturer at Johns Hopkins University, so it is not surprising that his views were close to those of British assurers.[34]

While Elderton and Pearson's study and the responses it provoked were not particularly influential, the focus on questions of method – experimental design, statistical analysis and interpretation – was significant. For Farrall this was a controversy *within* eugenics, which was 'at the same time a science and a social philosophy'; the study was attacked as a statement of the latter when its authors had expected a discussion of the former.[35] Keynes was also a member of the Eugenics Education Society, for example, but other members supported Elderton and Pearson. It seems equally true, however, that the statistical study *was* criticized as science – statistical and physiological – given the development of these different approaches to the study of alcohol.

A similar method and research design informed the last of the studies considered here, though this would prove to be more significant.

Moderation and the J-shaped curve

Our third study is Raymond Pearl's *Alcohol and Longevity*, published in 1926.[36] Pearl, an American biologist at Johns Hopkins, is well known in public health for the 'J-shaped curve', which suggested that those who drank little or no alcohol might live shorter lives than moderate drinkers, though mortality then increased with excessive consumption. This non-linear relationship between consumption and mortality was later confirmed by public health researchers.[37]

Framing *Alcohol* as a study of 'the effect of alcohol upon the duration of life of the individual', Pearl reviewed arguments based on insurance data under a wider heading of 'propaganda against alcohol' which simply supported pre-existing conclusions.[38] His assessment of the UKT's evidence was more positive, acknowledging that 'what the most reliable of the insurance experience has established beyond reasonable doubt is that abstainers, as a class, have a lower mortality than non-abstainers as a class'. His problem was with the General section, because it was not known how much those policyholders drank, or whether their consumption stayed unchanged over their life. If the data from the General section could not be trusted, then a valid comparison could not be made between the sections, and the conclusions which had been drawn since the 1860s 'can at the best be regarded as only suggestive of what may be the truth'.[39] Abstinence might be healthier, for this selected population at least, but the risks associated with moderate consumption were still to be established to Pearl's satisfaction.

Pearl's own analysis, using actuarial and other statistical methods, found that 'moderate steady' drinkers – who drank frequently, rather than occasionally, but in moderation – had a longer life expectancy than either abstainers or excessive drinkers. Pearl's quantification of moderate consumption matched that of the Medical Research Council's second edition of the CCB's report – a 'daily pint or two of beer, or a daily bottle of claret, or a few glasses of whiskey and soda' – though survey respondents were classed as moderate if they said that they never became intoxicated.[40] Given these definitions, Pearl's 'moderate steady' category was equally, if not more, likely to conceal excessive drinkers as those assured by the UKT, though this was not discussed. Pearl was an enthusiastic drinker himself, and Elazar Barkan concluded that 'the historian could perhaps not be blamed for evaluating the impact of Pearl's drinking habits on his conclusion as more meaningful than the eventual scientific validation'.[41] Pearl's criticisms of the limitations of life assurance records also applied to his own research design, in other words.

Returning to questions of context, it is worth noting that Pearl's political convictions were similar to Pearson's. The two were friends, Pearl studying biometrics at UCL in 1905–6, and Pearl's earlier work cited Elderton and Pearson's 1910 report. Shortly after the publication of *Alcohol*, Pearl began to publicly criticize eugenics for its cruder expressions of class and race prejudice, which he felt would harm the status of eugenics as a science. However, Barkan notes 'his earlier wholehearted support for eugenics did not fundamentally change', informing racist and antisemitic views expressed in private, and Margo Peyton has argued that Pearl's interpretation of differences in the prevalence of cancers between white and Black Baltimoreans was shaped by white supremacist ideas of biological difference.[42]

Pearl's *Alcohol* was published during Prohibition, and its influence grew after Repeal, when a broad consensus about the safety of moderate drinking began to develop in the US and Britain. Statistical work was important to this consensus, and life assurance remained relevant to the debate, with the UKT's experience examined by the CCB and Pearl. The 'new moderation' was also appealing to the British state, as an extension of wartime controls, and to US federal and state governments after Prohibition. In the UK in particular it also followed the downward trend in per capita alcohol consumption. The publication of Pearl's work provided support for moderation from a different direction, as abstinence was once again questioned. While some late twentieth-century doctors recommended a daily glass of red wine as protection from heart disease, this was not quite the same as the marginal position adopted by Granville in the 1890s; still, it ran counter to the arguments of the UKT and of temperance more generally. Encouraged by this suspicion of abstinence and the acceptance of moderation, the question for the twentieth century would be: how much drink is enough and how much is too much? As Vance Thompson put it in 1915, 'you may have met this important person, the moderate drinker. In the discussion of the good and ill of alcohol, no one is more conspicuous. A library of books has been written about him. He is the whetstone of every argument'.[43] The moderate drinker would only grow in importance after 1918.

Temperance lives: A summary

The archives of temperance life assurance firms demonstrate that ordinary temperance institutions, lives, ideas and material things were not always or only part of the political campaigns of groups like the UK Alliance or the 'crusades' of Christian reformers. They indicate that the ideas of reform that animated these firms, societies, and individuals may not have been moral or evangelical, including instead self-improvement, the desire to tame an uncertain future, or virtuous investment. Some of the individuals and groups who engaged with these institutions also had links to Radical and progressive initiatives which are not always mentioned in contemporary assessments of the wider movement. These connections are less surprising in the early days of the movement, animated by Chartism and Reform and inheriting some of the energies of Abolition, but they are also there at the end of the period covered by this book in the teetotal conscientious objectors of Huddersfield and elsewhere who lost their liberty during the War. Wartime patriotism had its teetotal supporters, too, while pacifist abstainers like John Burns shared Pearl's antisemitism; temperance shaped and was shaped by widely different political positions.

These records also allow something more to be learned about the geography of temperance, beyond a simple opposition between the moderationist metropolis and a teetotal industrial North. Local societies prospered or suffered in relation to local social and political currents, and the ubiquity of drink meant that while 'total temperance communities' were rare, 'alternative worlds' of temperance existed even in apparently hostile settings like Devon. Sceptre assured working- and lower-middle-class Londoners, while teetotal savings built homes on the Temperance and Permanent Building Society's 'Maine-law estate' at Stratford. Particularly in London, those temperance sites – along with memorials like the UKT's fountain, banished to Clapham Common – seem to have become invisible, through a combination of familiarity and forgetting. As temperance became ordinary, the material traces it left on British landscapes became harder to see; the names of Manchester, Chorley and

Torquay's Temperance Streets, and the Teetotal Street in St. Ives, Cornwall, probably prompt little recognition and reflection today.

The archives of the UKT also provide a sense of the experimental nature of this initiative. It was founded to fill a gap in the market, a gap created by existing insurantial and medical understandings. In time the firm came to be seen as an experiment, designed from the start to test the idea that abstinence was healthier than moderation. At the time of its founding, though, teetotalism had driven a wedge between respectable moderationists and working-class abstainers, while life assurance was plagued by spectacular frauds; the stability of the firm was threatened by the shaky finances and reputations of its guarantors, fraudulent agents and the caution of the teetotalers they courted. The company's survival depended on the taking up of existing networks, of local temperance societies and individual champions, and the strengthening of connections between them, from newspaper advertisements to travelling agents, directors and materials. Trust in the firm emerged from the successful management of these networks, which were also used to scrutinize applicants and agents; the UKT actively created truths and trust.

After two decades of work, it became possible to use the UKT's experience to compare the longevity of abstainers and moderate drinkers. These comparisons came to constitute a new way of understanding drinking, as part of a wider turn to statistical understandings of social problems, as 'moral statistics' and 'moral geographies'. These arguments circulated widely, and in the twentieth century they were taken up by the British state, with some qualifications. However, work was needed to convert people into facts, and life assurance forms presented a response to the problems and possibilities of managing life at a distance. The form travelled more easily than the applicant, though its use also required that other elements of the network be properly trained and disciplined. The creation of policies that were linked to, but distinct from, the lives they assured also created unexpected outcomes, like the speculation on the life of Jabez Balfour.

To build its network the UKT's board had to find local agents and medical referees they could trust and then hold this network together, which meant a lot of tinkering and careful instruction. Agents and referees kept a watchful eye on one another, supervised by the office and its travelling representatives; the firm and local societies scrutinized the men and women who applied for policies. Beyond the affluent men on its board, the UKT's network seems to have been largely made up of men from relatively modest positions in society, at least in its first decades, and its agents seem representative of early and mid-Victorian temperance. Its early medical referees were often outsiders in their profession, though it is likely that others were more interested in the fees than arguments about abstinence. The UKT also kept its eye on other goals, for example assuring longstanding teetotalers whose lives might well have been substandard by assurance standards. This in turn suggests the company was interested in a broad set of meanings of 'improvement', including moral reform, a promise of hope and security, a virtuous circle of investment and the sensible and profitable observance of the natural laws of the market and of human mortality. In a world thoroughly suffused by alcohol, though, the business of temperance could have unexpected outcomes; drinking fountains had to be moved and the UKT ended up owning at least one pub.

The Sceptre sample provides a clearer sense of who its late Victorian teetotalers were. The small number of gentlemen and professionals is not surprising, given that these groups were less supportive of temperance and more likely to assure with a longer-established firm. The relatively modest nature of the merchants in the sample presents a contrast with Brian Harrison's Alliance subscribers, though, and while the predominance of the lower middle class in the sample is again to be expected, it does include some more straightforwardly working-class lives. Focusing upon the lower-middle-class bulk of the sample, it seems likely that the political journey taken by this class may well have been affected by changing attitudes to both Liberalism and Toryism, with this group providing recruits for both parties into the twentieth century, as well as both drinkers and teetotalers.

Doctors moved from an initial hostility to abstinence, or at best support for anti-spirits moderationism, to accepting that teetotal lives could be healthy ones. The Alliance did not stifle research into the effects of drinking, and the UKT's experience and methods became increasingly influential, representing a third alternative to the tacit knowledge of the gentlemanly physician and to experimental physiology. Life assurance learned from both statistical and physiological work, adopting Anstie's limit as a measure of moderation. By the 1890s mainstream medical opinion accepted the safety of both abstinence and moderate consumption, and this would be further strengthened as part of the 'new moderationism' that characterized both medical research and state strategy in the first decades of the twentieth century. While new research continued to demonstrate the value of the statistical approach pioneered by the UKT and the GRO, it also reopened arguments about the safety of abstinence.

Reviewing these findings, it seems important to consider three final points. The first considers the nature of temperance life assurance as an experiment; the second, its nature as ordinary temperance; and the third as a sign of changes to the nature and meanings of temperance at the turn of the nineteenth century. Taken together, these points allow us to assess the significance of temperance life assurance in this period.

Temperance life assurance: An assessment

The injunctions of researchers in science and technology studies to avoid a priori understandings, coupled with historians' wariness of teleological explanations, remind us that every act is, in a sense, an experiment, though this threatens to rob the term of any value. Historical developments are not explained by their origins or endpoints, or perhaps it is better to say that those origins and endpoints are not explanations but themselves questions that require examination. Hindsight might suggest that temperance life assurance was bound to succeed because it harnessed the aspirations of an emerging lower middle class who would come to be important within British social and political history, but that is not how it felt to Robert Warner and his fellow directors in the 1840s, or how they remembered it forty or fifty years later. Those men were relatively wealthy, but the road they took was far from being the path of least resistance, and there were failures and reversals along the way. The most obvious of these was the UKT's opening of a General section to assure moderate drinkers, of course, a decision taken a year before the most significant moderationist organization, the British and Foreign Temperance Society, had 'disappeared from view', as Brian Harrison put it.[44] The B&FTS, which had provided the UKT with many of its core directors, was replaced by national teetotal organizations just as the UKT allowed moderate drinkers to become members. From one perspective the UKT failed – as a business assuring only teetotalers, at least – after seven short years, which in itself is a valuable reminder of the contingency of developments like these, and of the many problems the firm had to face.

What emerged from this failure, though, was something much more like an experiment in a more literal sense, where the firm's experience became an increasingly persuasive source of information on the relative longevity, and by implication general health, of abstainers and moderate drinkers. It took more than a decade for these figures and claims to begin circulating, however, suggesting that this was not a possibility many had anticipated in 1847. The idea that the UKT had proved to be an experimental test of the relative safety of drinking and abstinence was clearly well established by 1884, when James Clark suggested that the Temperance Hospital could instruct medicine much as the UKT had influenced life assurance. Arguments about the value of that experience – whether the abstainers assured by these firms were genuinely representative of all teetotalers or simply 'more than usually prudential', as T. E. Young had put it, or whether their General section contained an enormous hidden reserve of excessive drinkers or 'reclaimed drunkards' – can also be seen as arguments about experimental design and method. Elderton, Pearson and Pearl faced similar questions and arguments. In that respect, the UKT became an experiment unexpectedly, but may have demonstrated the appeal of this kind of work all the same.

The second conclusion that can be drawn about temperance life assurance is that much of it, and many of the people involved in it, could be described as ordinary or unremarkable. Recent histories of temperance have tended to focus on its religious, moral and above all political dimensions, but the materials associated with the business of temperance life assurance offer a different perspective. We might take James Dawson Burns as an example. Where Anthony Dingle saw Burns as a representative of the Alliance, and more recently Christopher Cook has considered him as a theologian, the Burns who wrote the UKT's unpublished history was acting as a company historian.[45] There is very little mention of either the Alliance or theology in the manuscript Burns wrote for the firm; the work he did in those areas went on elsewhere. Temperance was not a singular movement, but a set of initiatives in different spheres of life, trying to achieve particular aims in a variety of ways. Sometimes those spheres and efforts connected with one another, but at other times they were kept apart or failed to engage; sometimes the connections that were made produced new tensions and conflicts. Burns's work for the Liberator building society and his kinship with its disgraced founder Jabez Balfour may have prompted him to offer his resignation as the UKT's auditor, for example.

One of the arguments of the book is that temperance became more ordinary between 1840 and 1918, and Dawson Burns can also help us understand this shift. Cook argues that Burns, like many late Victorian teetotal clergymen, encouraged total abstinence from alcoholic drink because it undermined faith through weakening the drinker's will; 'while his work may have been motivated by his understanding of scripture, the foundation of his argument was situated solidly in the ground of human reason'.[46] Similarly Dominic Erdozain has argued that temperance demonstrated the 'secularization of sin' in the late nineteenth century, as churches put the reform of society before evangelism. 'If formal theology winced at the extravagance of the teetotal agenda' in the middle of the century, 'an emerging social theology quietly nodded in agreement. Drink and drunkenness were facts; and the facts suggested that an inebriated populace was unreachable'.[47] From this perspective, then, while British churches became increasingly supportive of temperance, that work was less concerned with sin and more with keeping Christians away from temptation; by the twentieth century, 'activism had triumphed over spirituality, on a national scale'.[48] Erdozain's characterization of this shift in the spiritual values and work of temperance is broadly persuasive. As it became more engaged in worldly efforts – campaigns for Local Option and pub closures, teetotal holidays and life assurance policies – temperance remained 'religious' in character but became less overtly concerned with salvation. A crusade became a mixture of social work and 'the institutionalised war on vice'.[49] It is hard to imagine what the Joseph Barker of the 1840s would have made of that. Religious temperance became harder to distinguish from other aspects of the movement; it became less distinctive and more ordinary as a result.

The growth of efforts to keep temptation at bay also made temperance more ordinary, as did the continued relevance of the 'drink question' in the 1890s and 1900s, and then through the war. As the search for the causes of intemperance and other social problems turned to questions of 'environment', and as the state began to expand its remit to cover these issues, what we now think of as 'social science' became more interested in drink. Researchers like Charles Booth and Joseph Rowntree investigated drink's relationship with poverty, while the Webbs considered the legacies of the licensing system as part of their examination of the limitations of local government. The development of a popular Conservatism interested in preserving the pub as a place of moderate consumption also increased the importance of drink, something to be managed rather than simply defended or annihilated. The labour movement had a long, if complicated, relationship with temperance, which meant that the three major political parties of the twentieth century had grown closer together in their evaluation of drink as a political and social issue, even if they continued to disagree about what to do about it. Despite – or because of – those disagreements, it seems likely that the reader of a national or local newspaper in the first decade of the twentieth century would have found something on temperance or drink to read in it; the drink question was hard to ignore, but unremarkable.

Temperance life assurance was also ordinary because it involved prosaic practices and relations: the paying of weekly, quarterly, or yearly premiums; some correspondence with the firm, usually at the start and end of the process; attention to the reporting of annual meetings and regular bonus payments; and an annual confirmation of abstinence from their temperance society. None of that would have seemed particularly exciting – hence the descriptions of the argument these materials made for abstinence as cool or cold, dull or prosaic, hard-headed or unprejudiced. While a policy might have promised security, it was probably not something the policyholder thought about very much; perhaps it made them *less* likely to think about the future. Alfred Marshall, who had criticized Elderton and Pearson's statistical method, described economics as the discipline pertaining to 'the ordinary business of life' on the first page of his influential *Principles of Economics*, and historians of economics have tended to take that 'business' to mean 'the production, distribution and consumption of wealth'.[50] If we think of the 'ordinary business of life' in a broader sense, though, as forms of practice, often done unconsciously, then engaging with temperance life assurance is clearly part of it in that respect too. The sense that the experience of temperance life assurance firms simply recorded and reported the outcomes of deeper causes – the laws of mortality and the market – might well have reinforced this further. Their figures promised to reveal the workings of these hidden laws; their outcomes could be harnessed to improve health and grow wealth.

Finally, temperance life assurance tells us a little more about what temperance might have meant to those engaged with it, and how that might have changed. Temperance life assurance was an experiment because it consciously set its face against medical and life assurance practice. Its institutions, employees and policyholders were also linked to many other initiatives, many of them more progressive than is often assumed of temperance. Temperance was part of a wider liberal, and sometimes Radical, Victorian culture, but that culture was highly heterogenous, with political and cultural currents mixing and clashing. The feuds that regularly split this apparently singular 'movement' either reflected existing tensions – between better-heeled moderationists and working-class teetotalers, for example – or allowed participants to create or refuse solidarities with other campaigns, as was the case when abstainers debated woman suffrage in the UK or segregated societies in the US. Thomas Hudson claimed 'there is no greater blunder committed by persons who … suppose that an energetic teetotaler is necessarily a man of only one idea', and that holds true for many of the more visible lives considered in this book.[51]

Beyond reminding us of the diverse and often progressive character of temperance, temperance life assurance also illustrates the ongoing strengths of the movement after the period studied by Brian Harrison's foundational study. The 1872 Licensing Act and 1874 election may have shown Liberals the danger of committing the party to the Alliance, with the Peel Commission further weakening the Alliance's influence in the 1890s, and the arguments over licensing in the 1900s signalled the end of Local Option (in England and Wales, at least.) The 1870s saw growing support from the established church and Wesleyans, however, with the formation of the British Women's Temperance Association and the arrival of Gospel Temperance. These campaigns largely called for moral, religious reform alongside support for prohibition, though, suggesting a further shift towards a familiar definition of temperance in this decade.

As has been argued throughout the book, however, this interpretation rests on the assumption that the Alliance *was* temperance, and that only the passing of Local Option would have counted as success. The Sceptre sample clearly shows the vitality of ordinary temperance between 1865 and 1881, the lives of some of those policyholders suggesting they lived in active temperance worlds. The number of new UKT policies established each year grew from the middle of the 1870s, after a gentle decline since the middle of the 1850s, and then showed steady growth until the mid-1890s (Figure 1.3). Significantly the 1870s also marked the high point of nineteenth-century alcohol consumption, one it would not return to until the end of the twentieth century. Increasing consumption may have prompted growing temperance activity, as a response to drunkenness or wasted funds. Premium money was reinvested in local authority improvement in this decade, too, and the 1870s also saw the founding and growth of the Temperance Hospital, the British Medical Temperance Association and the *Medical Temperance Journal*. These developments survived into the twentieth century, and the UKT was selling abstainers' policies into the 1950s at least.

Conclusions

This book has hopefully demonstrated that these materials allow us to ask new questions about familiar themes in the study of drink and temperance in Britain, with implications for other places where life assurance and temperance could both be found. The lives made visible by these records allow us to tell different stories about what politics might have meant to lower-middle-class teetotalers like James Theophilus Davis, for example (Chapter 7). If we are to have political histories of temperance, might they address these questions, for example the changing significance of drink and temperance in late Victorian and Edwardian popular Conservatism, or the way the movement influenced and was shaped by the shift from the radical Liberalism of the 1840s to the 'fanaticism' of the 1890s? These contexts may also have been strongly localized; historical-geographical studies working with local collections as well as the archives of national firms and organizations would show just how different local temperance worlds could be, from Lancashire to Devon, Cardiff to Chester, Nottingham to Poplar, Padstow to Walton-on-the-Naze.

Ultimately, though, this book has considered life assurance as a particular instance of temperance work. The greatest achievement of temperance life assurance lay in its proof – to the satisfaction of many within life assurance and medicine, at least – that abstinence did not threaten health and life. Given that the UKT was said to owe its existence to the assumption that Robert Warner's life was inferior to that of a moderate drinker, this was a victory. In many ways, though, temperance life assurance anticipated the 'new moderationism' that emerged in the twentieth century. Firms like the UKT promoted teetotalism, but also urged greater caution in the assessment of moderate drinkers; most firms were already concerned with 'excessive' drinking by the middle of the century, but this became a more pressing concern as temperance offices tightened definitions of excess and others lost money to hidden intemperance. The industry began to see publicans, and even grocers, as bad lives. Separating out the abstainers courted by the UKT and the excessive drinkers that no firm wanted revealed a large population of moderate drinkers who were probably drinking significantly less than their Victorian counterparts. While it had been established to promote total abstinence, the UKT had been more successful in encouraging life assurance offices to address drinking and teetotalism. Opening the General section made it possible to compare mortality rates, but it also meant that a firm run by teetotalers was now admitting moderate drinkers. The *British Medical Journal*'s 1891 editorial condemning Granville's plea for more drinking had observed that twenty years of temperance work had demonstrated 'the happy healthy lives which can be passed innocent of all contact with alcohol', emphasizing the positive aspects of the movement as well as its criticisms of alcohol. The author credited teetotalers with encouraging 'a general habit of greater moderation in drink even where total abstinence is not accepted'.[52] A campaign for total abstinence had ended up encouraging moderation in the general population. Ryosuke Yokoe suggests 'the advent of the First World War marked a decisive shift in the national conversation on drink, steering many temperance campaigners and other actors away from their earlier promotion of abstinence towards a more nuanced encouragement of moderate drinking by the 1920s', but the UKT had already, somewhat reluctantly, begun encouraging both moderation and abstinence by 1847.[53]

It seems likely that this reflected a sense – in medicine, government and certainly in life assurance – that drinking was something that should be managed, because it was proving hard to eradicate. Life assurance allowed uncertain consequences of drinking to be converted into calculable risks. The Sceptre's treatment of grocers provides an excellent example. Instead of rejecting the application of Benjamin Outred (Chapter 7), Sceptre simply charged him an extra premium to cover the additional risk, retaining the policy even after their medical examination decided his life had been damaged by his trade. Crucially, while these firms depended upon the socialization of risk – any loss from Outred's early death would be shared with the Sceptre's other moderate drinkers – and on the surveillance and discipline of local temperance societies, the decision to establish life assurance was still an individual choice. It was too late for Benjamin Outred to stop drinking, or change occupations, but temperance life assurance offered a chance for applicants to reflect on their attitude to drink. One moderate drinker might sign the pledge and take an abstainer's policy; another might see the Abstainers' section as proof of the firm's prudence and join the General section. Temperance life assurance offered a *choice* and might have encouraged people to change their practice through offering a financial incentive – what we might now call a 'nudge'. Private companies intervened in the conduct of conduct, in other words, shaping attitudes to drinking by making abstinence more attractive.

To conclude, it is worth considering the legacy of temperance life assurance in the light of the larger questions about finance with which this book began. It would seem quite possible to conclude that this business represented the 'capture' of temperance by Victorian finance capitalism, for example. Brian Harrison's suggestion that Livesey's influential *Malt Lecture* was a defence of property has been cited in more recent work, for example in Marianna Adler's conclusion that 'the movement offered a moral platform legitimating the demand for security of property, a disciplined labor force, and an expanded home market'.[54] When Livesey told 'capitalists' that 'the Temperance Society is an insurance for the safety of every man's property. Drunkenness and disorder are sure to drive capital away', he probably was not thinking of insurance in its literal sense.[55] As Harrison goes on to make clear, however, 'commercial and industrial capital was never monolithic', and temperance was also an *attack* on the property of the breweries and publicans who would lose pubs to either Local Option or market forces. While Robert Dundas Thomson would have agreed that temperance was a cure for pauperism and thus a means to cut the Poor Rate, many of the lives assured by these firms would not have owned property and would have sought more modest forms of security. Some of those ordinary teetotalers may have been Samuel Smiles–style strivers, aspirational members of the lower middle class and labour elite, making temperance life assurance a vehicle for both capital accumulation and bourgeois self-fashioning; but it has to be remembered that nearly a quarter of the policies established by the Sceptre sample lapsed within five years. Aspirations were not always realized. Considering this, it might make just as much sense to argue that temperance 'captured' capitalism. Markets were put to work to explore the value of abstinence, just as the 'improved' public house can be seen as another market arrangement that emerged in response to the new moderationism that had been encouraged by temperance.

Ultimately, perhaps temperance life assurance was closest to what Callon called a 'problematization' of drinking.[56] The UKT and its rivals presented themselves as the solution to a series of problems other actors were struggling with. Temperance life assurance allowed a statistical comparison of the longevity of drinkers and abstainers, for example, which meant it could compare rival medical approaches. It encouraged abstainers to remain teetotal and to look to the future, while a policy might provide them with security for a loan. It provided work for agents prepared to enrol their own social circles, as well as additional income for doctors struggling to survive in an overcrowded medical market. It also generated large capital sums through investment, in turn allowing local government organizations to borrow money to pay for improvement. These firms might not have been an 'obligatory point of passage', in Callon's terms, because they were not necessarily indispensable; other ways of measuring the consequences of drink or saving money continued to exist, and the claims of these firms were never universally acknowledged. They were still extraordinarily *productive*, though, generating security, hope, current and future incomes, capital for investment – as other assurance firms did – as well as knowledge about drinking, forms of networked community amongst abstainers, virtuous or perhaps ethical investment and more. Most importantly, perhaps, it offered a model for managing drinking, by rewarding abstainers, tolerating moderate drinkers and refusing the intemperate. Sceptre's additional charge for grocers presented a model for the new moderationism. Excessive drinkers were not to be encouraged, while teetotalers were given a financial incentive for abstinence, and moderate drinkers created funds to pay for any losses from their own intemperance.

The *reasons* for doing this could be purely financial, as this suggests, though it seems likely many of the people involved with these firms were genuinely trying to promote abstinence. Robert Warner may have established the firm because he was told he would pay more for life assurance as a teetotaler, but the firm ended up resembling the Albion Hotel, the pub he owned in Walton-on-the Naze, with its unlicensed temperance rooms and fully licensed hotel divided by a wall. Warner's hotel served both abstainers and drinkers; the company he had helped to found did the same. The success of these assurance firms may have depended upon the zeal of its agents, and the faith of men like William Bingham, but at the same time it was a business like any other. The success of these firms did not depend on belief in the healthiness of abstinence or the rightfulness of a Christian campaign for prohibition; ultimately, they would be evaluated on the size of their invested capital, the bonuses they paid and the ratio between income and expenses, like any other assurance company. The experiment had become a rather ordinary success story.

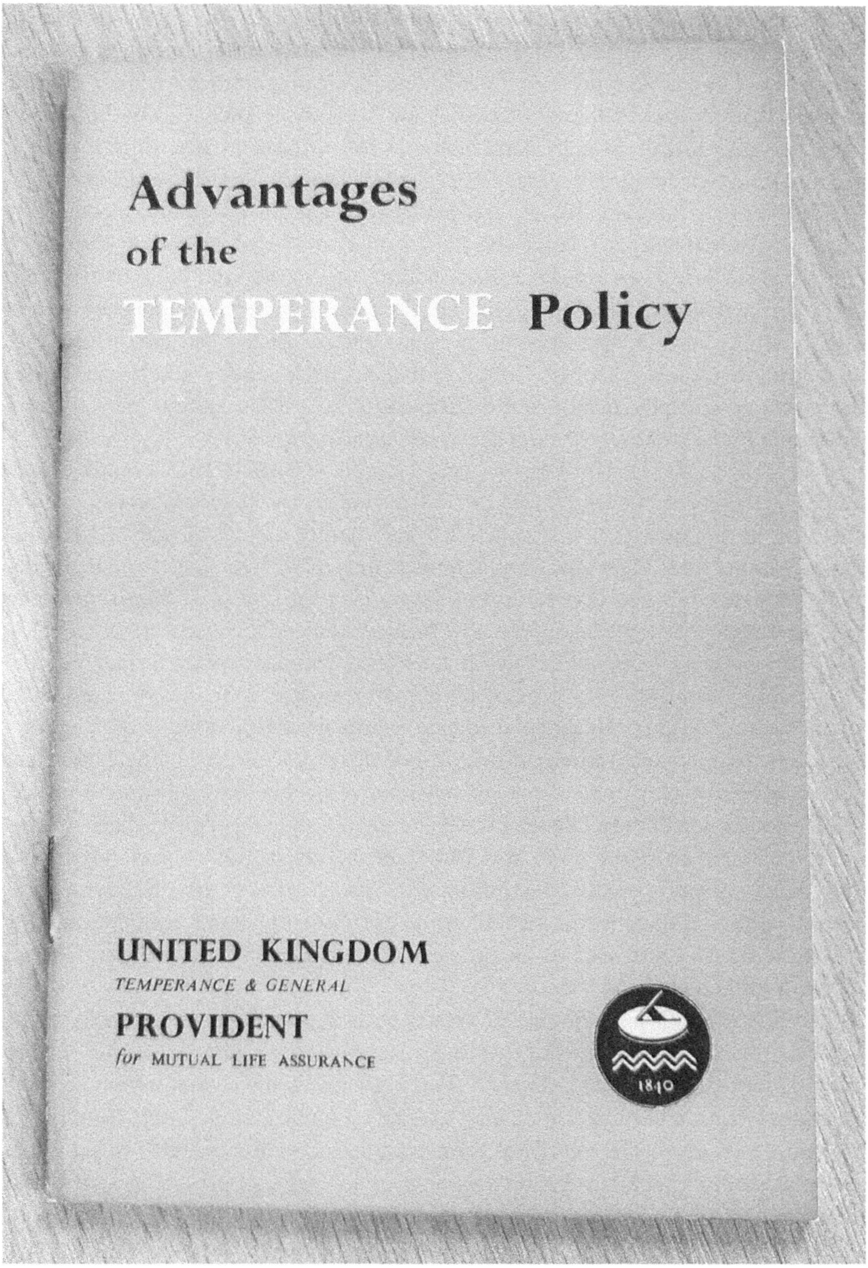

Figure 9.1 UKT prospectus, 1952.

Source: Courtesy of the Livesey Collection, UCLan.

In 1952 the Temperance section prospectus of the UKT revisited the story of Warner's 'bright idea' (Figure 9.1). The firm's directors included Trevor Roberts, second Baron Clwyd and Liberal peer; Sir Ernest Benn, uncle of Anthony Wedgwood Benn; and Isaac Foot, MP and father of future Labour Party leader Michael Foot. Both Benn and Foot were Liberals, from the kind of nonconformist background which remained so important for twentieth-century temperance, though Ernest Benn's liberalism was of a strongly individualist, laissez-fair character and the board also included the Conservative MP and later home secretary (and Baron) Henry Brooke. The UKT's radicalism was largely a distant memory, and its business was solid but unremarkable. Forty per cent of the firm's whole life and long-term endowment policies were in the Abstainers' section, and while the firm now offered discounted motor insurance premiums to teetotal members, its pitch had not changed for a century: 'In the experience of several generations the Temperance Policy has come to be associated with *better health and longevity and distinct financial advantages*.'[57]

One reviewer of Hartley Withers's 1951 *Pioneers of British Life Assurance*, which featured a chapter on the UKT, explained that teetotalers were expected to pay an extra premium for life assurance and concluded 'it is hardly surprising that in 1840 one Robert Warner with other abstainers founded [the UKT]'.[58] The idea that abstinence might be dangerous had become extraordinary over the course of the firm's life; in fact, the suspicion Warner had faced now seemed strange. The discovery of two time capsules containing temperance materials during the demolition of the former National Temperance Hospital in 2017 prompted a similar response, with one heritage adviser saying 'the routine use of alcohol in medicine sounds absurd today but in the Victorian age it was commonplace'; a journalist described this as a reminder of 'the days before doctors quizzed their patients on how many units of alcohol they consumed a week'.[59] While the question of the relationship between alcohol and longevity had been opened up in the twentieth century, the idea that medicine would value abstinence and be wary of intemperance remained unremarkable. The *agencement* the UKT created had been so successful in its recruitment of elements from temperance, medicine and life assurance, transforming each in the process, that it was now hard to imagine these things in a different configuration.

As Michel Callon pointed out, 'successful translation quickly makes us forget its history', as the new arrangement becomes a 'black box' – a singular, taken-for-granted thing rather than a complex network.[60] That black box – the idea of temperance life assurance – has not been all that difficult to open up again, though doing that requires two things: access to the records of these firms, which are vulnerable to the usual problems confronting archives, and a willingness to challenge prevailing ideas about what temperance was.

Notes

1. George B. Wilson, 'A Statistical Review of the Variations during the Last Twenty Years in the Consumption of Intoxicating Drinks in the United Kingdom, and in Convictions for Offences Connected with Intoxication, with a Discussion of the

Causes to Which These Variations May Be Ascribed', *Journal of the Royal Statistical Society* 75, 2 (1912), 183–247.

2. Beckingham and Watkins, 'Temperance Lives and Landscape'.
3. Fahey, 'Worrying', 12.
4. Citing Greenaway, *Drink and British Politics*, 80, and see Paul Jennings, '"Grasping a Nettle": The 1904 Licensing Act', in *Biographies of Drink; A Case Study Approach to Our Historical Relationship with Alcohol*, edited by Mark Hailwood and Deborah Toner (Newcastle upon Tyne: Cambridge Scholars Publishing, 2015), 30–48.
5. Gutzke, *Pubs and Progressives*.
6. Woolley and Johnson, *Temperance Progress*, 379.
7. 1904 [Cd. 2186] Inter-Departmental Committee on Physical Deterioration, Appendix to the report of the Inter-Departmental Committee on Physical Deterioration, Vol. III, Appendix and general index; 1904 [Cd. 2210] Inter-Departmental Committee on Physical Deterioration, Minutes of evidence taken before the Inter-Departmental Committee on Physical Deterioration, Vol. II, List of witnesses and minutes of evidence; and 1909 [Cd. 4746] Board of Education, Syllabus of lessons on 'temperance' for scholars attending public elementary schools.
8. Woiak, 'Medical Cromwell'.
9. Ibid., 361.
10. Ibid., 360.
11. Ryosuke Yokoe, *Alcohol and Liver Cirrhosis in Twentieth-Century Britain* (Switzerland: Springer, 2023), 77.
12. Central Control Board (Liquor Traffic) Advisory Committee, *Alcohol: Its Action on the Human Organism* (London: HM Stationery Office, 1918), ii.
13. Ibid., 114, 115–16.
14. Ibid., 117.
15. Ibid., 117–18.
16. Thomas P. Whittaker, 'Alcoholic Beverages and Longevity', collected in *Institute of Actuaries Life Assurance Tracts* 13 (1903–4), 19, emphasis added.
17. T. E. Young, 'Drinking and Drunkenness', *The Times*, 19 September 1891, 7.
18. 'Drinking and Drunkenness', *British Medical Journal* 703.
19. CCB, *Alcohol*, 125.
20. Ibid., 133.
21. 'Science and Alcohol', *Times*, 1 March 1918, 7; 'The Drink Problem', *Western Times*, 16 February 1918, 2.
22. Ethel M. Elderton and Karl Pearson, *A First Study of the Influence of Parental Alcoholism on the Physique and Ability of the Offspring* (London: Dulau, 1910).
23. Joe Cain, 'Publications Produced by the Francis Galton Laboratory for National Eugenics', *The Library* 22, 4 (2021), 523–48. Lyndsay Andrew Farrall, *The Origins and Growth of the English Eugenics Movement, 1865–1925*, STS Occasional Papers number 9 (London: UCL Department of Science and Technology Studies, 2019).
24. Rosaleen Love, '"Alice in Eugenics-Land": Feminism and Eugenics in the Scientific Careers of Alice Lee and Ethel Elderton', *Annals of Science* 36, 2 (1979).
25. Farrall, *English Eugenics Movement*, 259–61.
26. W. F. Bynum, 'Alcoholism and Degeneration in 19th Century European Medicine and Psychiatry', *British Journal of Addiction* 79 (1984).
27. Norman Kerr, *Inebriety: Its Etiology, Pathology, Treatment and Jurisprudence* (London: H. K. Lewis, 1888), 390; see Virginia Berridge, 'Society for the Study of Addiction', *British Journal of Addiction* 85 (1990), 987–1077, and Mariana Valverde,

Diseases of the Will: Alcohol and the Dilemmas of Freedom (Cambridge: Cambridge University Press, 1998).

28. Allen, *Medical Examinations*, first edition, 10; Brockbank, *Life Insurance*, 132.
29. Alborn, 'Insurance against Germ Theory'.
30. John Maynard Keynes, 'Influence of Parental Alcoholism', *Journal of the Royal Statistical Society* 73 (1910), 769–73; Karl Pearson and Ethel M. Elderton, *A Second Study of the Influence of Parental Alcoholism on the Physique and Ability of Offspring* (London: Dulau, 1911); and see Cuttings on Eugenics & Alcoholism 1910–11, Galton Collection, MS GALTON/2/13/1/13, UCL Special Collections.
31. Mary Sturge and Victor Horsley, 'On Some of the Biological and Statistical Errors in the Work on Parental Alcoholism by Miss Elderton and Professor Karl Pearson, F.R.S.', *British Medical Journal* 1, 2611 (14 January 1911), 72–82. See Farrall, *English Eugenics Movement*, 271–8, and Michael S. Dunnill, 'Victor Horsley (1857–1916) and the Temperance Movement', *Journal of Medical Biography* 20 (2012), 25–31.
32. Arthur MacNalty, 'Sir Victor Horsley: His Life and Work', *British Medical Journal* 1, 5024 (20 April 1957), 915.
33. Victor Horsley and Mary Sturge, *Alcohol and the Human Body: An Introduction to the Study of the Subject, and a Contribution to National Health* (London: Macmillan, 1907), 349, 353.
34. Arthur Newsholme, *Public Health and Insurance: American Addresses* (Baltimore, MD: The Johns Hopkins University Press, 1920).
35. Farrall, *English Eugenics Movement*, 281.
36. Raymond Pearl, *Alcohol and Longevity* (New York: Alfred A. Knopf, 1926).
37. Michael G. Marmot, M. J. Shipley, Geoffrey Rose and Briony J. Thomas, 'Alcohol and Mortality: A U-Shaped Curve', *The Lancet* 317, 8220 (1981), 580–3.
38. Pearl, *Alcohol*, 16, 27–8, 141, 35.
39. Ibid., 165.
40. Ibid., 73.
41. Elazar Barkan, *The Retreat of Scientific Racism: Changing Concepts of Race in Britain and the United States between the World Wars* (Cambridge: Cambridge University Press, 1991).
42. Barkan, *Retreat*, 214; Margo A. Peyton, 'Segregated in Life and Death: Arnold R. Rich and the Racial Science of Tuberculosis', *Bulletin of the History of Medicine* 98, 2 (2024), 214.
43. Thompson, *Drink and Be Sober*, 41.
44. Harrison, *Drink*, 138.
45. Dingle, *Campaign for Prohibition*; Christopher C. H. Cook, *Alcohol, Addiction and Christian Ethics* (Cambridge: Cambridge University Press, 2006).
46. Cook, *Alcohol, Addiction and Christian Ethics*, 123.
47. Dominic Erdozain, 'The Secularisation of Sin in the Nineteenth Century', *Journal of Ecclesiastical History* 62, 1 (2011), 76.
48. Ibid., 84–5.
49. Ibid., 87.
50. Roger E. Backhouse, *The Ordinary Business of Life: A History of Economics from the Ancient World to the Twenty-First Century* (Princeton, NJ: Princeton University Press, 2024), 4.
51. Hudson, *Temperance Pioneers*, 125.
52. 'Drinking and Drunkenness', *British Medical Journal* 703.

53. Ryosuke Yokoe, 'New Moderationism: Medical Discourses on Alcohol and the Decline of Drunkenness in Interwar Britain', *Modern British History* 36, 1 (2025), 2.
54. Marianna Adler, 'From Symbolic Exchange to Commodity Consumption: Anthropological Notes on Drinking as a Symbolic Practice', in *Drinking: Behavior and Belief in Modern History*, edited by Susanna Barrows and Robin Room (Berkeley: University of California Press, 1991), 386.
55. Cited in Harrison, *Drink*, 93.
56. Callon, 'Sociology of an Actor-Network'.
57. UKT, 'Advantages of the Temperance Policy', 1.
58. 'History of Life Insurance', *The Economist* 161 (15 September 1951), 623.
59. Valentine Low, 'Time Capsules Make for Sobering News', *Times*, 31 October 2017, 25.
60. Callon, 'Sociology of an Actor-Network', 28.

Appendix: The Sceptre sample and notes on method

Five of the Sceptre office's ledgers survive at the London Archives, covering 18,000 policies drawn up (but not necessarily issued) issued between March 1865 and August 1885 (MS SC04/01/01–SC04/01/05). A sample of 959 abstainers' policies (covering 967 lives, as eight policies were jointly held by two people) was created from these ledgers, recording every tenth abstainers' policy – or, if that was blank, the next full record of that kind – in the years 1865, 1870, 1871, 1877 and 1881. The sample is weighted towards the middle years of the period covered by the ledgers – 1870–1, 1877, and 1881 – as explained below (Table A.1).

The ledgers collate information from policy forms that were completed in a given year, and then track changes to the policy and its final outcome. Applications that were declined by the firm are not recorded in these ledgers, and policies that took months to complete might be entered into the next year's records. Some applications proceeded far enough to be given policy numbers but were then not taken up, leading to crossed-out or blank entries.

This information included the number of the policy – the life's key identifier – and the type of policy, the name of the person who would be the policy's beneficiary if that was not the policyholder themselves, the sum assured and date of issue, and the agent who brought the life to the office. The policyholder's details included their full name and address – this was rarely updated, suggesting a separate record may have been kept, given what we know about the mobility of nineteenth-century renters. The first ledger (only) records the place of birth of the policyholder. Occupation, age, and date of birth would have been used to calculate premiums and additional risks; notes about risks and changes of premiums were also recorded, as well as bonuses paid and loans established, as well as the outcome – whether the policy was claimed, lapsed or surrendered.

Table A.1 The sceptre sample

Year	Ledgers	Abstainers recorded	All policies issued that year
1865	One	61	824
1870	Two	198	873
1871	Two	70	744
1877	Three and four	275	859
1881	Four and five	355	1,169
Total		959	3,300

The forms themselves would always have been the key reference documents for a life, which might explain why some important information is occasionally missing from the ledgers. Clerks would have been able to consult the original forms, as well as minutes of meetings, when questions arose about premiums, charges or claims, though it seems likely the ledgers would have been their main resource.

A number of issues with the Sceptre ledgers make the sample rather uneven in terms of coverage. First of all, they cover only the first twenty years of the company's existence, when it survived for another thirty-two before being absorbed into the Eagle and British Dominions office in 1917 (Chapter 1). The office became increasingly dominated by abstainers' policies after 1885, so the sample gives us a picture of the office at a moment when teetotalers formed a sizeable minority, rather than the majority, of the lives assured each year. Within the twenty-year period covered by the ledgers, the years 1870–1, 1877 and 1881 account for 93.6 per cent of the lives in the sample, meaning that the sample is almost entirely a record of a much shorter period, 1870–81. This is largely the result of issues with the ledgers. The original intention had been to use five years: the first, 1865; 1871 and 1881, to allow cross-checking with the censuses; the midpoint between censuses, 1875 or 1876; and finally 1885. However, no teetotal policies were recorded between July 1871 and June 1876, suggesting this was recorded elsewhere for this period. 1870 and the first six months of 1871 were then considered together as the midpoint between the censuses. 1877 was chosen as the first full year of records of abstainers' policies after 1870.

Taken together 1870 and 1871 contribute almost as many records (268) to the sample as 1877 (275), these years providing 56.6 per cent of these policies. The records for 1865 make a smaller contribution to the sample, as ledger one begins in March 1865. Ledger five ends in August 1885, and there are only 204 abstainer's policies recorded in that year in total, so 1885 does not form part of the final sample.

The vagaries of accounting practices and archival survival have created further problems. Some are relatively minor; I have assumed that 'L' records a lapsed policy, especially when the policy number has also been struck through in red ink, for example; where there is no 'surr.', 'L', or claim marked, it is presumed that a claim was made, probably after 1885. Similarly, it is not always clear whether the date of a claim refers to the death of the life assured, or the arrival of a death certificate to support the claim. Other issues are more confusing. Policies were not entered in chronological order, for example, and it seems likely that while policy numbers were allocated when a policy was provisionally approved, there could be a long wait before it was finally issued. Emily Nuttall's policy (number 20) is dated October 1865 in the first ledger, for example, though it appears in the ledger amongst a run of policies from March and April of that year. The numbering also stops and starts as decisions were taken about new products and new forms of record-keeping. Policies 201–300 were kept in the Industrial Register, which does not survive, with ledger one starting again at 301; the recording of industrial policies becomes more complicated after that.

Crucially for this study, this messy account-keeping also extended to the identification of abstainers' policies. Though the directors agreed in 1866 that 'a special section and separate account be kept for Total Abstainers', this was not reflected in the ledgers.[1] A red ink 'T' is marked next to some policies, while others are marked 'Abstainer' or 'Total Abstainer', particularly in the later ledgers. As the premiums for these policies seem to be cheaper than unmarked policies of a comparable age, it seems safe to assume these would have been part of the firm's Abstainers' section. However the last 'T' is marked in July 1871 (ledger two) and there is then a gap until June 1876 (ledger three), suggesting either that no policies of this kind were issued for five years, or that they were not marked as such. The first suggestion seems unlikely, given the absence of any discussion of a policy change in the firm's minute books; the firm's representatives promoted the principle of temperance saving at a public meeting in Cardiff in 1870, in the presence of temperance worthies like Ebenezer Beavan (see Chapter 7). In addition, damage to the margins of pages in ledgers two and four means that some abstainers' policies might well have been missed, as this was where this information was most commonly marked.

Taken together, these issues suggest that the number of Sceptre abstainers' policies issued in these years might well have been significantly higher. The unevenness of the abstainers' policies in the five ledgers can be seen below in Table A.2. It's also worth noticing that this sampling strategy, driven by necessity, has resulted in a sample of 959 abstainers' policies of the 3,415 that are clearly identifiable in these ledgers, or 28.1 per cent of the number issued by the firm between March 1865 and August 1885.

Perhaps 300 of the sample of 959 lives were then cross-referenced with digitized sources, chiefly the census, trade directories, and newspaper archives, and with the temperance histories and biographies produced by Harrison, Winskill, and others. A study of working-class investors using savings bank ledgers notes that 'considerable challenges exist in linking bank accounts to basic biographical information via the census or other extant records that are likely to capture working-class individuals. This makes even the most rudimentary sketch of an individual's circumstances difficult to establish'.[2] However the Sceptre ledgers seem to include more details than these bank records, and while the firm did assure working-class lives beyond their Industrial section, many were better described as lower middle class or artisans (Chapter 7). Those lives are more likely to be recorded in digitized sources. Of course, because Winskill and other temperance historians concentrated on those who were more active in the movement, there is a risk that working-class lives look politically quiescent in comparison. The more ordinary the teetotaler, in other words, the harder it has been to find out anything about them beyond the fact that they established a policy with Sceptre.

Table A.2 Abstainers' policies by ledger

Ledger	Period covered	Abstainers' policies	All policies
One	1865–8	365	3,982
Two	1868–72	729	3,324
Three	1872–7	71	3,508
Four	1877–81	254	3,348
Five	1881–5	1,996	3,838
Total		3,415	18,000

Notes

1. Board Meeting, 14 September 1866, Sceptre Minute book 1.
2. Linda Perriton and Josephine Maltby, 'Working-Class Households and Savings in England, 1850–1880', *Enterprise and Society* 16, 2 (2015), 439.

Bibliography

Primary sources

Manuscripts

Aviva Archives

Copy of letter from H. Rickman to Robert Warner, December 1840, FL357.
'Drink and Death' Card, UKT, 1889? Specimen literature, UKP/07/01/01.
James Dawson Burns, manuscript company history, 1896, FL368.
Joseph T. Mitchell, *Report of the Medical Director to the Directors of the Temperance and General Provident Institution*, 16 September 1856, FL293.
Letter from Robert Warner to Thomas Cash, 27 January 1896, FL368.
Reference letters 1–249, Norwich Union Life 1809, NU5191.
Theodore Compton, 'Early Days of the Temperance Provident Institution', reprinted from 'The Temperance Record', 30 June 1881, single printed sheet, FL367.
Theodore Compton, 'The Temperance Provident Institution. Copied from the Weekly Record of Nov 8th, 1862', FL361.
UKT Board of Directors, Minute Book 1, FL108.
UKT Board of Directors, Minute Book 12, FL119.
UKT Board of Directors, Minute Book 15, FL122.
UKT Prospectus, 1897, showing 1 Adelaide Place, Specimen literature, UKP/07/01/01.
UKT Prospectus, 1908, showing 196, the Strand, Specimen Literature, UKP/07/01/01.
UKT Standing Committee, Minute Book 1, FL436.
UKT Standing Committee, Minute Book 2, FL437.
United Kingdom Temperance & General Provident Institution Annual Reports and Balance Sheets 1840–1910, FL1232.
Working Man's Section Card, Specimen Literature, FL387.

Bristol Record Office

Bristol Temperance Herald, MS 41001/WTL/J/1/1.

Essex Record Office

Becontree Brewster Sessions, 1882, MS P/B Mc4.
Committees of Quarter Sessions Minutes of Licensing Committee, 1873–1907, Essex County Licensing Committee, 1893–, MS Q/ACm 36.
Deeds of Bath House Hotel and Albion Hall, Walton-le-Soken, with correspondence, 1873–1904, MS D/DU 408/11.
Valuer's Notebook, MS D/DB B20.

Hertfordshire Record Office

County Hailstorm Insurance Company, letter to shareholders, 1 May 1848, MS 7257/1.

Institute and Faculty of Actuaries Library

Prospectus, 'The United Kingdom Total Abstinence Life Association', volume of prospectuses of Assurance Societies sent by the Clerical, Medical and General Life Assurance Society, MS R826-G.

Library of the Society of Friends

Barker, Arthur G. *The Temperance Century in the West* (Bristol: Printed by T. O. Elworthy and Son, 1937), 058.6 BAR.

Friends' Quarterly Examiner.

Friends Temperance Union lantern slides relating to medical aspects of temperance, 85L/2801–2808.

Memoir of Robert Charleton: Compiled Chiefly from His Letters, edited by Anna F. Fox (London: Samuel Harris, 1876), second edition, MS SR 092.3 CHA/FOX 2.

Memorials of Samuel Bowly, Born March 23, 1802, Died March 23, 1884 Compiled by His Daughter, Maria Taylor (Gloucester: Privately published, 1884), SR 092.3 BOW/TAY.

Senter, M. J., and A. M. Senter. *Walton-on-the-Naze: The Warner story* (Colchester: M. J. & A. M. Senter, 1997), box 127/3.

Sessions, Frederick. *The Life Story of Samuel Bowly: A Champion of Freedom, Progress and Temperance* (London: Friends Tract Association, 1903), box 289/3.

Suffolk Record Office. *Ipswich Remembered 2: Photographs of Victorian and Edwardian Ipswich* (Ipswich: Suffolk Record Office, 1979), 097 [Hist. 13/21].

Livesey Collection, University of Central Lancashire

Advantages of the temperance policy, United Kingdom Temperance and General Provident Institution, Prospectus, 1952, MS C Uni.

British and Foreign Temperance Society, 1832–47 (Annual Reports 1832–47), MS T33 C Bri.

New British and Foreign Temperance Intelligencer, MS J Bri.

London Archives

Eagle Star Abstainers' Section Prospectus, second edition, 1 January 1918, MS SC04/01/03/001.

National Life Assurance Society, Medical Reports, MS34418.

National Life Assurance Society, Proposal Form, MS 34431.

Revenue account for 5 years 1 January 1914–31 December 1918, Valuation accounts and statements of the Sceptre Fund of the Eagle Star & British Dominions Insurance Co. Ltd, 1918, Sceptre Fund, statements of account, quinquennial valuations and drafting papers, MS SC4/1/7/1/1.

Royal Farmers, Minute Book 3, MS 14989 3.

Royal Farmers, Minute Book 5, MS 14989/001.

Royal Farmers, Minute Book 14, MS 14989/14.
Sceptre Life Association, Board of Directors, Minute Book 1, MS SC01/05/01/001.
Sceptre Life Association, Board of Directors, Minute Book 3, MS SC01/05/01/003.
Sceptre Life Association, Board of Directors, Minute Book 4, MS SC01/05/01/004.
Sceptre Life Association Limited Policy Ledger 1, MS SC04/01/01.
Sceptre Life Association Limited Policy Ledger 2, MS SC04/01/02.
Sceptre Life Association Limited Policy Ledger 3, MS SC04/01/03.
Sceptre Life Association Limited Policy Ledger 4, MS SC04/01/04.
Sceptre Life Association Limited Policy Ledger 5, MS SC04/01/05.
Sceptre Life Association Limited Reports of Directors to Annual Meetings of Shareholders, 1872, 1886–90, 1903–4, 1914–17, MS SC 1/8/1/1.
Sceptre Life Association Limited Reports of proceedings at AGMs, 1887–91, MS SC1/7/2/1.
Summaries of the Whittington's accounts, policies, shares, investments etc, 1892–4, compiled in an audit by accountants for the National Life Assurance Society, with related correspondence, National Mutual Life Assurance Society, MS34412.
Whittington Life Assurance Company, Proposals in support of policy applications, 1885, MS 34430.
Whittington Life Assurance Company Prospectuses 1867–91, MS 34427/001 and MS 34427/002.

Lowewood Museum

Anthony Warner. *John Warner. Some Notes on His Family*, compiled 1990.

Greater Manchester County Record Office

Minutes, Manchester and Salford Temperance Society, March 1851, MS M136/2/3/1166.
Shareholders' report of fourth annual general meeting, The Manchester Temperance Hotels Company Ltd, MS M618/1/1.
Shareholders' report of fifth annual general meeting, The Manchester Temperance Hotels Company Ltd, MS M618/1/2.

National Archives

WO 12/9310 Commissary General of Musters Office and successors, General Muster Books and Pay Lists, Infantry, 91st Foot 1st Battalion.
WO 97 – Chelsea: Pensioners British Army Service Records 1760–1913, Box 2438, Box record number 33.
WO 121 – Chelsea: Pensioners' Discharge Documents 1760–1887, Reference WO 121, Box 0253.

National Art Library

Cassell's Illustrated Family Paper Exhibitor: Containing about Three Hundred Illustrations, with Letter-Press Descriptions of All the Principal Objects in the International Exhibition of 1862 (London: Cassell, Petter and Galpin, 1862), MS A.17.11.

University College London Hospital Archives

First Annual Report of the London Temperance Hospital, National Temperance Hospital Annual Reports, 1874–84, MS NTH/11/1.
Minute Book One, National Temperance Hospital Board of Management Minutes 1873–85, MS NTH/1/1.
Minute Book Two, National Temperance Hospital Board of Management Minutes 1885–8, MS NTH/1/1.
Sixth Annual Report of the London Temperance Hospital, National Temperance Hospital Annual Reports, 1874–84, MS NTH/1/1.

University of Leicester Special Collections Online

Historical Directories of England and Wales.

Prudential Archives

Agents' instructions: 1B Special for superintendents, 1870–1922, MS 1314.
Minute Book 1, 21 April 1847–7 October 1852.
Minute Book 4, 25 January 1872–14 January 1875.
Minute Book 24, 20 February 1896–29 July 1897.
Policy 94, 11 December 1864, Life Policies, 1855–, MS 3545.

Torquay Museum

Edward Vivian Letters.

Wellcome Library Special Collections

Alcoholism ephemera, EPH 568.
Professional and other correspondence, Thomas Barlow Letters, PP/BAR/C.
Testimonials, Thomas Barlow Letters, PP/BAR/K.

UCL Special Collections

Cuttings on Eugenics & Alcoholism 1910–11, Galton Collection, MS GALTON/2/13/1/13.

Government Papers

1892 (186) Life assurance companies, Statements of account and of life assurance and annuity business, and abstracts of actuarial reports deposited with the Board of Trade, under 'the Life Assurance Companies Act, 1870', during the year ended 31st December 1891.
Board of Education, Syllabus of lessons on 'temperance' for scholars attending public elementary schools, 1909 [Cd. 4746].

Census of England and Wales, 1881, Preliminary report, and tables of the population and houses enumerated in England and Wales, and in the Islands in British Seas on 4th April 1881 BPP 1881 XCVI [C.2955].
Inter-Departmental Committee on Physical Deterioration, Appendix to the report of the Inter-Departmental Committee on Physical Deterioration, vol. III, Appendix and general index, 1904 [Cd. 2186]
Inter-Departmental Committee on Physical Deterioration, Minutes of evidence taken before the Inter-Departmental Committee on Physical Deterioration, vol. II, List of witnesses and minutes of evidence, 1904 [Cd. 2210].
Report from the Select Committee on Inquiry into Drunkenness, with Minutes of Evidence, and Appendix, 1834, 19th Century House of Commons Sessional Papers, 1834 (559).
Return from Harbour Authorities of Cost of Works, Loans and Scale of Dues, 1883, vol. 62, 302 and 684, 19th Century House of Commons Sessional Papers, 1883 (313).
Sixteenth annual report of the Local Government Board, 1886–87, 19th Century House of Commons Sessional Papers, C.5131, vol. 36, LXIX.

Newspapers, journals and periodicals

Aberdeen Weekly Journal.
Abstainer's Journal.
Anti-Slavery Reporter.
Atchison Globe.
Auckland Star.
Bath Chronicle and Weekly Gazette.
Belfast News-Letter.
Bendigo Independent.
Birmingham Daily Post.
Blackburn Standard and North East Lancashire Advertiser.
Boston Daily Advertiser.
Bradford Observer.
Bristol Mercury (also *Bristol Mercury and Daily Post*).
Bristol Temperance Herald.
British Journal of Addiction.
British Medical Journal.
British Women's Temperance Journal.
Bury and Norwich Post, and Suffolk Standard (also *The Bury and Norwich Post, and East Anglian*).
Cambrian (later Cambrian News and Merionethshire Standard).
Chelmsford Chronicle.
Cheshire Observer.
Christian Investigator and Evangelical Reformer.
Cork Examiner.
Cornhill Magazine.
Cornwall Royal Gazette, Falmouth Packet and Plymouth Journal.
Daily Gazette.
Daily Gazette for Middlesborough.
Daily Inter Ocean.

Daily Mail.
Daily News.
Daily Picayune.
Daily Telegraph.
Derby Mercury.
Derbyshire Times and Chesterfield Herald.
Devon and Exeter Daily Gazette.
Edinburgh Review.
The Era.
Essex Review.
Essex Standard, West Suffolk Gazette, and Eastern Counties' Advertiser.
Evening Star.
Evening Telegraph.
Financial Times.
Friends' Quarterly Examiner.
Gloucester Citizen.
Gloucester Journal.
Good Templars' Watchword.
Good Words.
Hampshire Advertiser.
Hampshire Telegraph and Sussex Chronicle.
Huddersfield Chronicle (later *The Huddersfield Chronicle and West Yorkshire Advertiser*).
Hull Daily Mail.
Hull Packet and East Riding Times.
Illustrated Police News.
Insurance Register.
Isle of Man Times and General Advertiser.
Isle of Wight Observer.
Journal of the American Medical Association.
Journal of the Institute of Actuaries.
Journal of the Statistical Society of London (later *Journal of the Royal Statistical Society*).
Lancashire Evening Post.
Lancaster Gazette and General Advertiser for Lancashire, Westmorland, and Yorkshire.
The Lancet.
Leeds Mercury.
Leeds Times.
Leicester Chronicle (later *Leicester Chronicle and the Leicestershire Mercury*).
Leicester Journal.
Leicestershire Mercury.
Licensed Victuallers' Mirror.
Liverpool Mercury.
Llangollen Advertiser, Denbighshire, Merionethshire, and North Wales Journal.
Lloyd's Weekly Newspaper.
London Gazette.
Manchester Courier and Lancashire General Advertiser.
Manchester Guardian.
Manchester Magazine.

Manchester Times.
Merthyr Telegraph, and General Advertiser.
Minutes of the Proceedings of the Institution of Civil Engineers.
Montreal Daily Witness.
Morning Post.
National Review.
National Temperance Chronicle and Temperance Recorder.
New York Times.
New York Tribune.
Newcastle Courant.
Nineteenth Century.
North-Eastern Daily Gazette.
Northern Echo.
Nottingham Evening Post.
Nottinghamshire Guardian.
The Observer.
The Owl.
Pembrokeshire Herald and General Advertiser.
Perry's Bankrupt and Insolvent Gazette.
Phrenological Journal and Life Illustrated.
Pittsburgh Press.
The Practitioner.
Preston Chronicle and Lancaster Advertiser.
Proceedings of the Association of Life Insurance Medical Directors of America.
Quiver.
Royal Cornwall Gazette.
Sheffield & Rotherham Independent.
Sherborne Mercury.
Shields Daily Gazette.
Shrewsbury Chronicle.
South Wales Daily Post.
Southampton Herald.
The Spectator.
The Standard.
Stirling Observer.
Temperance Gazette.
The Times.
Trewman's Exeter Flying Post (also *Trewman's Exeter Flying Post or Plymouth and Cornish Advertiser)*
Wanganui Chronicle.
Weekly Mail.
Western Daily Press And Bristol Mirror.
Western Gazette.
Western Mail.
Western Times.
Wings.
Woolmer's Exeter and Plymouth Gazette.
Worcestershire Chronicle.

Wrexham Advertiser, Denbighshire, Flintshire, Shropshire, Cheshire & North Wales Register (also *The Wrexham Advertiser, and North Wales News)*
Y Genedl Cymreig.
York Herald.

Printed primary literature

Allen, Jonathan Adams. *Medical Examinations for Life Insurance*, first edition. Chicago: Horton and Leonard, 1867.
Allen, Jonathan Adams. *Medical Examinations for Life Insurance*, sixth edition. New York: J H and C M Goodsell, 1870.
'An Anti-Alcohol Congress. Extraordinary Debate', *Birmingham Daily Post*, 17 August 1893, 8.
Anstie, Francis. 'On the Physiological and Therapeutical Action of Alcohol'. *The Lancet* 86, 2195 (23 September 1865), 343–5.
Anstie, Francis. *Stimulants and Narcotics, Their Mutual Relations: With Special Researches on the Action of Alcohol, Aether, and Chloroform, on the Vital Organism.* London: Macmillan, 1864.
Anstie, Francis Edmund. 'Alcohol. Is It Food, Medicine, or Poison?' *Cornhill Magazine* 5 (1862), 707–16.
Anstie, Francis Edmund. 'Does Alcohol Act as Food?' *Cornhill Magazine* 6 (1862), 319–29.
Anstie, Francis Edmund. 'Final Experiments on the Elimination of Alcohol by the Body'. *Practitioner* 13 (1874), 15–28.
Anstie, Francis Edmund. 'Lectures on the Prognosis and Treatment of Certain Acute Diseases, with Special Reference to the Indications Afforded by the Graphic Study of the Pulse', first part, *The Lancet* 90, 2289 (13 July 1867), 35–6.
Anstie, Francis Edmund. 'Lectures on the Prognosis and Treatment of Certain Acute Diseases, with Special Reference to the Indications Afforded by the Graphic Study of the Pulse', second part, *The Lancet* 90, 2294 (17 August 1867), 189–91.
Anstie, Francis Edmund. 'The Medical Declaration Respecting Alcohol'. *The Lancet* 98, 2522 (30 December 1871), 931.
Anstie, Francis Edmund. 'The Medical Declaration Respecting Alcohol'. *The Practitioner* 8, January 1872, 45–8.
Anstie, Francis Edmund. 'On the Diurnal Fluctuations of the Pulse-Form, and on Certain Cautions Necessary to be Observed in Sphygmography'. *The Lancet* 68, 2267 (9 February 1867), 170–2.
Anstie, Francis Edmund. *On the Uses of Wines in Health and Disease*. New York: J. S. Redfield, 1870.
'The Anti-Alcohol Congress', *Leeds Mercury*, 17 August 1893, 8.
Barker, Arthur G. *The Temperance Century in the West*. Bristol: T. O. Elworthy and Son, 1937.
Beavan, Ebenezer. *History of the Welsh Sunday Closing Act*. Cardiff: Daniel Owen, 1885.
Billings, J. S., C. W. Eliot, H. W. Fortune, J. L. Greene and F. G. Peabody. *The Liquor Problem. A Summary of Investigations Conducted by the Committee of Fifty 1893–1903.* Boston: Houghton Mifflin, 1905.
Bingham, William J. P. *Alcohol and Life Assurance*. London: United Kingdom Alliance, 1922.

Boase, Frederic. 'Joseph Mortimer Granville'. In *Modern English Biography, Volume V*, 478–9 (1912, reproduced London: Frank Cass, 1965).
Brinton, William. *On the Medical Selection of Lives for Assurance*, first edition. New York: John Hopper, 1863.
Brockbank, Edward Mansfield. *Life Insurance and General Practice*. London: Henry Frowde, Hodder and Stoughton, 1908.
Burns, James Dawson. 'Some Remarks on Temperance Statistics'. In *Proceedings of the International Temperance and Prohibition Convention, 1862*, edited by J. C. Street, F. R. Lees and D. Burns, 281–6. London: Job Caudwell, 1862.
Burns, James Dawson. *Temperance History. A Consecutive History of the Rise, Development, and Extension of the Temperance Reform. Volume I. 1826–1842*. London: National Temperance Publication Depot, 1889.
Burns, James Dawson. *The Vital Statistics of Total Abstinence*. LSE Selected Pamphlets. London: National Temperance Publication Depot, 1883.
Cardew, George Arthur. *Echoes and Reminiscences of Medical Practitioners in Cheltenham of the Nineteenth Century*. Cheltenham: E. J. Burrow, 1906.
Caverly, R. B., and George Nugent Bankes. *Leading Insurance Men of the British Empire*. London: Index Publishing, 1892.
Census of England and Wales, 1881, Preliminary Report, and Tables of the Population and Houses Enumerated in England and Wales, and in the Islands in British Seas on 4th April 1881, BPP 1881 XCVI [C.2955].
Central Control Board (Liquor Traffic) Advisory Committee. *Alcohol: Its Action on the Human Organism*. London: HM Stationery Office, 1918.
Clay, John. 'Observations on the Annual Statistical Reports of the Gaol at Preston, in Lancashire, for the Last Four Years, Prepared by the Chaplain the Rev. John Clay'. *Proceedings of the Statistical Society of London* 1, 9 (1836–7), 246–60.
Cokayne, George E. *Complete Baronetage*. Exeter: W. Pollard, 1900.
'Congress about Alcohol. Attitude Taken by the Doctors. Extraordinary Debate', *Auckland Star* 24, 250 (21 October 1893), 4.
Cruikshank, G. *The Bottle. In Eight Plates. Designed and Etched by George Cruikshank*. London: Spottiswoode and Shaw, 1847.
De Havilland Hall, Francis. *The Medical Examination for Life Insurance. With Remarks on the Selection of an Office*, third edition. Bristol: John Wright, 1903.
Dickinson, William Howship. 'Alcohol as a Cause of Renal Disease', *British Medical Journal* 2, 621 (23 November 1872), 573–5.
Dickinson, William Howship. 'The Morbid Effects of Alcohol', *British Medical Journal* 2, 622 (30 November 1872), 605.
'Drinking and Drunkenness', *British Medical Journal*, 26 September 1891, 702.
Drysdale, Charles R. *The Length of Life of Total Abstainers and Moderate Drinkers Compared: As Taken from the Records of Insurance Companies and Benefit Societies*. London: National Temperance Publication Depot, 1884.
Duckworth, Dyce. 'An Address on Collective Investigation of Disease'. *British Medical Journal* 1, 1201 (1884), 4–5.
Duckworth, Dyce. 'Address in Medicine. The Prognosis of Disease'. *British Medical Journal*, 1 August 1896, 251–8.
Duckworth, Dyce. 'An Address on Some Insufficiently Recognized Points in the Diagnosis of Disease', *British Medical Journal*, 20 March 1909, 701–3.
Duckworth, Dyce. 'Moderate Drinking and Total Abstinence', *Journal of the American Medical Association* 37, 21 (1901), 1396.

Duckworth, Dyce. 'On the Medical Injunction of Stimulants in Disease and in Health'. *British Medical Journal* 2, 880 (10 November 1877), 660–2.

Duckworth, Dyce. 'Some Observations on Medical Examinations for Life Assurance: Being the Presidential Address delivered before the Life Assurance Medical Officers' Association on Jan. 27th, 1904', *The Lancet* 163, 4197 (6 February 1904), 355–6.

Duckworth, Dyce. *Views on Some Social Subjects*. London: George Allen & Unwin, 1915.

'E. Cahill & Sons'. In *Twentieth Century Impressions of Ceylon: Its History, People, Commerce, Industries and Resources*, edited by A. Wright, 452. London: Lloyd's Greater Britain Publishing, 1907.

Elderton, Ethel M., and Karl Pearson. *A First Study of the Influence of Parental Alcoholism on the Physique and Ability of the Offspring*. London: Dulau, 1910.

Elliott, T. R. 'Thomas Barlow. 1845–1945'. *Obituary Notices of Fellows of the Royal Society* 5, 14 (1945), 158–67.

Felkin, W. 'Moral Statistics of a District Near Gray's Inn, London, in 1836'. *Journal of the Statistical Society of London* 1 (1839), 541–2.

Felkin, W. 'Moral Statistics of a Section of the City of Norwich'. *Journal of the Statistical Society of London* 1 (1839), 540–1.

Fisk, Eugene Lyman. *Alcohol: Its Relation to Human Efficiency and Longevity*. New York: Funk and Wagnalls, 1917.

Fox, Anna F., ed. *Memoir of Robert Charleton: Compiled Chiefly from His Letters*. London: S. Harris, 1876.

General Board of Health Medical Council. *Report of the Committee for Scientific Inquiries in Relation to the Cholera Epidemic of 1854*. London: Eyre and Spottiswoode, 1855.

Granville, Joseph Mortimer. *Common Mind Troubles*. London: David Bogue, 1878.

Granville, Joseph Mortimer. 'Drink: Ethical Considerations, and Physiological'. *National Review* 18, 104 (1891), 160–76.

Granville, Joseph Mortimer. 'Drinking and Drunkenness'. *The Times*, 15 September 1891, 8.

Granville, Joseph Mortimer. 'Fish as Food and Physic'. *Good Words* 22 (1881), 676–7.

Granville, Joseph Mortimer. *Gout in Its Clinical Aspects: An Outline of the Disease and Its Treatment for Practitioners*. London: J. & A. Churchill, 1885.

Granville, Joseph Mortimer, *Minds and Moods: Gossiping Papers on Mind-Management and Morals*. London: Renshaw, 1878.

Granville, Joseph Mortimer. *Nerve-Vibration and Excitation as Agents in the Treatment of Functional Disorder and Organic Disease*. London: J. & A. Churchill, 1883.

Granville, Joseph Mortimer. 'Nightcaps'. *Huddersfield Daily Chronicle*, 12 December 1883.

Granville, Joseph Mortimer. 'Seasonable Wish'. *Moonshine*, 12 January 1884, 24.

Granville, Joseph Mortimer. 'Worry'. *Nineteenth Century: A Monthly Review* 10, 55 (1881), 423–9.

Greene, Charles Lyman. *The Medical Examination for Life Insurance and Its Associated Clinical Methods, with Chapters on the Insurance of Substandard Lives and Accident Insurance*, second edition. London: Rebman, 1905.

Groves, John Percy. *History of the 91st Princess Louise's Argyllshire Highlanders*. Edinburgh: W. & A. K. Johnston, 1894.

Harben, Henry A. *A Dictionary of London*. London: H. Jenkins, 1918. www.british-history.ac.uk/no-series/dictionary-of-london, accessed 6 September 2023.

Hawes, C. W. *Hawes' Handbook of Temperance Hotels 1888*, new edition. London: National Temperance Publication Depot, 1888.
History of Teetotalism in Devonshire. Devonport: W. Hunt and J. Pasco, 1841.
'History of Life Insurance', *The Economist* 161, 15 September 1951, 623.
Hollingshead, John. 'The City of Unlimited Paper'. *Household Words* 17, 12 December 1857, 1–4.
Horsley, Victor, and Mary Sturge. *Alcohol and the Human Body: An Introduction to the Study of the Subject, and a Contribution to National Health*. London: Macmillan, 1907.
The House of Jarrolds 1823–1923: A Brief History of One Hundred Years. Norwich: Jarrolds, 1924.
Hoyle, William. *Our National Resources; And How They Are Wasted. An Omitted Chapter in Political Economy*. London: Simpkin, Marshall, 1871.
Hudson, Thomas. *Temperance Pioneers of the West*. London: National Temperance Publication Depot, 1888.
Hunter, Arthur. 'The Medico-Actuarial Investigation of the Mortality of American and Canadian Life Assurance Companies'. *Journal of the Institute of Actuaries* 48, 2 (1914), 186–97.
Hunter, Arthur, and Oscar H. Rogers. 'Ratings for the Principal Impairments'. In *Proceedings of Association of Life Insurance Medical Directors of America*, 121–67. New York: Knickerbocker Press, 1922.
'In Memoriam: Francis Edmund Anstie', *The Lancet* (19 September 1874), 427.
Kerr, Norman. *Inebriety: Its Etiology, Pathology, Treatment and Jurisprudence*. London: H. K. Lewis, 1888.
Keynes, John Maynard. 'Influence of Parental Alcoholism'. *Journal of the Royal Statistical Society* 73 (1910), 769–73.
Kirton, John W. *The Life of Joseph Harrap of Leicester*. Leicester: Richard Lawrence, 1873.
'Law Intelligence', *Journal of the Institute of Actuaries & Assurance Magazine* 22, 1 (1879), 20–4.
Lister, Thomas David. *Medical Examination for Life Insurance*. London: Edward Arnold, 1921.
Lynas, George. 'Why will ye die?' *Wings*, 1 July 1893, 219–20.
MacLaren, James Paterson. *Medical Insurance Examination: Modern Methods and Rating of Lives, for Medical Practitioners, and Insurance Officials*. London: Baillière, Tindall and Cox, 1927.
Macmillan, Alistair, ed. *Mauritius Illustrated: Historical and Descriptive, Commercial and Industrial Facts, Figures, & Resources*. London: W. H. and L. Collingridge, 1914.
Mason, Griselda Fox. *Sleigh Ride to Russia*. York: Sessions, 1985.
McCall Anderson, Thomas, Alfred G. Barrs, William H. Bennett, James Crichton-Browne, W. E. Dixon, Dyce Duckworth, Thomas R. Fraser, T. R. Glynn, W. R. Gowers, W. D. Halliburton, Jonathan Hutchinson, Robert Hutchinson, Edmund Owen, P. H. Pye-Smith, Fred. T. Roberts and Edgcombe Venning. 'The Use of Alcoholic Beverages'. *The Lancet* 169, 4361 (30 March 1907).
'Medical Declaration Respecting Alcohol', *British Medical Journal* (23 December 1871), 737–8.
The Methodist's Who's Who. London: Charles H. Kelly, 1912.
'Moderate Drinking and Total Abstinence', *Journal of the American Medical Association* 37, 21 (1901), 1396.
Moinet, Francis W. *Guide to Medical Examination for Life Insurance*. Edinburgh: Maclachlan and Stewart, 1876.

Moir, Henry. 'Address by the President, Henry Moir. State and National Enterprise'. *Transactions, Actuarial Society of America* 21, 63–64 (1920), 1–15.
Moore, Benjamin. *History of Wesleyan Methodism in Burnley and East Lancashire*. Burnley: Gazette Printing Works, 1899.
'The Morbid Effects of Alcohol', *British Medical Journal* 2, 621 (23 November 1872), 583–4.
Mowatt, James Alexander. 'Life Insurance and Moderate Drinking – Facts!' *Phrenological Journal and Life Illustrated* 57, 5 (1 November 1873), 304–5.
Mudge, Henry. *Exposure of Odd Fellowship*. London: Whittaker and Son, 1845.
Mudge, Henry. *Physiology, Health, & Disease, Demanding Abstinence from Alcoholic Drinks, and Prohibition of Their Common Sale: Being a Course of Five Lectures*. London: William Tweedie, 1859.
Neison, Francis G. P. *Contributions to Vital Statistics*, third edition. London: Simpkin, Marshall, 1857.
Newsholme, Arthur. 'The Possible Association of the Consumption of Alcohol with Excessive Mortality from Cancer'. *Journal of the Institute of Actuaries* 38, 4 (1904), 347–53.
Newsholme, Arthur. *Public Health and Insurance: American Addresses*. Baltimore, MD: Johns Hopkins University Press, 1920.
'Obituary: Francis Edmund Anstie', *The Lancet* (19 September 1874), 433–4.
Parkes, Edmund. 'Letter re the Medical Declaration Respecting Alcohol'. *The Practitioner* 8, February 1872, 82–5.
Parkes, Edmund. *Manual of Practical Hygiene*, first edition. London: John Churchill and Sons, 1864.
Parkes, Edmund. *Manual of Practical Hygiene*, eighth edition. London: J. A. Churchill, 1891.
Parkes, Edmund. *On Personal Care in Health*. London: Society for Promoting Christian Knowledge, 1876.
Parkes, Edmund, and Cyprian Wollowicz. 'Experiments on the Effect of Alcohol (Ethyl Alcohol) on the Human Body'. *Proceedings of the Royal Society London* 18 (1869–70), 362–93.
Pearl, Raymond. *Alcohol and Longevity*. New York: Alfred A. Knopf, 1926.
Pearson, Karl, and Ethel M. Elderton. *A Second Study of the Influence of Parental Alcoholism on the Physique and Ability of Offspring*. London: Dulau, 1911.
Pollock, James Edward, and Chisholm, James. *Medical Handbook of Life Assurance for the Use of Medical and other officers of Companies*, fourth edition. London: Cassell, 1895.
'Poor-Law Medical Officers' Association and the Late Dr. Anstie', *The Lancet* 104, 2668 (17 October 1874), 568–9.
Price, Seymour J. *From Queen to Queen: The Centenary Story of the Temperance Permanent Building Society 1854–1954*. London: Franey, 1954.
'Proceedings of the Statistical Society', *Journal of the Statistical Society of London* 28, 4 (1865), 538–9.
The Proceedings of the World's Temperance Convention, Held in London, August 4th, and Four Following Days. London: World's Temperance Convention, 1846.
Quetelet, M. A. *A Treatise on Man and the Development of his Faculties*, translated by Robert Knox. Edinburgh: William and Robert Chambers, 1842.
Ransome, Edwin R. 'Bygone Ipswich Friends'. *Friends' Quarterly Examiner* 42 (1908), 308–20.
Ridge, J. James. 'Medical Declarations re Alcohol'. *British Medical Journal* 1 (1888), 1033.

Rowntree, Joseph, and Arthur Sherwell. *The Temperance Problem and Social Reform*. London: Hodder and Stoughton, 1899.

Sessions, Frederick. *The Life Story of Samuel Bowly: A Champion of Freedom, Progress and Temperance*. London: Friends Tract Association, 1903.

Sieveking, Edward Henry. *The Medical Adviser in Life Insurance*, second edition. London: J & A Churchill, 1882.

Smiles, Samuel. *Thrift*. London: John Murray, 1875.

Snowden, Philip. *An Autobiography. Volume I, 1864–1919*. London: Ivor Nicholson and Watson, 1934.

'Statistics. Medical Examinations in Scotland for Life Assurance Companies', *Edinburgh Medical Journal* 1, 6 (1855), 553–4.

Sturge, Mary, and Victor Horsley. 'On Some of the Biological and Statistical Errors in the Work on Parental Alcoholism by Miss Elderton and Professor Karl Pearson, F.R.S.'. *British Medical Journal* 1, 14 January 1911, 72–82.

Taylor, Maria. *Memorials of Samuel Bowly, Born March 23, 1802, Died March 23, 1884 Compiled by His Daughter, Maria Taylor*. Gloucester: Privately published, 1884.

Temperance, Longevity, Insurance. A Tract for the Times. Toronto: Canada Citizen Publishing, 1884.

'Temperance Notes and News', *Quiver* 908 (January 1902), 207–8.

Thompson, Vance. *Drink and Be Sober*. New York: Yard, 1915.

Thomson, Robert Dundas. *Digestion: The Influence of Alcoholic Fluids on that Function, and on the Value of Health and Life. With a Scheme for Rendering the Working Classes Independent of Parish Relief*. London: John Snow, 1841.

Wagg, Henry J. *A Chronological Survey of Work for the Blind*. London: Pitman and Sons, 1932.

Walford, Cornelius. 'History of Life Assurance in the United Kingdom, 5. Life Assurance 1825 to 1843'. *Journal of the Institute of Actuaries* 26 (1886–7), 302–15.

Warne, Eliza. *A Memoir of the Life and Ministry of Edmund Warne, Lately an Itinerant Preacher in the Bible Christian Connexion*, revised by James Thorne. Devon: S. Thorne, 1830.

Watkins, Henry. *The Art of Gerald Moira. With Some Notes and Thoughts on Decorative Art by Gerald Moira*. London: E. W. Dickens, 1922.

Whittaker, Thomas P. 'Alcoholic Beverages and Longevity'. *Institute of Actuaries Life Assurance Tracts* 13 (1903–4), 19.

Whittaker, Thomas. *Brighter England and the Way to It*. London: Hodder and Stoughton, 1891.

Whittaker, Thomas. *Life's Battles in Temperance Armour*, third edition. London: Hodder and Stoughton, 1888.

Wilson, George B. 'A Statistical Review of the Variations during the Last Twenty Years in the Consumption of Intoxicating Drinks in the United Kingdom, and in Convictions for Offences Connected with Intoxication, with a Discussion of the Causes to Which These Variations May Be Ascribed', *Journal of the Royal Statistical Society* 75 (1912), 183–247.

Winskill, Peter T. *The Comprehensive History of the Rise and Progress of the Temperance Reformation from the Earliest Period to September 1881*. Warrington: P.T. Winskill, 1881.

Winskill, Peter T. *The Temperance Movement and Its Workers: A Record of Social, Moral, Religious, and Political Progress*, vol. 1. London: Blackie, 1891.

Winskill, Peter T. *The Temperance Movement and Its Workers: A Record of Social, Moral, Religious, and Political Progress*, vol. 2. London: Blackie, 1891.
Winskill, Peter T. *The Temperance Movement and Its Workers: A Record of Social, Moral, Religious, and Political Progress*, vol. 3. London: Blackie, 1892.
Winskill, Peter T. *The Temperance Movement and Its Workers: A Record of Social, Moral, Religious, and Political Progress*, vol. 4. London: Blackie, 1892.
Winskill, Peter T. *Temperance Standard Bearers of the Nineteenth Century. A Biographical and Statistical Temperance Dictionary*, vol. 1. Liverpool: Winskill, 1897.
Winskill, Peter T. *Temperance Standard Bearers of the Nineteenth Century. A Biographical and Statistical Temperance Dictionary*, vol. 2. Liverpool: Winskill, 1898.
Woolley, John Granville, and William E. Johnson. *Temperance Progress in the Century*. London: Linscott Publishing, 1903.

Secondary sources

Adler, Marianna. 'From Symbolic Exchange to Commodity Consumption: Anthropological Notes on Drinking as a Symbolic Practice'. In *Drinking: Behavior and Belief in Modern History*, edited by Susanna Barrows and Robin Room, 376–98. Berkeley: University of California Press, 1991.
Alborn, Timothy. 'Insurance against Germ Theory: Commerce and Conservatism in Late-Victorian Medicine'. *Bulletin of the History of Medicine* 75 (2001), 406–45.
Alborn, Timothy. 'Quill-Driving: British Life-Insurance Clerks and Occupational Mobility, 1800–1914'. *Business History Review* 82 (2008), 31–58.
Alborn, Timothy. *Regulated Lives: Life Insurance and British Society, 1800–1914*. Toronto: University of Toronto Press, 2009.
Amoore, Louise. 'Security and the Incalculable'. *Security Dialogue* 45 (2014), 423–39.
Andersen, Lisa M. F. *The Politics of Prohibition*. Cambridge: Cambridge University Press, 2013.
Anderson, Gregory. *Victorian Clerks*. Manchester: Manchester University Press, 1976.
Andersson, Peter K. 'How Civilized Were the Victorians?' *Journal of Victorian Culture* 20, 4 (2015), 439–52.
Armstrong, W. A. 'The Use of Information about Occupation'. In *Nineteenth-Century Society*, edited by Edward A. Wrigley, 191–310. Cambridge: Cambridge University Press, 1972.
Aspin, Richard. 'Barlow, Sir Thomas, First Baronet (1845–1945)'. In *Oxford Dictionary of National Biography*. Oxford University Press, 2004. www.oxforddnb.com/view/article/30595, accessed 5 February 2013.
Backhouse, Roger E. *The Ordinary Business of Life: A History of Economics from the Ancient World to the Twenty-First Century*, new edition. Princeton, NJ: Princeton University Press, 2024.
Bailey, Adrian R., David C. Harvey and Catherine Brace. 'Disciplining Youthful Methodist Bodies in Nineteenth-Century Cornwall'. *Annals of the Association of American Geographers* 97, 1 (2007), 142–57.
Bailey, Peter. 'White Collars, Gray Lives? The Lower Middle Class Revisited'. *Journal of British Studies* 38 (1999), 273–90.
Bailey, Peter. '"Will the Real Bill Banks Please Stand up?" Towards a Role Analysis of Mid-Victorian Working-Class Respectability'. *Journal of Social History* 12, 3 (1979), 336–53.

Bailey, Victor. 'In Darkest England and the Way Out'. *International Review of Social History* 92 (1984), 133–71.

Bailey, Victor. 'Salvation Army Riots, the "Skeleton Army" and Legal Authority in the Provincial Town'. In *Order and Disorder in Modern Britain: Essays on Riot, Crime, Policing and Punishment*, 16–33. London: Breviary Stuff, 2014.

Baldwin, Arthur D. 'Anstie's Alcohol Limit. Francis Edmund Anstie 1833–1874'. *American Journal of Public Health* 67, 7 (1977), 679–81.

Barkan, Elazar. *The Retreat of Scientific Racism: Changing Concepts of Race in Britain and the United States between the World Wars*. Cambridge: Cambridge University Press, 1991.

Barker, Hannah. *Family and Business during the Industrial Revolution*. Oxford: Oxford University Press, 2016.

Beckingham, David. *The Licensed City: Regulating drink in Liverpool*. Liverpool: Liverpool University Press, 2017.

Beckingham, David. 'The Press and the Pledge: Father Theobald Mathew's 1843 Temperance Tour of Britain'. *Historical Geography* 42 (2014), 93–110.

Beckingham, David. 'Private Spirits, Public Lives: Sober Citizenship, Shame and Secret Drinking in Victorian Britain'. *Journal of Victorian Culture* 26, 3 (2021), 419–34.

Beckingham, David, and Charles Watkins. 'Temperance Lives and Landscape: Lady Elizabeth Biddulph, Lady Henry Somerset, and Late Nineteenth-Century Ledbury'. *Rural History* (2024), 1–22.

Bell, E. Moberly. *Storming the Citadel: The Rise of the Woman Doctor*. London: Constable, 1953.

Bentham, Jeremy. *The Works of Jeremy Bentham*, vol. 1. New York: Russell and Russell, 1962.

Bergquist, Ann-Kristin, and Liselotte Eriksson. 'Sober Business: Shared Value Creation between the Insurance Industry and the Temperance Movement'. *Business History* 61, 2 (2019), 322–42.

Berridge, Virginia. *Demons: Our Changing Attitudes to Alcohol, Tobacco, and Drugs*. Oxford: Oxford University Press, 2013.

Berridge, Virginia. 'Opium Eating and Life Insurance'. *British Journal of Addiction* 72 (1977), 371–7.

Berridge, Virginia. 'Society for the Study of Addiction'. *British Journal of Addiction* 85 (1990), 987–1077.

Black, Ian S. 'Spaces of Capital: Bank Office Building in the City of London, 1830–1870'. *Journal of Historical Geography* 26, 3 (2000), 351–75.

Black, Ros. *Scandal, Salvation and Suffrage: The Amazing Women of the Temperance Movement*. Kibworth Beauchamp: Matador, 2015.

Boase, G. C. 'Charleton, Robert (1809–1872)', rev. K. D. Reynolds. In *Oxford Dictionary of National Biography*. Oxford University Press, 2004. www.oxforddnb.com/view/article/5156, accessed 9 January 2013.

Bonea, Amelia, Melissa Dickson, Sally Shuttleworth and Jennifer Wallis. 'The Woman Secret Drinker in the Late Nineteenth-Century Press'. In *Anxious Times: Medicine and Modernity in Nineteenth-Century Britain*, 119–48. Pittsburgh, PA: Pittsburgh University Press, 2019.

Booth, Kate, and Andrew Harwood. 'Insurance as Catastrophe: A Geography of House and Contents Insurance in Bushfire-Prone Places'. *Geoforum* 69 (2016), 44–52.

Bouk, Dan. *How Our Days Became Numbered: Risk and the Rise of the Statistical Individual*. London: University of Chicago Press, 2015.

Bowser, Alfred T. 'Temperance Sections in Life Offices', *The Spectator* 15, 5 (1 November 1875).

Brantlinger, Patrick. *Fictions of State: Culture and Credit in Britain, 1694–1994*. Ithaca, NY: Cornell University Press, 1996.

Brendon, Piers. 'Cook, Thomas (1808–1892), Travel Agent'. In *Oxford Dictionary of National Biography*. Oxford University Press, 2008. www.oxforddnb.com/view/10.1093/ref:odnb/9780198614128.001.0001/odnb-9780198614128-e-6152.

Bressey, Caroline. *Empire, Race and the Politics of Anti-Caste*. London: Bloomsbury, 2015.

Brockett, Allan. *Nonconformity in Exeter, 1650–1875*. Manchester: Manchester University Press, 1962.

Bynum, W. F. 'Alcoholism and Degeneration in 19th Century European Medicine and Psychiatry'. *British Journal of Addiction* 79 (1984), 59–70.

Cain, Joe. 'Publications Produced by the Francis Galton Laboratory for National Eugenics'. *The Library* 22, 4 (2021), 523–48.

Çalişkan, Koray, and Michel Callon. 'Economization, Part 2: A Research Programme for the Study of Markets'. *Economy and Society* 39, 1 (2010), 1–32.

Callon, Michel. *Markets in the Making: Rethinking Competition, Goods, and Innovation*, translated by Olivia Custer. Brooklyn, NY: Zone Books, 2021.

Callon, Michel. 'The Sociology of an Actor-Network: The Case of the Electric Vehicle'. In *Mapping the Dynamics of Science and Technology*, edited by Michel Callon, John Law and Arie Rip, 19–34. London: Palgrave Macmillan, 1986.

Chapman, Johnathan. 'Interest Rates, Sanitation Infrastructure, and Mortality Decline in Nineteenth-Century England and Wales'. *European Historical Economics Society Working Paper No. 218*, October 2021. https://ehes.org/wp/EHES_218.pdf.

Chapman, S. D. 'Felkin, William (1795–1874)'. In *Oxford Dictionary of National Biography*. Oxford University Press, 2004. www.oxforddnb.com/view/article/53532, accessed 2 August 2016.

Clark, Geoffrey W. *Betting on Lives: The Culture of Life Insurance in England, 1695–1775*. Manchester: Manchester University Press, 1999.

Clarke, Richard. 'Self-Help, Saving and Suburbanization: The Birkbeck Freehold Land and Building Societies, Their Bank, and the London Mechanics' Institute 1851–1911'. *London Journal* 40, 2 (2015), 123–46.

Clement, Mark. 'Mudge, Henry (1806–1874)'. In *Oxford Dictionary of National Biography*. Oxford University Press, 2004. www.oxforddnb.com/view/article/19483, accessed 9 January 2013.

Clow, Miranda. 'The Design of Trust, Past and Present: A Dialogue between "Design for Trust" in Contemporary Design Practice and the Fire Insurance Industry in England 1680–1914', PhD thesis, Royal College of Art, 2020.

Cockerell, Hugh A. L., and Edwin Green. *The British Insurance Business: History and Archives*. Sheffield: Sheffield Academic Press, 1994.

Cook, Christopher C. H. *Alcohol, Addiction and Christian Ethics*. Cambridge: Cambridge University Press, 2006.

Cordery, Simon. *British Friendly Societies, 1750–1914*. New York: Palgrave, 2003.

Crook, Tom. 'Suspect Figures: Statistics and Public Trust in Victorian England'. In *Statistics and the Public Sphere: Numbers and the People in Modern Britain, c. 1800–2000*, edited by Tom Crook and Glen O'Hara, 179–98. London: Routledge, 2011.

Crossick, Geoffrey, ed. *The Lower Middle Class in Britain, 1870–1914*. London: Croom Helm, 1977.

Cullen, Michael John. *The Statistical Movement in Early Victorian Britain*. Hassocks: Harvester Press; New York: Barnes and Noble, 1975.

Curtis, Bruce. 'Social Investment in Medical Forms: The 1866 Cholera Scare and Beyond'. *Canadian Historical Review* 81, 3 (2000), 347–79.

Daunton, Martin. *Coal Metropolis. Cardiff 1870–1914*. Leicester: Leicester University Press, 1977.

Davison, Andrew. '"Try the Alternative": The Built Heritage of the Temperance Movement'. *Brewery History* 123 (2006), 92–109.

de Certeau, Michel. *The Practice of Everyday Life*, translated by Steven Rendall. Berkeley: University of California Press, 1984.

Defert, Daniel. '"Popular Life" and Insurance Technology'. In *The Foucault Effect: Studies in Governmentality*, edited by Graham Burchell, Colin Gordon and Peter Miller, 211–33. Hertfordshire: Harvester Wheatsheaf, 1991.

Dennis, Richard. *English Industrial Cities of the Nineteenth Century*. Cambridge: Cambridge University Press, 1984.

Dennis, Richard. 'The Geography of Victorian Values: Philanthropic Housing in London, 1840–1900'. *Journal of Historical Geography* 15, 1 (1989), 40–54.

Dias-Lewandowska, Dorota, and Pam Lock. 'Women, Home, and Alcohol: Constructed Façades and Social Norms in Nineteenth-Century Polish and British Representations of Female Drinking Practices'. *Journal of Victorian Culture* 28, 2 (2023), 227–42.

Digby, Anne. *Making a Medical Living: Doctors and Patients in the English Market for Medicine, 1720–1911*. Cambridge: Cambridge University Press, 1994.

Dingle, Anthony E. *The Campaign for Prohibition in Victorian England: The United Kingdom Alliance 1872–1895*. London: Croom Helm, 1980.

Dingle, Anthony E. 'Drink and Working-Class Living Standards in Britain, 1870–1914'. *Economic History Review* second series, 25 (1972), 608–22.

Driver, Felix. 'Moral Geographies: Social Science and the Urban Environment in Mid-Nineteenth Century England'. *Transactions of the Institute of British Geographers* 13, 3 (1988), 275–87.

Duncan, Robert. *Pubs and Patriots: The Drink Crisis in Britain during World War One*. Liverpool: Liverpool University Press, 2013.

Dunnill, Michael S. 'Victor Horsley (1857–1916) and the Temperance Movement'. *Journal of Medical Biography* 20 (2012), 25–31.

Dupree, Marguerite W. 'Other than Healing: Medical Practitioners and the Business of Life Assurance during the Nineteenth and Early Twentieth Centuries'. *Social History of Medicine* 10, 1 (1997), 79–103.

Durie, Alistair. 'Almost Twins by Birth: Hydropathy, Temperance and the Scottish Churches 1840–1914'. *Scottish Church History Society* 32 (2002), 143–63.

Earles, M. P. 'Anstie, Francis Edmund (1833–1874)'. In *Oxford Dictionary of National Biography*. Oxford University Press, 2004. www.oxforddnb.com/view/article/583, accessed 12 August 2013.

Edensor, Tim. 'Entangled Agencies, Material Networks and Repair in a Building Assemblage: The Mutable Stone of St Ann's Church, Manchester'. *Transactions of the Institute of British Geographers* 36 (2011), 238–52.

Erdozain, Dominic. 'The Secularisation of Sin in the Nineteenth Century'. *Journal of Ecclesiastical History* 62, 1 (2011), 59–88.

Ewald, Francois. 'Insurance and Risk'. In *The Foucault Effect: Studies in Governmentality*, edited by Graham Burchell, Colin Gordon and Peter Miller, 197–210. Hertfordshire: Harvester Wheatsheaf, 1991.

Fahey, David M. 'Arthur Sherwell (1863–1942): Temperance Reformer and Liberal MP'. *Social Science Review* 98, 2 (2002). https://issr.ung.edu/articles/3.

Fahey, David M. 'Pope, Samuel (1826–1901)'. In *Alcohol and Temperance in Modern History: An International Encyclopedia*, edited by Jack S. Blocker, Jr., David M. Fahey and Ian R. Tyrrell, vol. 2, 486. Oxford: ABC-CLIO, 2003.

Fahey, David M. 'Temperance and the Liberal Party – Lord Peel's Report, 1899'. *Journal of British Studies* 10 (1971), 132–59.

Fahey, David M. *Temperance Societies in Late Victorian and Edwardian England*. Newcastle upon Tyne: Cambridge Scholars, 2020.

Fahey, David M. 'Worrying about Drink'. *Brewery History* 166 (2016), 2–19.

Farrall, Lyndsay Andrew. *The Origins and Growth of the English Eugenics Movement, 1865–1925*. STS Occasional Papers number 9. London: UCL Department of Science and Technology Studies, 2019.

Finn, Margot C. *The Character of Credit: Personal Debt in English Culture, 1740–1914*. Cambridge: Cambridge University Press, 2003.

Fisher, Fiona, and Rebecca Preston. 'Light, Airy and Open: The Design and Use of the Suburban Public-House Garden in England between the wars'. *Studies in the History of Gardens & Designed Landscapes* 39 (2019), 5–21.

Fladeland, Betty. *Abolitionists and Working-Class Problems in the Age of Industrialisation*. London: Macmillan, 1984.

French, Shaun, and James Kneale. 'Excessive Financialisation: Insuring Lifestyles and Everyday Geographies of Social Excess'. *Environment and Planning D: Society and Space* 27, 6 (2009), 1030–53.

French, Shaun, and James Kneale. 'Speculating on Careless Lives: Annuitising the Biofinancial Subject'. *Journal of Cultural Economy* 5, 4 (2012), 391–406.

Garrod, A. E. 'Duckworth, Sir Dyce, First Baronet (1840–1928)', rev. Patrick Wallis. In *Oxford Dictionary of National Biography*. Oxford University Press, 2004. www.oxforddnb.com/view/article/32912, accessed 27 July 2012.

Geison, Gerald. *Michael Foster and the Cambridge School of Physiology: The Scientific Enterprise in Late Victorian Society*. Princeton, NJ: Princeton University Press, 1978.

Gilbert, Pamela K. *Mapping the Victorian Social Body*. Albany: SUNY Press, 2004.

Girouard, M. 'A Hundred Years of Free Water'. *Country Life* 125, 3246 (2 April 1959), 700–1.

Gosden, P. H. J. H. *The Friendly Societies in England, 1815–1875*. Manchester: Manchester University Press, 1961.

Gramsci, Antonio. 'Rationalisation of Production and Work'. In *Selections from the Prison Notebooks of Antonio Gramsci*, edited and translated by Quintin Hoare and Geoffrey Nowell Smith, 385–9. New York: International Publishers, 1971.

Greenaway, John. *Drink and British Politics since 1830: A Study in Policy-Making*. Basingstoke: Palgrave Macmillan, 2003.

Greenaway, John. 'The "Improved" Public House, 1870–1950: The Key to Civilised Drinking or the Primrose Path to Drunkenness?' *Addiction* 93 (1998), 173–81.

Gregory, James. 'Hoyle, William (1832–1886)'. In *Alcohol and Temperance in Modern History: An International Encyclopedia*, edited by Jack S. Blocker, Jr., David M. Fahey and Ian R. Tyrrell, vol. I, 302. Oxford: ABC-CLIO, 2003.

Gregory, James. *Of Victorians and Vegetarians: The Vegetarian Movement in Nineteenth-Century Britain*. London: Tauris, 2007.

Gregory, James "'Zealously Affected in a Good Thing': The Publishing Career and Life of William Horsell (1807–1863)' (online, 2013).

Grierson, Janet. *Temperance, Therapy and Trilobites: Dr Ralph Grindrod, Victorian Pioneer*. Cora Weaver: Malvern, 2001.

Groth Lyon, Eileen. 'Barker, Joseph (1806–1875)'. In *Oxford Dictionary of National Biography*. Oxford University Press, 2004.

Gunn, Simon. *The Public Culture of the Victorian Middle Class*. Manchester: Manchester University Press, 2007.

Gutzke, David W. *Pubs and Progressives: Reinventing the Public House in England, 1896–1960*. DeKalb: Northern Illinois University Press, 2005.

Hacking, Ian. *The Taming of Chance*. Cambridge: Cambridge University Press, 1990.

Hankins, Richard. 'Pen Portraits of Presidents. Robert Dundas Thomson, MD, CM, FRS'. *Weather* 53 (1998), 266–8.

Harris, Bernard, and Andrew Hinde. 'Sanitary Investment and the Decline of Urban Mortality in England and Wales, 1817–1914'. *History of the Family* 24, 2 (2019), 339–76.

Harrison, Brian. 'The British Prohibitionists 1853–1872: A Biographical Analysis'. *International Review of Social History* 15, 3 (1970), 375–467.

Harrison, Brian. *Dictionary of Temperance Biography*. Coventry: Society for the Study of Labour History, 1973.

Harrison, Brian. *Drink and the Victorians*. London: Faber, 1971.

Harrison, Brian. 'Teetotal Chartism'. *History* 58, 193 (1973), 193–217.

Harrison, Brian, and Barry Trinder. *Drink and Sobriety in an Early Victorian Country Town: Banbury 1830–1860*. Harlow: Longmans, 1969.

Harvey, David C., Catherine Brace and Adrian R. Bailey. 'Parading the Cornish Subject: Methodist Sunday Schools in West Cornwall, c. 1830–1930'. *Journal of Historical Geography* 33, 1 (2007), 24–44.

Henry, Nancy. '"Ladies Do It?" Victorian Women Investors in Fact and Fiction'. In *Victorian Literature and Finance*, edited by Francis O'Gorman, 111–31. Oxford: Oxford University Press, 2007.

Henry, Nancy, and Cannon Schmitt, eds. *Victorian Investments: New Perspectives on Finance and Culture*. Bloomington: Indiana University Press, 2009.

Herbert, Christopher. 'Filthy Lucre: Victorian Ideas of Money'. *Victorian Studies* 44, 2 (2002), 185–213.

Hodder, Jake. 'On Absence and Abundance: Biography as Method in Archival Research', *Area* 49, 4 (2017), 452–59.

Hosgood, Christopher P. 'The "Knights of the Road": Commercial Travellers and the Culture of the Commercial Room in Late-Victorian and Edwardian England'. *Victorian Studies* 37, 4 (1994), 519–47.

Hosgood, Christopher P. 'The "Pigmies of Commerce" and the Working-Class Community: Small Shopkeepers in England, 1870–1914'. *Journal of Social History* 22, 3 (1989), 439–60.

Huxley, Margo. 'Geographies of Governmentality'. In *Space, Knowledge and Power: Foucault and Geography*, edited by Stuart Elden and Jeremy Crampton, 185–204. Oxford: Routledge, 2007.

Ischei, Elizabeth. *Victorian Quakers*. Oxford: Oxford University Press, 1970.

Ismay, Penelope. 'Between Providence and Risk: Odd Fellows, Benevolence and the Social Limits of Actuarial Science, 1820s–1880s'. *Past & Present* 226 (2015), 115–47.

Ivy, James D. 'Sons of Temperance'. In *Alcohol and Temperance in Modern History. An International Encyclopedia*, edited by Jack S. Blocker, Jr., David M. Fahey, and Ian R. Tyrrell, vol. 2, 572–4. Oxford: ABC-CLIO, 2003.

Jackson, Gordon, and Charles Munn. 'Trade, Industry and Commerce'. In *Glasgow. Volume II: 1830–1912*, edited by W. Hamish Fraser and Irene Maver, 52–95. Manchester: Manchester University Press, 1996.

Jennings, Paul. '"Grasping a Nettle": The 1904 Licensing Act'. In *Biographies of Drink; A Case Study Approach to Our Historical Relationship with Alcohol*, edited by Mark Hailwood and Deborah Toner, 30–48. Newcastle upon Tyne: Cambridge Scholars Publishing, 2015.

Jeremy, David J. *Capitalists and Christians: Business Leaders and the Churches in Britain, 1900–1960*. Oxford: Clarendon Press, 1990.

Jones, Charlotte. 'An Historical Geography of the Turkish Bath in Victorian Britain'. PhD thesis, University College London, 2017.

Jones, Stephen G. 'Labour, Society and the Drink Question in Britain, 1918–1939'. *Historical Journal* 30, 1 (1987), 105–22.

Joyce, Patrick. *Work, Society and Politics: The Culture of the Factory in Later Victorian England*. Brighton: Harvester Press, 1980.

Joyce, Patrick, and Chandra Mukerji. 'The State of Things: State History and Theory Reconfigured'. *Theory & Society* 46 (2017), 1–19.

Jureidini, Ray and Kevin White. 'Life Insurance, the Medical Examination and Cultural Values'. *Journal of Historical Sociology* 13 (2000), 190–214.

King, Elspeth. *Scotland Sober and Free: The Temperance Movement, 1829–1979*. Glasgow: Glasgow Museums and Art Galleries, 1979.

Kneale, James. 'The Battle of Torquay: The Late Victorian Resort as Social Experiment'. In *Coastal Cultures of the Long Nineteenth Century*, edited by Matthew Ingleby and Matthew Kerr, 79–97. Edinburgh: University of Edinburgh Press, 2018.

Kneale, James. 'Consumption'. In *Alcohol in the Age of Industry, Empire and War*, edited by Deborah Toner, 43–63. London: Bloomsbury, 2021.

Kneale, James. 'Dr Granville's Thunderbolt: Drink and the Public in the Life of One Nineteenth-Century Doctor'. *Social History of Alcohol and Drugs* 28, 2 (2014), 120–42.

Kneale, James. 'Good, Homely, Troublesome or Improving? Historical Geographies of Drinking Places, c. 1850–1950'. *Geography Compass* 15, e12557.15 (2021).

Kneale, James. 'Numbering Babylon? Failed Attempts to Map British Drinking, 1817–1914'. In *Narcotic Cities. Counter-Cartographies of Drugs and Spaces*, edited by M. Germes, L. Klaus and S. Höhne, 42–53. Berlin: Jovis, 2023.

Kneale, James. 'The Place of Drink: Temperance and the Public, 1856–1914'. *Social and Cultural Geography* 2 (2001), 43–59.

Kneale, James. '"A Problem of Supervision": Moral Geographies of the Nineteenth Century British Public House',. *Journal of Historical Geography* 25, 3 (1999), 333–48.

Kneale, James. '"These Are the Cases Who Call Themselves 'Moderate Drinkers', Because They Are Never Seen Embracing a Lamp-Post." The Problem of Moderate Drinking in Nineteenth- and Early Twentieth-Century Britain'. In *Just Enough: The History, Culture and Politics of Sufficiency*, edited by Matthew Ingleby and Samuel Randalls, 77–9. London: Palgrave Macmillan, 2019.

Kneale, James, and Shaun French. 'Mapping Alcohol: Health, Policy and the Geographies of Problem Drinking in Britain'. *Drugs: Education, Prevention, and Policy* 15, 3 (2008), 233–49.

Kneale, James, and Shaun French. 'Moderate Drinking before the Unit: Medicine and Life Assurance in Britain and the US c.1860–1930'. *Drugs: Education, Prevention and Policy* 22, 2 (2015), 111–17.

Kneale, James, and Shaun French. '"The Relations of Inebriety to Insurance": Geographies of Medicine, Insurance and Alcohol in Britain, 1840–1911'. In *Intoxication: Problematic Pleasures*, edited by Jonathan Herring, Ciaran Regan, Darin Weinberg and Phil Withington, 87–109. Basingstoke: Palgrave Macmillan, 2013.

Kneale, James, and Samuel Randalls. 'Imagined Geographies of Climate and Race in Anglophone Life Assurance, c.1840–1930'. In *Weather, Climate and the Geographical Imagination: Placing Atmospheric Knowledges*, edited by Martin Mahony and Samuel Randalls, 115–31. Pittsburgh, PA: University of Pittsburgh Press, 2020.

Kneale, James, and Samuel Randalls. 'Invisible Atmospheric Knowledges in British Insurance Companies, 1830–1914'. *History of Meteorology* 6 (2014), 35–52.

Kneale, James, and Samuel Randalls. 'Making Climate Risks Work: Governmentality and "Foreign Residence" in British Life Assurance, 1840–1940'. *Transactions of the Institute of British Geographers* 45, 4 (2020), 833–48.

Krasnick, Cheryl L. '"Because There Is Pain": Alcoholism, Temperance and the Victorian Physician'. *Canadian Bulletin of Medical History/Bulletin canadien; histoire de la médecine* 2 (1985), 1–22.

Lambert, David. 'Reflections on the Concept of Imperial Biographies'. *Geschichte und Gesellschaft* 40 (2014), 22–41.

Latham, Alan and Jack Layton. 'Social Infrastructure and the Public Life of Cities: Studying Urban Sociality and Public Spaces', *Geography Compass* 13, e12444 (2019).

Latour, Bruno. *Pandora's Hope*. Cambridge, MA: Harvard University Press, 1999.

Latour, Bruno. 'Technology Is Society Made Durable'. In *A Sociology of Monsters: Essays on Power, Technology, and Domination*, edited by John Law, 103–31. London: Routledge, 1991.

Latour, Bruno. *We Have Never Been Modern*. New York: Harvester Wheatsheaf, 1993.

Law, John, and Evelyn Ruppert. 'The Social Life of Methods: Devices'. *Journal of Cultural Economy* 6 (2013), 229–40.

Lawrence, Christopher. 'Incommunicable Knowledge: Science, Technology and the Clinical Art in Britain 1850–1914'. *Journal of Contemporary History* 20, 4 (1985), 503–20.

Lawrence, Jon. 'Class and Gender in the Making of Urban Toryism, 1880–1914'. *English Historical Review* 108, 428 (1993), 629–52.

Laybourn, Keith. *Philip Snowden: A Biography 1864–1937*. Aldershot: Temple Smith, 1988.

Le Messurier, B. *A History of the Mint Methodist Church, Exeter*. Exeter, 1962.

Lehtonen, Turo-Kimmo. 'Picturing How Life Insurance Matters'. *Journal of Cultural Economy* 7, 3 (2014), 308–33.

Levine, Harry Gene. 'The Committee of Fifty and the Origins of Alcohol Control'. *Journal of Drug Issues* 13 (1983), 95–116.

Levitt Ian, ed. *Joseph Livesey of Preston: Business, Temperance and Moral Reform*. Preston: University of Central Lancashire, 1996.

Liddington, Jill, and J. Norris. *One Hand Tied behind Us: The Rise of the Women's Suffrage Movement*. London: Virago, 1978.

Livingstone, David N. *Putting Science in Its Place: Geographies of Scientific Knowledge*. Chicago: University of Chicago Press, 2003.

Lobo-Guerrero, Luis. '*Uberrima Fides*, Foucault and the Security of Uncertainty'. *International Journal for the Semiotics of Law* 26 (2013), 23–37.

Longmate, Norman. *The Waterdrinkers: A History of Temperance*. London: Hamish Hamilton, 1968.

Love, Rosaleen. '"Alice in Eugenics-Land": Feminism and Eugenics in the Scientific Careers of Alice Lee and Ethel Elderton'. *Annals of Science* 36, 2 (1979), 145–58.

MacNalty, Arthur. 'Sir Victor Horsley: His Life and Work'. *British Medical Journal* 1, 5024 (20 April 1957), 910–16.

Magnusson, Mamie. *A Length of Days: The Scottish Mutual Assurance Society 1883–1983*. London: Henry Melland, 1983.

Malleck, Dan. *Try to Control Yourself: The Regulation of Public Drinking in Post-prohibition Ontario, 1927–44*. Vancouver: University of British Columbia Press, 2012.

Mark-Lawson, Jane, Mike Savage and Alan Warde. 'Gender and Local Politics: Struggles over Welfare Policies'. In *Localities, Class and Gender*, edited by The Lancaster Regionalism Group, 195–215. Pion: London, 1985.

Marmot, Michael G., M. J. Shipley, Geoffrey Rose and Briony J. Thomas. 'Alcohol and Mortality: A U-Shaped Curve'. *The Lancet* 317, 8220 (1981), 580–3.

Martin, Janette L. 'Popular Political Oratory and Itinerant Lecturing in Yorkshire and the North East in the Age of Chartism'. PhD Thesis, University of York, 2010.

McAllister, Annemarie. 'The Alternative World of the Proud Non-Drinker: Nineteenth-Century Public Displays of Temperance'. *Social History of Medicine and Drugs* 28, 2 (2014), 161–79.

McAllister, Annemarie. *Demon Drink: Temperance and the Working Class*. 2014.

McAllister, Annemarie. 'Giant Alcohol – A Worthy Opponent for the Children of the Band of Hope'. *Drugs: Education, Prevention and Policy* 22, 2 (2015), 103–10.

McAllister, Annemarie. 'Picturing the Demon Drink: How Children Were Shown Temperance Principles in the Band of Hope'. *Visual Resources* 28, 4 (2012), 309–23.

McAllister, Annemarie. *Writing for Social Change in Temperance Periodicals: Conviction and Career*. New York: Routledge, 2023.

McCrae, Niall. 'The Beer Ration in Victorian Asylums'. *History of Psychiatry* 15, 2 (2004), 155–75.

McDowell, Linda, and Doreen Massey. 'A Woman's Place?' In *Geography Matters! A Reader*, edited by Doreen Massey and John Allen, 128–47. Cambridge: Cambridge University Press, 1984.

McFall, Liz. *Devising Consumption: Cultural Economies of Insurance, Credit and Spending*. London: Routledge, 2019.

McFall, Liz, and Francis Dodsworth. 'Fabricating the Market: The Promotion of Life Assurance in the Long Nineteenth-Century'. *Journal of Historical Sociology* 22 (2009), 30–54.

McKie, David. *Jabez. The Rise and Fall of a Victorian Rogue*. London: Atlantic Books. 2004.

McLeod, Kari S. 'Our Sense of Snow: The Myth of John Snow in Medical Geography'. *Social Science & Medicine* 50 (2000), 923–35.

McWilliam, Rohan. 'The Gaiety Girl and the Matinee Idol: Constructing Celebrity, Glamour and Sexuality in the West End of London, 1890–1914'. *Transactions of the Royal Historical Society* 1 (2023), 69–93.

McWilliam, Rohan. *The Tichborne Claimant: A Victorian Sensation*. London: Continuum, 2007.

Midgley, Clare. 'Slave Sugar Boycotts, Female Activism and the Domestic Base of British Anti-slavery Culture', *Slavery & Abolition* 17, 3 (1996), 137–62.

Midgley, Clare. *Women against Slavery: The British Campaigns, 1780–1870*. London: Routledge, 1995.

Millward, Robert, and Sally Sheard. 'The Urban Fiscal Problem, 1870–1914: Government Expenditure and Finance in England and Wales', *Economic History Review* XLVIII (1995), 501–35.

Mitchell, Rosemary. 'Brewster, Patrick (1788–1859)'. In *Oxford Dictionary of National Biography*. Oxford University Press, 2004. www.oxforddnb.com/view/article/3374, accessed 5 December 2013.

Mooney, Graham. 'Diagnostic Spaces: Workhouse, Hospital, and Home in Mid-Victorian London'. *Social Science History* 33, 3 (2009), 357–90.

Moore, Francesca. '"A Band of Public-Spirited Women": Middle-Class Female Philanthropy and Citizenship in Bolton, Lancashire before 1918'. *Transactions of the Institute of British Geographers* 41 (2016), 149–62.

Morris, John Hogan. 'Decentring Ingenuity: Calculation, Intuition and Atmospheres in the Bank of England's Financial Literacy Assemblages'. *Geoforum* 90 (2018), 45–54.

Murphy, Sharon Ann. *Investing in Life: Insurance in Antebellum America*. Baltimore, MD: Johns Hopkins University Press, 2010.

Musson, Albert Edward. *Trade Union and Social History*. London: Frank Cass, 1974.

Newton, Robert. *Victorian Exeter, 1837–1914*. Leicester: Leicester University Press, 1968.

Nicholls, James. *The Politics of Alcohol: A History of the Drink Question in England*. Manchester: Manchester University Press, 2009.

O'Gorman, Francis. 'Introduction'. In *Victorian Literature and Finance*, edited by Francis O'Gorman, 1–16. Oxford: Oxford University Press, 2007.

O'Malley, Pat. 'Imagining Insurance: Risk, Thrift and Industrial Life Insurance in Britain'. *Connecticut Insurance Law Journal* 5 (1999), 676–705.

O'Malley, Pat, and Alex Roberts. 'Governmental Conditions for the Economization of Uncertainty'. *Journal of Cultural Economy* 7 (2014), 253–72.

Ogborn, Miles. *Global Lives: Britain and the World 1550–1800*. Cambridge: Cambridge University Press, 2008.

Ogborn, Miles. *Indian Ink: Script and Print in the Making of the English East India Company*. Chicago: The University of Chicago Press, 2007.

Olsen, Gerald Wayne. 'From Parish to Palace: Working- Class Influences on Anglican Temperance Movements, 1835–1914', *Journal of Ecclesiastical History* 40, 2 (1989), 239–52.

Olsen, Gerald Wayne. '"Physician Heal Thyself": Drink, Temperance and the Medical Question in the Victorian and Edwardian Church of England, 1830–1914', *Addiction* 89 (1994), 1167–76.

Olsen, Stephanie. *Juvenile Nation: Youth, Emotions and the Making of the Modern British Citizen, 1880–1914*. New York: Bloomsbury, 2014.

Pearce, Cyril. 'A Landscape of Dissent: Topography and Identity in Three Pennine Valleys'. *Landscapes* 3, 2 (2002), 84–102.

Pearce, Cyril. *Comrades in Conscience: The Story of an English Community's Opposition to the Great War*, second edition. London: Francis Boutle, 2014.

Pearce, Cyril, and Helen Durham. 'Patterns of Dissent in Britain during the First World War'. *War & Society* 34, 2 (2015), 140–59.

Pelling, Henry. *Social Geography of British Elections 1885–1910*. London: Macmillan, 1967.

Pennybacker, Susan D. *A Vision for London, 1889–1914: Labour, Everyday Life and the LCC Experiment*. London: Routledge, 1995.

Perriton, Linda, and Josephine Maltby. 'Working-Class Households and Savings in England, 1850–1880'. *Enterprise and Society* 16, 2 (2015), 413–45.

Peterson, M. Jeanne. *The Medical Profession in Mid-Victorian London*. Berkeley: University of California Press, 1978.

Peyton, Margo A. 'Segregated in Life and Death: Arnold R. Rich and the Racial Science of Tuberculosis'. *Bulletin of the History of Medicine* 98, 2 (2024), 205–34.

Plunkett, John, and Jill A. Sullivan. 'Fetes, Bazaars and Conversaziones: Science, Entertainment and Local Civic Elites'. In *Popular Exhibitions, Science and Showmanship, 1840–1910*, edited by Joe Kember, John Plunkett and Jill A. Sullivan, 41–60. Pittsburgh, PA: University of Pittsburgh Press, 2015.

Poovey, Mary. 'Economics and Finance'. In *The Cambridge History of Victorian Literature*, edited by K. Flint, 388–404. Cambridge: Cambridge University Press, 2012.

Poovey, Mary (ed.). *The Financial System in Nineteenth-Century Britain*. New York: Oxford University Press, 2003.

Poovey, Mary. *Making a Social Body: British Cultural Formation, 1830–1864*. Chicago: University of Chicago Press, 1995.

Porter, Theodore. 'Life Insurance, Medical Testing, and the Management of Mortality'. In *Biographies of Scientific Objects*, edited by Lorraine Daston, 226–46. Chicago, IL: University of Chicago Press, 2000.

Porter, Theodore. *Trust in Numbers: The Pursuit of Objectivity in Science and Public Life*. Princeton, NJ: Princeton University Press, 1995.

Price, Robin. 'Hydropathy in England 1840–70'. *Medical History* 25, 3 (1981), 269–80.

Purvis, Martin. 'Popular Institutions'. In *Atlas of Industrializing Britain, 1780–1914*, edited by John Langton and R. J. Morris. London: Routledge, 1986, 194–7.

Quinn, John F. *Father Mathew's Crusade: Temperance in Nineteenth-Century Ireland and Irish America*. Amherst: University of Massachusetts Press, 2002.

Randalls, Samuel, and James Kneale. 'A Fragile Network: Effecting Hail Insurance in Britain, 1840–1900'. *Enterprise & Society* 22, 3 (2020), 739–69.

Rappaport, Erika. 'Sacred and Useful Pleasures: The Temperance Tea Party and the Creation of a Sober Consumer Culture in Early Industrial Britain'. *Journal of British Studies* 52, 4 (2013), 990–1016.

Reinarz, Jonathan, and Rebecca Wynter. 'The Spirit of Medicine: The Use of Alcohol in Nineteenth-Century Medical Practice'. In *Drink in the Eighteenth and Nineteenth Centuries*, edited by Susanne Schmid and Barbara Schmidt-Haberkamp, 127–40. London: Pickering and Chatto, 2014.

Rintala, Marvin. 'Taking the Pledge: H. H. Asquith and Drink'. *Biography* 16, 2 (1993), 103–35.

Robb, George. 'Ladies of the Ticker: Women, Investment, and Fraud in England and America, 1850–1930'. In *Victorian Investments: New Perspectives on Finance and Culture*, edited by Nancy Henry and Cannon Schmitt, 120–40. Bloomington: Indiana University Press, 2009.

Robb, George. *White-Collar Crime in Modern England: Financial Fraud and Business Morality, 1845–1929*. Cambridge: Cambridge University Press, 1992.

Rose, R. B. 'John Finch, 1784–1857: A Liverpool Disciple of Robert Owen', *Transactions of the Historic Society of Lancashire and Cheshire* 109 (1957), 159–84.

Rose, Sonya O. *Limited Livelihoods: Gender and Class in Nineteenth Century England*. London: Routledge, 1992.

Ross, Duncan M. '"Penny Banks" in Glasgow, 1850–1914'. *Financial History Review* 9, 1 (2002), 21–39.

Ross, Duncan M. 'Savings Bank Depositors in a Crisis: Glasgow 1847 and 1857'. *Financial History Review* 20, 2 (2013), 183–208.

Schrad, Mark Lawrence. *The Political Power of Bad Ideas: Networks, Institutions, and the Global Prohibition Wave*. Oxford: Oxford University Press, 2010.

Schweber, Libby. *Disciplining Statistics: Demography and Vital Statistics in France and England, 1830–1885*. Durham, NC: Duke University Press, 2006.

Seth, Suman. 'Race, Specificity, and Statistics in Victorian Medicine'. *Journal of Victorian Culture* 27, 2 (2022), 370–83.

Shapiro, Susan P. 'The Social Control of Impersonal Trust'. *American Journal of Sociology* 93, 3 (1987), 623–8.

Shiman, Lilian Lewis. *Crusade against Drink in Victorian England*. London: Macmillan, 1988.

Shortt, Samuel E. D. 'Physicians, Science, and Status: Issues in the Professionalization of Anglo-American Medicine in the Nineteenth Century'. *Medical History* 27, 1 (1983), 51–68.

Slinn, Judy. 'Shaen, William (1821–1887)'. In *Oxford Dictionary of National Biography*. Oxford University Press, 2004. www.oxforddnb.com/view/article/50082, accessed 13 October 2013.

Snow, Stephanie J. 'John Snow MD, (1813–1858). Part II. Becoming a Doctor – His Medical Training and Early Years of Practice'. *Journal of Medical Biography* 8 (2000): 71–7.

Sournia, Jean-Charles. *A History of Alcoholism*, translated by Nick Handley and Gareth Stanton. Oxford: Basil Blackwell, 1990.

Spencer, Steven. '"The Fatal Gaze of This Moral Basilisk": The Salvation Army's War on Drink in Victorian Britain'. *Social History of Alcohol and Drugs* 33, 2 (2019), 230–56.

Stedman Jones, Gareth. *Outcast London: A Study in the Relationship between Classes in Victorian Society*. London: Penguin, 1992.

Stedman Jones, Gareth. 'Working-Class Culture and Working-Class Politics in London, 1870–1900: Notes on the Remaking of a Working Class'. In *Languages of Class: Studies in English Working Class History 1832–1982*, 179–238. Cambridge: Cambridge University Press, 1984.

Steedman, Carolyn. *Landscape for a Good Woman: A Story of Two Lives*. New Brunswick: Rutgers University Press, 1997.

Storch, Robert D. 'The Plague of the Blue Locusts: Police Reform and Popular Resistance in Northern England 1840–1857'. *International Review of Social History* 20 (1975), 61–90.

Storch, Robert D. 'The Policeman as Domestic Missionary: Urban Discipline and Popular Culture in Northern England, 1850–1880'. *Journal of Social History* 9, 4 (1976), 481–509.

Strange, Julie-Marie. *Death, Grief and Poverty in Britain, 1870–1914*. Cambridge: Cambridge University Press, 2005.

Suffolk Record Office. *Ipswich Remembered 2: Photographs of Victorian and Edwardian Ipswich*. Ipswich: Suffolk Record Office, 1979.

Summerson, John. 'The Victorian Rebuilding of the City of London'. *London Journal* 3, 2 (1977), 163–85.

Taylor, James. 'Numbers, Character and Trust in Early Victorian Britain: The Independent West Middlesex Fire and Life Assurance Company Fraud'. In *Statistics and the Public Sphere: Statistics and the People in Modern Britain, c.1800–2000*, edited by Tom Crook and Glen O'Hara, 185–202. New York: Routledge, 2001.

Thévenot, Laurent. 'Rules and Implements: Investment in Forms'. *Social Science Information* 23, 1 (1984), 1–45.

Thrift, Nigel. 'Driving in the City'. *Theory, Culture & Society* 21, 4–5 (2004), 41–59.
Thrift, Nigel. *Non-representational Theory: Space, Politics, Affect*. London: Routledge, 2008.
Townend, Paul A. *Father Mathew: Temperance and Irish Identity*. Dublin: Irish Academic Press, 2002.
Tregoning, David, and Hugh Cockerell. *Friends for Life: Friends' Provident Life Office 1832–1982*. London: Melland, 1982.
Valverde, Mariana. *Diseases of the Will: Alcohol and the Dilemmas of Freedom*. Cambridge: Cambridge University Press, 1998.
Valverde, Mariana. *Law's Dream of a Common Knowledge*. Princeton, NJ: Princeton University Press, 2003.
Vaughan, Laura. *Mapping Society: The Spatial Dimensions of Social Cartography*. London: UCL Press, 2015.
Vieira Paisana, J. M. 'Tipplers, Drunkards and Backsliders: The Temperance Movement in England 1830–72, Including a Case Study of Lincoln'. PhD thesis, Universidade do Minho, Braga, 2002.
Warner, John Harley. 'Physiological Theory and Therapeutic Explanation in the 1860s: The British Debate on the Medical Use of Alcohol'. *Bulletin for the History of Medicine* 54 (1980), 235–57.
Waters, Chris. *British Socialists and the Politics of Popular Culture, 1884–1914*. Stanford, CA: Stanford California Press, 1990.
Webb, W. W. 'Thomson, Robert Dundas (1810–1864)', rev. Richard Hankins. In *Oxford Dictionary of National Biography*. Oxford University Press, 2004. www.oxforddnb.com/view/article/27322, accessed 17 November 2009.
Webster, Ian. 'The Public Works Loan Board and the Growth of the State in Nineteenth-Century England'. *Economic History Review* 71 (2018), 887–908.
Weinbren, Daniel. 'The Good Samaritan, Friendly Societies and the Gift Economy'. *Social History* 31, 3 (2006), 319–36.
Williams, Sarah E. 'The Use of Beverage Alcohol as Medicine, 1790–1860'. *Journal of Studies on Alcohol* 41, 5 (1980), 543–66.
Winlow, Heather. 'Mapping Moral Geographies: W. Z. Ripley's Races of Europe and the United States'. *Annals of the Association of American Geographers* 96, 1 (2006), 119–41.
Wise, M. Norton, and Crosbie Smith. 'Work and Waste: Political Economy and Natural Philosophy in Nineteenth Century Britain (III)'. *History of Science* 28 (1990), 221–61.
Withers, Hartley. *Pioneers of British Life Assurance*. London: Staples Press, published for the UK Provident Institution, 1951.
Woiak, Joanne. '"A Medical Cromwell to Depose King Alcohol": Medical Scientists, Temperance Reformers, and the Alcohol Problem in Britain'. *Social History* 54 (1994), 337–65.
Yeomans, Henry. *Alcohol and Moral Regulation: Public Attitudes, Spirited Measures and Victorian Hangovers*. Bristol: Policy Press, 2014.
Yokoe, Ryosuke. *Alcohol and Liver Cirrhosis in Twentieth-Century Britain*. Switzerland: Springer, 2023.
Yokoe, Ryosuke. 'New Moderationism: Medical Discourses on Alcohol and the Decline of Drunkenness in Interwar Britain'. *Modern British History* 36, 1 (2025), 1–17.
Zakim, Michael. 'Paperwork'. *Raritan* 33, 4 (2014), 34–56.
Zelizer, Viviana A. *Economic Lives: How Culture Shapes the Economy*. Princeton, NJ: Princeton University Press, 2011.
Ziegler, Garrett. 'The City of London, Real and Unreal'. *Victorian Studies* 49, 3 (2007), 431–55.

Index of individuals

Index

Note: For the purposes of the index, English towns and cities are categorized by their nineteenth-century counties, with the exceptions of London, Bristol and Manchester which are indexed separately. London is broadly understood as its post-1888 boundaries. Locations in Wales, Scotland and Ireland are indexed under their respective nations

www.ingramcontent.com/pod-product-compliance
Ingram Content Group UK Ltd.
Pitfield, Milton Keynes, MK11 3LW, UK
UKHW020241290926
15470UKWH00002B/672

9 781350 529717